BY THE EDITORS OF
CONSUMER GUIDE®

HOME REMEDIES HEALTH

HANDBOOK

100s of Solutions for Common Ailments

**With John H. Renner, M.D., and the
Consumer Health Information
Research Institute**

CONSULTANT:

John H. Renner, M.D., is the president and medical director of the Consumer Health Information Research Institute (CHIRI), a nonprofit organization dedicated to providing reliable and accurate patient health education for preventive care, wellness, and self-help. Dr. Renner also serves as a member of the Board of Directors of the National Council Against Health Fraud; as clinical professor of family practice at the University of Missouri in Kansas City, Missouri; and as an adjunct professor of preventive medicine at the University of Kansas Medical School in Kansas City, Kansas.

CONTRIBUTING WRITERS:

Sue Berkman is a veteran science/health writer who writes for a variety of consumer and professional publications, including *Woman's Day, Good Housekeeping, Health,* and *Women's Health and Fitness News.* She has also coauthored two books on health.

Linda J. Brown is a freelance writer specializing in health and the environment. She writes an environmental column for *Good Housekeeping,* and her articles have appeared in *Self, Omni,* and other national magazines.

Jenny Hart Danowski researches and writes consumer articles for newsletters and magazines in the areas of health, fitness, and psychology. Her work has appeared in Whittle Communications' health and living publications, *Woman's Day,* and *Men's Health.*

Bobbie Hasselbring is the former editor of *Medical SelfCare* and has authored five books on health and psychology. She currently writes a column for the *Oregonian* and has become a nationally recognized health writer. The American Heart Association awarded her its 1991 Award for Media Excellence.

Susan G. Hauser is a freelance writer who works as a contributing writer to the *Wall Street Journal* and as a special correspondent to *People Magazine.*

Susan Nielsen writes regularly on health and consumer issues for such magazines as *Good Housekeeping* and *Family Circle Magazine.* She has been an associate health editor of *Redbook Magazine,* as well as a senior editor for "The Better Way" section of *Good Housekeeping.*

Brianna L. Politzer is a freelance writer specializing in health, medicine, and nutrition. She has worked as a newspaper reporter and an editor. She has contributed to many health publications, including *Medical Tribune News Service, American Health,* and *AIDS-Patient Care.*

Diana Reese is a medical writer who has written for such national publications as *American Health, Health, Longevity, HealthWatch,* and *Physician's Weekly.* She was previously senior editor on health publications at Whittle Communications.

Contents

CONTENTS

FOREWORD

Home Remedies Health Handbook is a comprehensive health advisory manual. It is holistic, in the correct sense of the word—it offers preventive medicine tips as well as sound nutrition, medical, mental, dental, and cosmetic advice.

The home remedies that are described in this book are not "miracle" cures or risky alternative therapies done over your doctor's objections, nor are they meant to take the place of the advice and treatments prescribed by your health-care providers. Rather, they are safe, practical actions that you can take to help yourself with your own health care. They are designed to help you prevent, cope with, and/or treat more than 80 common health problems. They can save you money on health-care costs. They can help to keep you healthy, wealthy, and wise.

How much this book helps you, however, depends on how you use it. As you read and use this book and as you take more responsibility for your own health care, keep the following important points in mind:

• There are no "secrets" in this book. All of the health-care providers openly and easily shared their recommendations without payment or promise. Discuss these ideas with your own doctor to see if he or she thinks these are valid for you. Use this book to improve communication with your health-care providers. This book is loaded with practical ideas. Your doctor will be interested in your use of them.

• Be careful of "self" diagnosis. Work with your doctor on your diagnosis. Even a doctor has a "fool for a patient" if he treats himself.

• Don't try every remedy listed for your condition on every condition you have. Especially, don't put everything listed *for*

7

your skin *on* your skin—you could end up with a new medication rash. Go slowly; use common sense.

• Heed the warnings included with the remedies. These warnings are carefully written to help you avoid harm or quackery. Pay special attention to the boxes labeled "Hello, Doctor?" These include special warnings and can help alert you to conditions and symptoms that require a doctor's attention.

Home Remedies Health Handbook has been carefully compiled. It contains information currently held to be true and helpful. As medicine and scientific experience grow, we may learn to do some things differently. Learn along with us. Continue to practice good, safe, self-help techniques based on scientific opinions and facts. Continue to maintain an open dialogue with your health-care providers. Continue to read, to ask questions, and to be an active, informed participant in your own health care.

John H. Renner, M.D.
President
Consumer Health Information Research Institute
Kansas City, Missouri

Acne

15 Skin-Clearing Solutions

A cne. If you're a teenager, you can't wait to get rid of it. If you're an adult, you can't believe it's back. Fortunately, improvements in acne treatments over the last decade mean you don't have to put up with it anymore.

The major determining factor in who gets acne is genes, according to Albert M. Kligman, M.D., Ph.D., emeritus professor of dermatology at the University of Pennsylvania School of Medicine in Philadelphia. In other words, you may have inherited a skin characteristic that makes you more likely to develop acne.

You have thousands of oil glands in the skin on your face, chest, and back that lubricate the skin by producing sebum, or oil, explains Alan D. Klein, M.D., a member of the teaching staff at Ventura County Medical Center in California and a spokesperson for the American Academy of Dermatology. "You have as many as 2,000 oil glands per square inch in the central part of your face," he says. The oil from the glands flows through tiny ducts to the skin surface.

Sometimes, these oil ducts become plugged with sebum, bacteria, and dead skin cells that are shed from the lining of the duct. That's acne. The condition often appears during adolescence because of changing hormone levels, which enlarge the oil glands and encourage them to produce more oil. Although the process is not well understood, the increase in oil appears to fuel acne, perhaps by stimulating the production of "sticky" skin cells that, when shed, tend to plug the duct. The situation usually settles down by the end of the teen years or during the early 20s.

ACNE GLOSSARY

Most of us think of pimples when we think of acne. But dermatologists have divided those annoying spots into the following categories:

Comedo (pl. comedones). An oil duct plugged up with oil, dead skin cells, and bacteria.

Whitehead. A closed comedo, or a comedo with skin covering the top. It looks like a tiny, white bump.

Blackhead. An open comedo, or a comedo that does not have skin covering it. It appears black not because it contains dirt, as is commonly believed, but because the material has been exposed to oxygen.

Papule. A ruptured comedo in which there is inflammation and secondary infection. It looks like a small, hard, red bump.

Pustule. A ruptured comedo in which there is inflammation and secondary infection. In contrast to the papule, the pustule has more pus near the surface, giving it a yellowish center.

Nodule (sometimes called a cyst). A ruptured comedo that is generally larger, deeper, and more painful than a pustule and is more likely to result in scarring. This type of lesion marks the most severe form of acne.

ACNE ROSACEA

If you're over 40 and suddenly develop severe acne, you could be suffering from acne rosacea, which is a different disease from acne vulgaris, the medical name for your garden variety of acne.

How can you tell the difference? Acne rosacea is characterized by redness, inflammation (swelling), and dilated blood vessels. Further clues: You don't have any blackheads, the acne is located mainly on the central part of your face (your nose and cheeks), and you have a lot of pustules (pus-containing pimples). You're more likely to suffer from this type of acne if you're light-skinned.

Unfortunately, there's not much you can do on your own for acne rosacea, says Vincent A. DeLeo, M.D., although you should be especially careful about avoiding the sun, since sun exposure can worsen the condition. It can, however, be treated by a dermatologist.

So why do adults develop acne? There are a variety of reasons, among them:

• **Hormones.** "Premenstrual acne is real," Kligman says. Pregnancy, changes during the menstrual cycle, and birth control pills can cause fluctuations in hormone levels and subsequent fluctuations in acne in women. In some women, low-dose oral contraceptives improve acne; in others, they make acne worse. If you have acne and menstrual irregularities, consult a physician to see if abnormal hormone levels are to blame.

• **Stress.** Dermatologists agree that high levels of stress can affect hormone levels.

• **Cosmetics.** Wearing heavy, oily makeup may clog pores and cause acne.

• **Occupational exposure.** If you're a mechanic or you're standing over the deep-fat fryer at the local fast-food joint, your face may be getting assaulted by oils, some of which may cause acne. Numerous chemicals in the workplace can also cause acne.

• **Certain medications.** Some drugs, such as Dilantin (which is used in the treatment of epilepsy), can cause acne, says Alan N. Moshell, M.D., director of the Skin Disease Program at the National Institute of Arthritis and Musculoskeletal and Skin Diseases.

No matter what's causing your acne, there are steps you can take to help clear up your skin.

DO NO HARM.

In other words, don't pick, press, rub, or otherwise manipulate those pimples, warns Kligman. "You risk spreading the bacteria and increasing the chances for scarring," explains Klein. Vincent A. DeLeo, M.D., assistant professor of dermatology at Columbia–Presbyterian Medical Center in New York, gets even more descriptive: The plug at the top of the pore is like a balloon. You can pop it, but below the surface, the sebum, bacteria, and skin cells may leak into the surrounding tissue, causing inflammation.

USE BENZOYL PEROXIDE.

A number of over-the-counter products contain this ingredient, which helps break up the plug of dead skin cells, bacteria, and oil in pores and cuts down on the bacteria as well. Start with the lowest concentration, and work your way up, especially if you have sensitive skin, because the higher the concentration, the more irritating it may be. Use it once or twice a day. If it dries the skin too much, Kligman suggests applying a mild moisturizer.

GIVE ONE OF THE OTHER OVER-THE-COUNTER PRODUCTS A SHOT.

Other acne products contain sulfur or resorcinol, which help unplug oil glands by irritating the skin, Klein says. Most dermatologists, however, believe that benzoyl peroxide is the most effective over-the-counter ingredient for acne.

APPLY OVER-THE-COUNTER PRODUCTS FOR PREVENTION.

"Don't just spot the product on existing acne," DeLeo says. "Put it on acne-prone areas." That can include your entire face (avoiding the lips and eyes, however), back, and chest.

GO EASY ON YOUR FACE.

"Kids with oily skin use hot water, a washcloth, and a drying soap and think they can wash their acne away," Kligman says. "But they can't." DeLeo points out, "You can wash your face ten times a day and still have acne. It has nothing to do with cleanliness." Washing removes oils from the surface of the skin, not from within the plugged ducts. And adults can certainly suffer from both acne and dry skin, says Klein. In fact, if you're too aggressive in your cleanliness, you may well end up drying out or irritating the sensitive skin on your face.

WASH PROPERLY.
How do you do that? Use a mild soap. DeLeo recommends Dove Unscented, Tone, Basis, or Neutrogena. Rub lightly with your fingertips and warm water. Do not use a washcloth. If your skin is oily, use a soap with benzoyl peroxide for its drying properties, suggests Klein. And wash once or twice a day.

DON'T EXFOLIATE.
That refers to removing the top layer of dead skin cells. Some dermatologists recommend using a rough washcloth or specially designed product to do just that. "But your skin is already irritated if you have acne," says Kligman. Don't use brushes, rough sponges, cleansers with granules or walnut hulls, or anything else of that nature on the delicate facial skin, says Klein. For the back and chest, where skin is less sensitive, you can try one of the acne scrub pads along with soap that contains benzoyl peroxide, he adds.

WATCH OUT FOR OILY PRODUCTS.
That goes for oily pomades on your hair, heavy oil-based moisturizers, and even oily cleansers. "The classic that I hear from women is that they use only cold cream on their face," says DeLeo. "They think they're avoiding wrinkles, but dry skin doesn't cause the skin to age, exposure to the sun does."

USE WATER-BASED MAKEUP.
If you're not sure—and DeLeo says some cosmetic labels are misleading—set the bottle of makeup on the counter. If it separates into water and powder, it's water-based, he says. If it doesn't, it contains oil. He also ad-

vises that you opt for powder blushes and loose powders. Eye makeup and lipstick are OK because you don't generally get acne in those areas.

FORGO THE FACIAL.

DeLeo warns that most people giving facials aren't trained to treat acne-prone skin properly and may end up doing more harm than good.

DON'T REST YOUR CHIN ON YOUR HANDS.

Try not to constantly touch your face. "People who do a lot of telephone work will get chin-line acne," DeLeo says. It causes trauma to acne, just like picking the pimples does. Tight sweatbands and chin straps from sports equipment can have the same effect.

SOAK UP THE OIL.

Some cosmetic companies make a paper product that can be pressed onto the skin to soak up oil, says Kligman. "It's a very simple procedure," he says. "It doesn't help the acne, but it helps relieve the oiliness, which is disagreeable."

SCREEN OUT THE SUN.

At one time, sun exposure was believed to help acne, says Klein. However, too much sun can lead to skin cancer and premature aging, making the risks outweigh the benefits. He suggests protecting the skin with a sunscreen that has a sun protection factor (SPF) of 15 or higher. "Look for one that's oil-free or noncomedogenic," he says. Unfortunately, many waterproof products are too likely to clog oil glands to use on the face, so you'll need to be diligent about reapplying the sunscreen often.

WHAT DOES A DOCTOR DO FOR ACNE?

With today's drugs, there is just no reason for anyone to put up with serious acne, says Albert M. Kligman, M.D., Ph.D.

"Persistent acne can affect self-esteem and confidence," Kligman says. "The psychological, social, and sexual effects of acne are very, very prominent, and the social consequences can be severe." He suggests children be treated fairly young if they start showing signs of acne, especially if their parents suffered from severe acne in their youth.

When should you see a dermatologist for your acne? Most dermatologists answer that by saying "when it bothers you." Severity is in the eye of the beholder in this case.

Vincent A. DeLeo, M.D., gives some additional guidelines for when professional treatment is called for. He advises that you see a dermatologist under the following conditions:

• If you use benzoyl peroxide products for six to eight weeks and still have problems

• If you have pustules larger than a match head

• If you have nodules the size of the end of your little finger

• If you have any scarring from your acne

It's extremely important to see a dermatologist before scarring occurs.

DON'T WORRY ABOUT DIET.

Chocolate, french fries, and other foods have not been proven to have anything at all to do with causing teenage acne. "It doesn't matter what you eat," says Kligman. Eating chocolate, nuts, or greasy foods is not to blame when it comes to the zits on your face. On the other hand, if you notice a correlation between something you eat and your face breaking out, most dermatologists agree that you should avoid the offending food. "Maybe 1 out of 100 or even 1,000 patients will have some relationship of acne to certain foods," says Moshell.

WATCH OUT FOR IODINE.

This is still somewhat controversial, but some doctors believe that high levels of iodine, found in some multiple vitamins and in iodized salt, may encourage acne.

Allergies

29 Ways to Feel Better

Spring's pollens. Summer's smog. Autumn's falling leaves. Winter's house dust. For millions of Americans, each change of season brings its own brand of allergens and irritants. For people with common hay fever and allergies, these pollutants can bring on symptoms ranging from a continuous, annoying postnasal drip to a full-scale, coughing-sneezing-itchy-eyed attack. For other allergy sufferers, such as those with allergic asthma or an allergy to bee stings, attacks can be fatal.

In many cases, allergy symptoms are difficult to differentiate from the symptoms of other disorders and illnesses, such as a cold, a deformity of the nose, or a food intolerance. For this reason, many doctors suggest that allergies be properly diagnosed by a board-certified allergist (a medical doctor who treats allergies) to avoid the self-administration of inappropriate medications or other remedies. Also, many allergy sufferers can benefit from today's wide range of available treatments, such as new prescription antihistamines that don't cause drowsiness, nasal corticosteroids, and allergy injections that can provide immunity to a specific allergen (an allergen is the name for any substance, such as pollen, that causes an allergic reaction). If you don't go to the doctor, you may be missing out on a treatment that may be of great help to you.

However, many mild allergies, such as seasonal hay fever or an allergy to cats, can be treated with a combination of properly used, over-the-counter antihistamines and a wide range of strategies to reduce or eliminate your exposure to particularly annoying allergens.

The following tips are designed to help reduce the discomfort caused by the most common allergies. They may be used in combination with an allergist's treatment or, if your allergies are mild, by themselves.

AVOID THE CULPRIT.

Sometimes, the best way to reduce the discomfort of an allergy is to avoid exposure to the allergen as much as possible, according to Edward J. O'Connell, M.D., professor of pediatrics at the Mayo Clinic in Rochester, Minnesota, and past president of the American College of Allergy and Immunology. "Take all practical measures,"

HELLO, DOCTOR?

If your allergies are causing you to cough, wheeze, and have trouble breathing, you should see an allergist, says Abba I. Terr, M.D., a clinical professor of medicine and director of the Allergy Clinic at Stanford University Medical Center in California. "You may have allergic asthma, which really has to be supervised by a doctor," he says. People with allergic asthma, which is sometimes mistaken for bronchitis, must often be prescribed inhalers and other medications. Trying to self-treat may be dangerous, Terr says.

he says. For example, if you are allergic to cats, avoid visiting the homes of friends who own them. If you must be around a cat, make the visit as short as possible and avoid touching or picking up the animal, he says.

RINSE YOUR EYES.
If your eyes are itchy and irritated and you have no access to allergy medicine, rinsing your eyes with cool, clean water may help soothe them, O'Connell says. This certainly can't do any damage, and it may help.

TRY A WARM WASHCLOTH.
If sinus passages feel congested and painful, a washcloth soaked in warm water may make things flow a little easier,
(Continued on page 22)

....

BUST THE DUST

The following tips from Edward J. O'Connell, M.D., can help you rid your bedroom of dust mites—microscopic insects that live in dusty, humid environments. The feces and corpses of the mites are thought to be the irritating components in dust. Allergists believe that since we spend most of our time at home in the bedroom, that's the most important place to allergy proof.

Encase pillows and mattresses. Invest in airtight, plastic or vinyl cases or special covers that are impermeable to allergens for your pillows and mattresses (except for water beds). Pillows and mattresses contain fibrous material that is an ideal environment for dust-mite growth. These cases are usually available at your local department store or through mail-order companies. You can also contact the Asthma and Allergy Foundation of America, Department CG, 1125 15th Street NW, Suite 502, Washington, D.C. 20005, for more information on where to purchase cases and covers.

Wash your bedding. Down, kapok, and feather comforters and pillows are out for people with allergies. The feathers have a tendency to leak and can wreak havoc with your respiratory tract. Comforters and sheets should be washed every seven to ten days in as hot water as they'll tolerate. Wash your mattress pads and synthetic blankets every two weeks.

Clean the bedroom once a week. Putting off cleaning for longer than this may allow an excessive amount of dust to collect, O'Connell says. However, since cleaning raises dust, it's best not to clean more than once a week. If necessary, you can spot dust with a damp cloth more often, he says.

Avoid overstuffed furniture. "If the bedroom's decor lends itself to it, add more wood and vinyl furniture and avoid overstuffed furniture," O'Connell says. Since carpeting makes an excellent dust-mite lair, opt instead for bare floors or ask your doctor about a prescription product for killing dust mites in carpets.

Choose washable curtains. If possible, invest in curtains that can be washed, since their fabric is often a place where dust mites hide.

Vacuum the venetians. The slats of venetian blinds are notorious dust collectors. If you can't replace your venetian blinds with washable curtains, at least run the vacuum lightly over them or dust them well during your thorough weekly cleaning.

Don't use the bedroom as storage space. Stored items tend to collect dust and have no place in an allergy-proof bedroom. The same goes for knickknacks and miscellaneous items kept on dressers and nightstands. If the bedroom is the only storage space you have, wrap items tightly in plastic garbage bags. Try to keep smaller items in drawers or cabinets.

Clean out your air conditioner and heating ducts. Every month or so, clean out the vents on your heating and air-conditioning units, or have someone clean them for you. These ducts are breeding grounds for mold, dust mites, and bacteria. If you let such nasties collect, they'll be blown into the room each time you turn on your air conditioner or heater.

CHOOSING AND USING AN OVER-THE-COUNTER ANTIHISTAMINE

If you've got your doctor's OK to use them, over-the-counter antihistamines can be an economical way to relieve your allergy misery. However, many people misuse these drugs, believing them to be an on-the-spot fix for whenever they feel itchy-eyed or sneezy.

"The problem with antihistamines is, most people wait until they're miserable, then take one and don't find they work," says Miles M. Weinberger, M.D., director of the Pediatric Allergy and Pulmonary Division at the University of Iowa Hospitals and Clinics in Iowa City. "If you have classical ragweed hay fever, you'll get the maximum benefit from antihistamines if you start taking them a week or two before the allergy season begins." (When the season begins depends on where you live.)

As for what type of antihistamine to use, Weinberger recommends chlorpheniramine maleate, which is found in many over-the-counter preparations. Chlorpheniramine maleate is one of the oldest, safest allergy drugs with a proven track record, he says. It can take care of symptoms

according to O'Connell. Put the washcloth over the nose and upper-cheek area and relax for a few minutes.

USE SALINE SOLUTION.
Irrigating the nose with saline solution may help soothe upper-respiratory allergies by removing irritants that become lodged in the nose, causing inflammation, ac-

such as sneezing; itchy, runny nose; and itchy eyes. (If you also have nasal stuffiness, says Weinberger, you might try a combination product that contains chlorpheniramine and pseudoephedrine, a nasal decongestant.) He suggests starting with a dose of perhaps one-fourth of what the package recommends, then slowly building up to 24 milligrams per day (12 milligrams in the morning and 12 milligrams in the evening), providing you can maintain that dosage without drowsiness. Since drowsiness tends to go away in a week or two, Weinberger recommends starting with evening doses, then adding a morning dose as you begin to tolerate the medication. (Be sure to avoid operating a motor vehicle or heavy machinery if the medication makes you drowsy.) "Approximately 75 percent of the people with pollen symptoms will get quite adequate relief with a 24 milligram dosage," he says.

Edward J. O'Connell, M.D., agrees that antihistamines work best when they are used as preventive medicine. For people with pet allergies who know they will be exposed to someone else's cat or dog, he recommends taking antihistamines beginning 10 to 14 days in advance.

cording to Anthony Montanaro, M.D., associate professor of medicine in the Division of Allergy and Immunology at Oregon Health Sciences University in Portland.

WASH YOUR HAIR.
If you've spent long hours outdoors during the pollen season, wash your hair after you come inside to remove

pollen, suggests Clifton T. Furukawa, M.D., clinical professor of pediatrics at the University of Washington School of Medicine in Seattle and past chairman of the Professional Education Council for the American Academy of Allergy and Immunology. The sticky stuff tends to collect on the hair, making it more likely to fall into your eyes.

TAKE A SHOWER.

If you wake up in the middle of the night with a coughing, sneezing allergy attack, a hot shower may wash off any pollen residues you've collected on your body throughout the day, says Furukawa. The warm water also relaxes you and helps you go back to sleep, he adds.

WEAR SUNGLASSES.

On a windy day in pollen season, a pair of sunglasses may help shield your eyes from airborne allergens, according to O'Connell. For extra protection, try a pair of sunglasses with side shields or even a pair of goggles.

BEWARE OF THE AIR.

"Air pollution may augment allergies and may actually induce people to have allergies," Montanaro says. He recommends staying outside as little as possible on smoggy days or wearing a surgical mask, especially if you exercise outside. "The mask won't remove everything, but it will help," he adds.

MAKE YOUR HOUSE A NO-SMOKING ZONE.

"Don't allow smoking in your house or apartment," O'Connell says. Tobacco smoke is a notorious irritant, either causing or aggravating respiratory allergies.

IS IT A FOOD ALLERGY?

Do you feel congested after you eat dairy products? Does red meat make you feel sluggish? Does sugar give you a headache? If you answered "yes" to any of these questions, you probably don't have a food allergy.

"There's a big difference between what the public perceives as a food allergy and what is really a food allergy," says Anthony Montanaro, M.D. "The distinction is important, since a real food allergy can kill you and a food intolerance can't."

If you are truly allergic to a food, the reaction will be almost immediate, occurring from within a few minutes to two hours after you eat it, according to Abba I. Terr, M.D. The most common symptoms, he says, are hives, diffuse swelling around the eyes and mouth, or abdominal cramps. A less common symptom is difficulty breathing. In severe cases, extremely low blood pressure, dizziness, or loss of consciousness may result. In these instances, a call for an ambulance or other emergency medical assistance is warranted.

KEEP THE WINDOWS SHUT.

Most Americans, except those with outdoor employment, are mostly indoors. During pollen season, this can be an advantage for those with pollen allergies. "The bottom line, for pollen allergies, is keeping the windows shut," O'Connell says. "Closed windows will keep pollen out of the house or apartment. For pollen sufferers, during the pollen season, there is really no such thing as fresh air." Air purifiers may help eliminate indoor pollen, but they tend to stir up dust, he adds.

FILTER YOUR VACUUM.

"It is very important to not recycle the allergy factors back into your home as you clean," says Furukawa. "For example, you're not doing much good if your vacuum cleaner allows small particles of dust to be blown back into the air as you vacuum." He recommends putting a filter on the exhaust port of your vacuum, if your machine is the canister type (uprights don't usually have an exhaust port). If dust really bothers you and you've got the money, you can invest in an industrial-strength vacuuming system, Furukawa says. Some allergists recommend a brand called Nilfisk, he adds, which has an excellent filtering system and retails for about $500. To find out where you can purchase filters or special vacuums, talk to your allergist or write to the Asthma and Allergy Foundation of America, Department CG, 1125 15th Street NW, Suite 502, Washington, D.C. 20005.

DUST WITH A DAMP CLOTH.

Dusting at least once a week is important—but if done improperly, it may aggravate respiratory allergies, O'Connell says. He recommends dusting with a damp cloth and avoiding feather dusters and dusting sprays.

DON'T DUST AT ALL.

If dusting aggravates your allergies, don't do it. Ask a family member or hire a housekeeper, O'Connell recommends.

DEHUMIDIFY.

"Dust mites (microscopic insects that are usually the allergy culprits in dust) grow very well in humid areas," O'Connell says. He recommends investing in a dehumidifier or using the air conditioner, which works equally well. A dehumidifier can also help prevent mold, another allergen, from growing. When cooking or showering, take advantage of the exhaust fan—another way to help keep humidity to a minimum.

THINK BEFORE YOU BURN.

Although it is common to burn household and construction refuse, this may not be such a wise idea, says Furukawa. "Wood that is treated with heavy metals or other chemical-laden materials will irritate everybody, but the person who is allergic or asthmatic will have proportionately more difficulty," he says. "Also, pay attention to what you are throwing in the fireplace." Of course, your best bet is to stay away from the fireplace when it's in use.

CUT THROUGH THE SMOKE.

Many people with respiratory allergies find that wood smoke poses a particular problem, Furukawa says. With wood stoves, the biggest problem is "choking down" the stove, or decreasing the amount of oxygen in order to cool down the fire, he explains. Choking down throws irritating toxins into the air, which will be breathed in by you and your neighbors.

LEAVE THE LAWN MOWING TO SOMEONE ELSE.

During pollen season, a grass-allergic person is better off letting someone else—anyone else—mow the lawn,

Montanaro says. "Find out when the pollination season in your area is," he advises. "Here in the Northwest, I tell people not to mow between May and the Fourth of July."

WASH YOUR PET.

A little-known trick for cat or dog owners who are allergic to fur: Bathe your pet frequently. "There is strong evidence that simply bathing the animal in warm water substantially reduces the amount of allergen on the animal's fur," Furukawa says. "Animals secrete substances from their sweat glands and their saliva—it is water soluble and you can rinse it off." If you're a cat owner and can't imagine bathing your pet for fear of being scratched to death, take heart: Furukawa says that in an informal survey that he conducted, he discovered that one out of ten cats will purr when bathed. If they are started as kittens, chances are higher that bath time will be a harmonious experience, he says. Bathe your pet in warm water, with no soap, once every other week.

In addition to bathing your pet, wash your hands soon after you've had direct contact with your furry friend.

MAKE SURE YOUR FINAL RINSE REALLY RINSES.

Chemicals in detergents and other laundry products can cause skin irritation in many people, O'Connell says. "There really are no mild detergents," he explains. "It's important that the final rinse cycle on your machine thoroughly rinses the detergent from your clothes."

CALL AHEAD.

When planning a vacation or business trip, call ahead to find a room that will be easier on your allergies. Ask for a room that's not on the lower level, because a room on the lower level may have been flooded in the past and may still be a haven for mold growth. Shop around for a hotel or motel that doesn't allow pets, so you won't be subject to the leftover dander of the last traveler's dog or cat. If possible, bring your own vinyl- or plastic-encased pillow.

Arthritis

44 Coping Strategies

An estimated 37 million Americans are caught in the grip of some form of arthritis or rheumatic disease. And few of us will make it to a ripe old age without joining the fold. If one of these diseases has a hold on you, read on. While there are no cures, there are steps you can take to ease discomfort and get back more control over your life. There are more than 100 different forms of arthritis and rheumatic disease, with a host of causes, according to the Arthritis Foundation in Atlanta. Among the more widely known afflictions are osteoarthritis, rheumatoid arthritis, gout, and lupus.

Osteoarthritis is primarily marked by a breakdown and loss of joint cartilage. Cartilage is the tough tissue that separates and cushions the bones in a joint. As cartilage is worn away and the bones begin to rub against each other, the joint becomes aggravated. In osteoarthritis, this breakdown of cartilage is accompanied by minimal inflammation, hardening of the bone beneath the cartilage, and bone spurs (growths) around the joints. "It will eventually affect virtually everyone in old age," says John Staige Davis IV, M.D., professor in the Division of Rheumatology at the University of Virginia School of Medicine in Charlottesville.

Rheumatoid arthritis, on the other hand, is not an inevitable aspect of aging. For reasons unknown, the synovial membrane, or lining, of a joint becomes inflamed, so pain, swelling, heat, and redness occur.

In the case of gout, needle-shaped uric acid crystals collect in the joints, due to a fault in the body's ability to metabolize, or process, purines. Purines are naturally occurring chemicals found in certain foods, such as liver, kidney, and anchovies. The disease primarily affects overweight, fairly inactive men over the age of 35.

Lupus, on the other hand, affects many more women than men. It is a condition in which the body's own immune system attacks healthy cells. The symptoms are wide-ranging, from joint pain to mouth sores to persistent fatigue.

Researchers are beginning to understand what may predispose some people to arthritis. One clue to the puzzle: "There are indications that collagen, which helps form the body's cartilage, may be defective in some people," says Arthur I. Grayzel, M.D., senior vice-president for Medical Affairs at the Arthritis Foundation.

While you cannot cure your condition, you can adopt a variety of coping techniques that will leave you more active and in control of your life.

EASING STIFFNESS AND DISCOMFORT

Here are some tips to help relieve discomfort and get you back into the swing of things.

KEEP MOVING.

Maintain movement in your joints as best you can. This can help keep your joints functioning better for a longer amount of time and, at the same time, brighten your outlook on life. "Every patient should keep active," says John R. Ward, M.D., professor of medicine at the University of Utah School of Medicine in Salt Lake City. "And remember that even small movements mean a lot. If all you can tolerate is a little housecleaning or gardening, for instance, that's OK, too."

EXERCISE, EXERCISE, EXERCISE.

"Exercises work best when inflammation has calmed down," notes Janna Jacobs, P.T., C.H.T., physical therapist, certified hand therapist, and president of the Section on Hand Rehabilitation of the American Physical Therapy Association (APTA).

There are a few different types of exercises that are used to help arthritis sufferers. The simplest, easiest exercises that can be done by almost any arthritis sufferer are called range-of-motion exercises. They help maintain good movement by putting the joints through their full range of motion. You'll find several range-of-motion exercises recommended by the Arthritis Foundation in "Exercises for Arthritis."

Isometrics, in which you create resistance by tightening a muscle without moving the joint, can help to strengthen muscles. Weight-bearing exercises, such as walking, also build muscle strength. While strengthening exercises can be beneficial for the arthritis sufferer, however, they should only be done under the supervision and care of a therapist or physician, says Grayzel. And, "anyone with any type of cardiovascular disease should not do multiple resistance exercises for a sustained amount of time," warns Ward.

Stretching, which helps make the muscles more flexible, is often recommended as the first step in any exercise regimen. Likewise, warming up your joints before beginning any exercise makes them more flexible. Massage your muscles and/or apply hot or cold com-

EXERCISES FOR ARTHRITIS

These exercises are recommended by the Arthritis Foundation. For best results, carry out the exercises in a smooth, steady, slow-paced manner; don't bounce, jerk, or strain. Don't hold your breath; breathe as naturally as possible. Do each exercise five to ten times, if possible. If any exercise causes chest pain, other pain, or shortness of breath, stop. When your joints are inflamed, it's best to skip the exercises and rest. If you have any questions, contact your therapist or physician. And remember: It may be some time before you feel the benefits of regular exercise, so be patient with yourself.

Shoulders: Lie on your back and raise one arm over your head, keeping your elbow straight. Keep your arm close to your ear. Return your arm slowly to your side. Repeat with the other arm.

Knees and hips: Lie on your back with one knee bent and the other as straight as possible. Bend the knee of the straight leg and bring it toward the chest. Extend that same leg into the air and then lower the straightened leg to the floor. Repeat with the other leg.

presses or both—whichever your health-care practitioner recommends or you prefer. A warm shower is another way to warm up. (See "Heat or Cold: Which Is Best?")

GIVE YOUR HANDS A WATER WORKOUT.

Try doing your hand exercises in a sink full of warm water for added ease and comfort, suggests Jacobs.

Hips: Lie on your back with your legs straight and about six inches apart. Point your toes up toward the ceiling. Slide one leg out to the side and then return to the starting position, keeping your toes pointing up. Repeat the exercise with the other leg.

Knees: Sit on a chair that's high enough so you can swing your legs. Keep your thigh on the chair and straighten out your knee. Hold a few seconds. Then bend your knee back as far as possible to return to the starting position. Repeat with the other knee.

Ankles: Sit on a chair and lift your toes off the floor as high as possible while keeping your heels on the floor. Then return your toes to the floor and lift your heels as high as possible. Repeat.

Fingers: Open your hand with your fingers straight. Bend all the finger joints except the knuckles. Touch the top of the palm with the tips of your fingers. Open your hand and repeat the exercise.

Thumbs: Open your hand with your fingers straight. Reach your thumb across your palm until it touches the base of the little finger. Stretch your thumb out again and repeat.

DON'T OVERDO IT.

Ward has come up with a "useful recipe" you can use to see if you've overdone your exercise routine. See how you feel a few hours after you exercise and then again after 24 hours. If your pain has increased considerably during that period of time, then it's time to cut back on the frequency and amount of exercise, he says. If the activity brought relief, you've found a worthwhile exercise. Tailor your routine to include the exercises that give you the most relief—and the most enjoyment.

PLAY IN A POOL.

If you find even simple movements difficult, a heated pool or whirlpool may be the perfect environment for exercise (unless you also have high blood pressure, in which case you should avoid whirlpools and hot tubs). Try a few of your simpler exercises while in the water. The buoyancy will help reduce the strain on your joints. And, "the warm water will help loosen joints and maintain motion and strength," says Ward. Even a warm bath may allow you some increased movement. In a pinch, a hot shower may do: Running the stream of water down your back, for instance, may help relieve back pain.

DON'T OVERUSE OVER-THE-COUNTER CREAMS.

These pain-relieving rubs give temporary relief by heating up the joints. However, "frequent use may activate enzymes that can break down the cartilage in the joints," says Davis.

PUT ON A SCARF.

Not around your neck, but around the elbow or knee joint when it aches. "A wool scarf is your best bet," says

Jacobs. Be careful not to wrap it too tightly, however; you don't want to hamper your circulation.

PULL ON A PAIR OF STRETCH GLOVES.

"The tightness caused by the stretchy kind may, in fact, reduce the swelling that often accompanies arthritis," says Ward. And the warmth created by covered hands may make the joints feel better. "Wearing thermal underwear may have the same warming effect on joints," says Grayzel.

GET ELECTRIC GLOVES.

Hunters use these battery-operated mitts to keep their hands toasty on cold mornings in the woods. "The gloves just may do the trick to keep your hands warm and pain-free," says Jacobs. She recommends keeping them on all night while you sleep.

TRY A WATER BED.

According to the National Water Bed Retailers' Association in Chicago, many owners claimed in a study that their rheumatoid arthritis "was helped very much by a water bed." And Earl J. Brewer, Jr., M.D., former head of the Rheumatology Division of Texas Children's Hospital in Houston, believes he knows why. "The slight motions made by a water bed can help reduce morning stiffness," he says. "And a heated water bed may warm the joints and relieve joint pain."

SLIP INTO A SLEEPING BAG.

If a water bed is out of the question, you might consider camping gear. "The cocoonlike effect of a sleeping bag traps heat, which can help relieve morning aches and pains," reports Brewer. He learned of its therapeutic effects when many of his patients told him that they got relief by sleeping in sleeping bags on top of their beds.

GET "DOWN."

Brewer tells the story of a doctor from Norway who happened to stay in a bed-and-breakfast while on business in New York. The doctor, who was suffering from arthritis pain, slept peacefully each night in the B&B's bed and

---

HEAT OR COLD: WHICH IS BEST?

There are no hard and fast rules when it comes to deciding which—heat, cold, or a combination of the two—will give you the best results. The bottom line, says John R. Ward, M.D.: "Do whichever feels the best." Here are some guidelines that may help you decide.

Heat relieves pain primarily by relaxing muscles and joints and decreasing stiffness. In some instances, however, heat may aggravate a joint that's already "hot" from inflammation, as is sometimes the case with rheumatoid arthritis. On the other hand, osteoarthritis causes minimal inflammation and may respond well to heat application. If you find that your compress cools down quickly, you may want to try methods that offer more consistent heating. An electric blanket or heating pad can provide sustained dry heat. A warm shower, bath, or whirlpool can keep the wet heat coming. And using some method of warmth to loosen up the muscles before exercise can help them perform better.

---

woke each morning pain-free. The bed was outfitted with a goose-down comforter and pillow. According to Brewer, the bedding's warmth and minute motion brought on the relief. For those who are allergic to down, an electric blanket may bring some relief.

WATCH YOUR WEIGHT.

Being overweight puts more stress on the joints. As a matter of fact, a weight gain of 10 pounds can mean an

Cold is ordinarily used to reduce pain in specific joints. Cold application should not be used with vasculitis (inflammation of the blood vessels) or Raynaud's phenomenon (a condition, characterized by spasms of the arteries in the fingers and toes, that may occur in conjunction with rheumatoid arthritis) without a doctor's approval, however. There are many ways to make a cold pack: Fill a plastic bag with crushed ice, use a package of frozen peas or frozen unpopped popcorn, or use a package of blue ice, for example. Apply the cold pack, wrapped in a thin towel, to only one or two joints at a time, so you don't get a chill.

You may find that alternating heat and cold gives you the most relief. For the best results, the Arthritis Foundation recommends the contrast bath: Soak your hands and feet in warm water (no more than 110 degrees Fahrenheit) for about three minutes, then soak them in cold water (about 65 degrees Fahrenheit) for about a minute. Repeat this process three times, and finish with a warm-water soak.

equivalent stress increase of 40 pounds on the knees. So if you are carrying excess pounds, losing some weight can help you to improve joint function. "People who lose weight can slow the progress of their osteoarthritis," says Grayzel.

QUESTION ANY CURE-ALL.

Frustrated by the chronic pain of arthritis, some sufferers pursue a litany of promises for 100 percent relief—whether from a so-called miracle drug, a newfangled diet, or another alternative treatment. Unfortunately, at this time, arthritis has no cure. So, before you jump at the next hot-sounding testimonial, proceed with caution. Get all the facts. Consult your physician or other healthcare provider. Even age-old techniques, such as wearing a copper bracelet, should be viewed with skepticism, agree most experts. And remember, if something sounds too good to be true, it probably is.

PROTECTING YOUR JOINTS

In addition to easing discomfort, you can learn to live well with arthritis by protecting your joints. What's more, with a little planning and reorganizing, you can learn to do daily tasks more efficiently, so that you'll have more energy to spend on activities you enjoy. Here are some tips from the Arthritis Foundation that can help.

PLAN AHEAD EACH DAY.

Prepare a realistic, written schedule of what you would like to accomplish each day. That way, you can carry out your most demanding tasks and activities when you think you'll have the most energy and enthusiasm—in the morning, for instance.

SPREAD THE STRAIN.

As a general rule, you want to avoid activities that involve a tight grip or that put too much pressure on your fingers. Use the palms of both hands to lift and hold cups, plates, pots, and pans, rather than gripping them with your fingers or with only one hand. Place your hand flat against a sponge or rag instead of squeezing it with your fingers. Avoid holding a package or pocketbook by clasping the handle with your fingers. Instead, grasp your goods in the crook of your arm—the way a football player holds the ball as he's running across the field—and you won't be tackled by as much pain.

AVOID HOLDING ONE POSITION FOR A LONG TIME.

Keeping joints "locked" in the same position for any length of time will only add to your pain and stiffness. Relax and stretch your joints as often as possible.

"ARM" YOURSELF.

Whenever possible, use your arm instead of your hand to carry out an activity. For example, push open a heavy door with the side of your arm rather than with your hand and outstretched arm.

TAKE A LOAD OFF.

Sitting down to complete a task will keep your energy level up much longer than if you stand.

REPLACE DOORKNOBS AND ROUND FAUCET HANDLES WITH LONG HANDLES.

They require a looser, less stressful grip to operate, so you'll put less strain on your joints.

BUILD UP THE HANDLES ON YOUR TOOLS.

For a more comfortable grip, tape a layer or two of thin foam rubber, or a foam-rubber hair curler, around the handles of tools such as brooms and mops.

CHOOSE LIGHTER TOOLS.

Lightweight eating and cooking utensils can keep your hands from getting heavy with hurt.

LET AUTOMATIC APPLIANCES DO THE WORK FOR YOU.

Electric can openers and knives, for instance, are easier to operate than manual versions. An electric toothbrush has a wider handle than a regular toothbrush.

DON'T OVERDO THE HOUSEWORK.

Plan on tackling only one major cleaning chore a day, whether it is doing the laundry or cleaning the kitchen.

KEEP YOUR STUFF WITHIN EASY REACH.

Adjust the shelves and racks in any storage area so that you don't have to strain to reach the items you need. Buy clothes with pockets to hold things you use often and need close by, like a pair of glasses. Use an apron with pockets to carry rags and lightweight cleaning supplies with you as you do your household chores. Store cleaning supplies in the area in which they will be used. Keep the same supplies in several places, such as the upstairs bathroom, downstairs bathroom, and kitchen.

USE A "HELPING HAND."

For those items you can't store nearby, buy a long-handled gripper, the kind used in grocery stores to grab items from top shelves, to extend your reach. Make household chores easier with a long-handled feather duster or scrub brush. Grab your clothes from the dryer with an extended-reach tool.

SAY NO TO SCRUBBING.
Spray pots and pans with nonstick cooking spray and/or use cookware with a nonstick surface. Consider getting a dishwasher, too, to save your joints some work.

VELCRO IS THE WAY TO GO.
Interlocking cloth closures on clothing and shoes can save you the frustration of buttoning and lacing.

WALK THIS WAY UP AND DOWN THE STAIRS.
Lead with your stronger leg going up, and lead with your weaker leg coming down.

BEND WITH YOUR KNEES.
When reaching for or lifting something that's low or on the ground, bend your knees and keep your back straight as you lift.

LET LOOSE WITH LOOPS.
You won't need quite as tight a grip if you put loops around door handles, such as those on the refrigerator and oven. Have loops sewn on your socks, too, then use a long-handled hook to help you pull them up.

DIG OUT THAT LITTLE RED WAGON.
Heavier loads will be out of your hands if you use a wagon or cart that glides along on wheels. Use it to tote groceries or baskets of laundry, for instance.

READ WITH EASE.
Lay your newspaper out on the table to read. Lay a book flat or use a book stand.

SIT ON A STOOL IN THE TUB.
A special stool can give you a steady place to bathe.

PLANT YOURSELF ON A STOOL IN THE GARDEN.
Sitting, rather than stooping, over your garden may help reduce the stress on your back and legs.

ASK FOR HELP.
Don't be afraid to ask your family members or friends for assistance. Many hands make light work.

CONTACT THE ARTHRITIS FOUNDATION.
The Arthritis Foundation can let you know of joint-friendly or energy-saving items for arthritis sufferers. Call the Arthritis Foundation Information Line at 800-283-7800, Monday through Friday, 9:00 A.M. to 7:00 P.M. Eastern time, to talk to a skilled operator who can answer your questions about arthritis.

Asthma

28 Ways to Breathe Easier

If you have asthma, you know the dreaded choking sensation, the faintness, the anxiety. It's as if someone made you run around the block, then pinched your nose shut and forced you to breathe through a straw. And you know all too well that once an asthma attack starts, it won't go away by itself.

About five to ten percent of the population have asthma. And while no two persons with asthma are alike in the subtle characteristics of the condition, they do have one thing in common: Trouble breathing properly. Their lungs are supersensitive and easily provoked into constriction by many factors, called triggers.

As you have probably discovered, perhaps the hard way, many things can set an asthma attack into motion—someone's perfume, a smoke-filled room, a friendly dog, a flowery garden, a strong wind, or even a good laugh. (Asthma, however, is a hereditary condition, so unless a person is genetically predisposed, nothing will make asthma happen.) Triggers can be allergic or nonallergic, and reactions can be immediate or delayed.

While there is no cure for asthma, the good news is that asthma—whether mild, moderate, or severe—can be managed. Doctors who specialize in treating asthma can be very helpful. Every patient with asthma should see a doctor to be sure another cause of wheezing is not present and, if true atopic asthma is present, to develop a therapeutic program for managing the disorder.

In addition to working with your doctor, you can take measures to help control your asthma. The key is to track down the triggers and, as completely as possible, eliminate them from your life. Here's how:

SMITE THE MITE.

"Dust mites are microscopic insects that thrive on food debris and high humidity," says Allan M. Weinstein, M.D., an asthma/allergy specialist in private practice in

Washington, D.C. "Since they are among the most common allergic asthma triggers, dustproofing is a must." His suggestions:

• Enclose your mattress in an airtight, dustproof cover, then cover it with a washable mattress pad. Keep a bedspread on the bed during the day.

• Wash your sheets in hot water every week, wash your mattress pads and synthetic blankets every two weeks, and wash your pillows every month.

• Use polyester or dacron pillows, not those made of kapok or feathers, and enclose them in airtight, dustproof covers.

• Avoid carpeting, which is difficult to clean; stick to bare floors with washable area rugs.

• Choose washable curtains instead of draperies.

• Avoid dust-catchers (such as knickknacks) all over the house, especially in the room where you sleep; the less clutter the better. If possible, avoid storing out-of-season clothing or bedding in the bedroom; never store things under the bed.

• Try not to do heavy cleaning, but if you must, use only a vacuum cleaner and damp cloth to clean; dust mops and brooms stir up the dust. Always use hot water. "Cold water is like a day in the sun to a dust mite," says Weinstein.

• Wear a mask over your mouth and nose while cleaning, and leave the room when you're done.

• Run an air conditioner or dehumidifier in warm weather, especially in spring and fall when mites multiply. Aim to keep the humidity level in your home under 40 percent but above 25 percent.

• Consider using an air purifier in the bedroom to keep the room free from dust particles.

MINIMIZE MOLD.

"Fungus is a parasite that can literally 'grow on you,'" says Stuart Young, M.D., an asthma/allergy specialist in New York. "It can grow on nonliving organic material, too, in several forms—mold, dry rot, and downy mildew." Fungi reproduce by producing spores. The spores are the real problem, as millions of them float through the air to be inhaled in every breath, touching off an allergic reaction that can contribute to asthma. To stave off the spores, Young advises you to:

• Keep your windows closed, because the mold spores can come right in through the windows even if the windows have screens.

• Stay out of attics, basements, and other dank, musty places.

• Wear a face mask and give your bathroom a going-over for signs of mold. (Better yet, have a nonallergic family member do this.) The most likely spots for mold growth: dark areas, such as the backs of cabinets and under the sink.

• Examine all closets regularly to see that molds have not set up housekeeping in unused shoes and boots.

• On a regular basis, have a family member or friend investigate the inner workings of air conditioners, humidifiers, and vaporizers in your home where molds like to grow.

• Periodically check houseplants for mold growth. In fact, getting rid of mold will help your plants, as well.

MAKE PEACE WITH POLLEN.

Pollen is released when plants are blooming—trees in the spring, grass in the late spring and early summer, ragweed from mid-August until the first frost. Plants that are pollinated by the wind are much more of a problem for asthmatics than are those pollinated by insects. "The goal is to learn how to live with pollen, not hide away from it," says Loomis Bell, M.D., chief of pulmonary–critical care medicine at St. Luke's–Roosevelt Hospital Center in New York. He recommends that you avoid cutting grass or even being outside while grass is being mowed. Keep your windows closed as much as possible—pollen can get through screens, too—and use an air conditioner to cool your home instead. Room air purifiers are also available that can purify recirculated air, removing particles of all sorts that are suspended in the air and further cleansing the air by passing it through a charcoal filter. After being outside in the midst of pollen, take off your clothes and wash them or at least run a vacuum over the articles of clothing. Wash yourself, too, and don't forget your hair.

DON'T PET A PET.

The best approach is to not have a pet that can trigger your asthma, advises Young. The problem is not the hair of the animal but the dander—the dead, dry skin that flakes off. The animal licks the skin, and the dander remains in its saliva. "If giving up a pet is impossible, the next logical step is to make very strict rules about living with an allergenic animal," Young warns. Do not allow your pet into the bedroom—ever. If the animal is in the bedroom at any time during the day, the dander will remain for hours. Leave the pet home if you are going for a car ride that would necessitate very close contact with the animal. If you do have direct contact with your pet (or any animal, for that matter), wash your hands right away. If you simply cannot keep your hands off your pet, at least keep your face away; kiss the air—your pet will still get the idea.

In addition, you can try bathing your dog or cat once every other week in warm water with no soap. Bathing the animal in this way significantly reduces the amount of allergen on your pet's fur, according to Clifton T. Furukawa, M.D., clinical professor of pediatrics at the University of Washington School of Medicine in Seattle.

KICK THE CIGARETTE HABIT.

Tobacco smoke can be an irritant that triggers asthma as well as an allergen that touches off an allergic response leading to asthma. Tobacco smoke is one of the worst irritants known: It paralyzes the tiny hairlike cilia along the mucous membranes of the respiratory tract. It also reduces immune response and leaves a smoker much more susceptible to upper-respiratory infection. "There is not a single redeeming feature to cigarette smoking," cautions Weinstein. "Given the known health risks associated with smoking, asthma patients should make every effort to stop smoking—either on their own or with the help of a smoking-cessation program."

Nonsmokers who live with a smoker are no better off. So if there's someone in your household who won't quit smoking, ask that individual to take his or her habit outdoors.

WEATHER THE WEATHER.

While each person responds to weather conditions and weather variations differently, some general trends may be noted. "Keep close watch on how the weather affects you," advises Young. (That means paying attention to factors including temperature, wind velocity, barometric pressure, and humidity.) "Then try to avoid conditions that cause you problems." For example, you should stay indoors when it is very cold, since a blast of cold air can cause a spasm in your bronchial tubes. Stay indoors if the wind is strong, too. While gusts of wind can blow pollution and smog away, they can also blow pollen in your direction. If you enjoy walking in the rain, you're in luck, because rain tends to wash away roving allergens, pollutants, and irritants.

WATCH WHAT YOU EAT.

The question of whether foods trigger chronic asthma has yet to be answered. Some foods, such as nuts, shellfish, milk, eggs, and strawberries, can result in an array of allergic responses, including asthma symptoms. Sulfites in wine can have a similar effect. "While the information available today suggests that the chances are small that food allergies are a trigger for chronic asthma in adults, it is still wise to reduce or eliminate your consumption of certain foods that you notice make your asthma worse. But consult your doctor if you think the foods are nutritionally necessary," says Weinstein.

Allergies to certain types of food, especially milk and wheat, are more often a trigger of asthma in children. If milk and wheat seem to be causing problems for your asthmatic child, eliminate these foods. Check labels, and avoid foods that list milk, milk solids, casein, whey, or caseinate as ingredients. (Talk to your doctor about alternate dietary sources of nutrients such as calcium.)

Eating away from home can sometimes be a problem, says Weinstein. If you are invited to dinner and don't know what dinner will be, eat something at home before you leave so you won't be left hungry. If you are eating in a restaurant, inquire about the ingredients in the dish you want to order as well as the method of preparation. No matter where you have your meal, common sense suggests that you avoid overeating, eating too fast, and talking while you are eating. Steer clear of alcohol, too, especially if you are taking medications for your asthma. One final reminder: Avoid so-called cytotoxicity tests and similar methods that promise to root out hidden food allergies and cure asthma (see "The Quack Comes Back").

THE QUACK COMES BACK

If you have gone from doctor to doctor in search of a remedy for your asthma, you may feel frustrated and be tempted to explore some "alternative" treatments— cytotoxicity testing, special diets, herbal preparations, massage, and vitamins, to name a few. As tempting as these promised solutions may sound, there is one problem: They rarely work.

Cytotoxicity, for instance, is based on the premise that if the allergenic extract of a food to which you are allergic is mixed with a drop of your blood, certain cells in your blood will attack the food. Your blood cells will, therefore, be altered and, when viewed under a microscope, will be distorted. "The Asthma and Allergy Foundation of America has evaluated this test and concluded that it is unreliable," says Stuart Young, M.D.

STAY HEALTHY.

A problem in the upper airways—such as a respiratory infection—can cause trouble in the lower airways—the bronchial tubes—and precipitate an asthma attack. "Everybody wants to be in a state of good health," says Bell. "For a person with asthma, maintaining good health can mean a dramatic lessening of symptoms." Bell suggests that you stay away from people who have a cold or the flu, drink plenty of fluids, and avoid getting overtired; otherwise, you will be more susceptible to infections. If, despite your best efforts, you do develop an infection, see your doctor; early use of antibiotics, when appropriate, can be quite helpful.

EXERCISE YOUR OPTIONS.

For years, people with asthma have been told to avoid exercise because it would induce attacks. Research has shown, however, that the more asthmatics exercise, the more exercise they can tolerate. "If you have asthma, you should partake in regular aerobic exercise," says Bell. He recommends that you start by warming up with light exercise before a more vigorous workout. (Young recommends using cromolyn sodium, a prescription medication, 15 to 20 minutes before aerobic exercise; discuss this with your doctor.) Begin with short workouts and gradually increase them. At least at first, keep a bronchodilator with you. If you feel tightness in your chest and can't work through it, use the device. If you are out in very cold or dry air, wear a scarf around your nose and mouth to heat the air before breathing it in. Cool down with light exercise at the end of your workout. If one type of exercise still brings on attacks, try another form of exercise. You may not be able to tolerate running, for example, but you may be able to swim on a regular basis.

AVOID ASPIRIN.

Aspirin and certain products that contain aspirin can trigger asthma attacks in certain people. "It's just wise to stay away from the whole family of aspirin products if you have asthma," says Weinstein. "This is especially true for patients with nasal polyps, for whom aspirin ingestion can be life threatening. Even if you have not experienced an asthma flare in the past, it could occur at any time." Weinstein encourages anyone with asthma to keep aspirin out of the medicine chest by checking labels on every over-the-counter drug that is purchased. (Avoid those that list "aspirin" and those that contain the initials "ASA," "APC," or "PAC"; ask your pharmacist if you are unsure whether the medication you want to purchase contains aspirin.) If you feel that you must take aspirin, get your doctor's approval.

According to an expert report from the National Asthma Education Program, people with asthma should also stay away from nonsteroidal anti-inflammatory agents (ibuprofen is one such medication) that have effects similar to aspirin's. Opt instead for such "usually safe alternatives" as acetaminophen, sodium salicylate, or disalcid. You may also need to avoid tartrazine (yellow food dye #5), which is found in a number of soft drinks, cake mixes, candies, and some medications, if it aggravates your asthma.

TAKE A DEEP BREATH.

Breathing exercises provide a form of relaxation and can be of benefit to some patients during an asthma attack. However, it would be a mistake to rely on breathing exercises alone to control an asthma flare, says Weinstein. As long as this rule is not broken, breathing exercises are fine for those patients who find them beneficial. "You can practice controlled breathing, which concentrates on slow inhalations through the nose rather than panting breathing through the mouth," says Weinstein. He suggests that before starting these breathing exercises, you blow your nose to make sure that your air passages are clear of all foreign matter. Then sit in a chair in a comfortable position. Take a deep breath and feel your breath going as far down as possible. Your abdomen should expand as you do this exercise. Exhale slowly, feeling your abdomen relax as your breath comes out of your nose. Repeat this exercise at least three times a day (but never right after eating).

KEEP YOUR WEIGHT DOWN.

"Unfortunately, some asthma medications can result in weight gain. An overweight person has to breathe more heavily, and the heart works harder to pump blood all around the body. Weight reduction is very important," says Bell. If you are overweight, you and your doctor should work together to establish a diet plan that will reduce your calorie intake without depriving you of necessary nutrients.

MIND YOUR MIND.

The notion that asthma is "all in your head" has gone the way of many medical myths. Asthma is an illness with both physical and emotional aspects. For example, asthma attacks can be triggered by emotional changes, such as laughing or crying, or by stress. "The human body interacts with the mind," says Young, "so by putting your mind at ease, you can dramatically reduce the panicky feeling that can make an already existing attack worse." He recommends developing an upbeat mind-set by committing yourself to feeling better. A positive attitude works wonders to enhance your other coping methods. In addition, be forthright about your asthma; others will respect your directness and, in most cases, try to make things easier for you.

LEARN TO RELAX.
Since stress and emotional upsets can trigger asthma attacks, try setting aside time each day—preferably the same time—to practice some form of relaxation.

Athlete's foot

21 Strategies to Beat Athlete's Foot

Blame the advertising man who misnamed it in the 1930s, but athlete's foot has nothing to do with athletes. It's a fungal infection of the feet. Also known as tinea pedis, or "ringworm of the feet," it has nothing to do with worms either. The Trichophyton fungus that causes the redness, itching, cracking, and scaling of athlete's foot can also infect the scalp, where it causes hair loss and scaly patches; the body, where it causes round, red, scaly patches that itch; and the groin, where the so-called "jock itch" causes itching and thickening of the skin.

Athlete's foot is the most common fungal infection of the skin. It affects more men than women, probably because men typically wear heavy, often airtight shoes, and the fungus loves hot, dark, moist environments.

Contrary to popular myth, athlete's foot fungus isn't just found in locker rooms, although the moist locker-room environment is perfect for fungal growth. "The fungus is probably present in your bathroom and in your shoes all the time," says Andrew Schink, D.P.M., a podiatrist in private practice and past president of the Oregon Podiatric Medical Association.

Frank Parker, M.D., professor and chairman of the Department of Dermatology at Oregon Health Sciences University in Portland, agrees. "There's no good way to avoid exposure to the athlete's foot fungus," he says, "because it's everywhere where there's moisture."

In fact, most people harbor the fungus on their skin, but it's kept in check by bacteria that live on the skin. So if the fungus is commonly present, why do some people develop an athlete's foot infection, while other people don't? Doctors aren't really sure, but they believe some people are genetically more prone to developing athlete's foot, and people with certain health conditions, such as eczema, asthma, and hay fever, have more difficulty getting rid of the infection. "Some people are simply more susceptible to getting it than others," explains James Shaw, M.D., chief of the Division of Dermatology at Good Samaritan Hospital and Medical Center in Portland, Oregon. "Some people have chronic athlete's foot problems and others are never bothered by it. It may have to do with genetic factors or with exposure— being in places where there are numerous feet in moist environments."

Most cases of athlete's foot cause only bothersome redness, itching, flaking, and scaling on the soles of the feet and between the toes. In severe cases, however, blisters form on the soles of the feet; fissures, or cracks, that weep fluid can also open between the toes. These fissures are vulnerable to secondary infection. When the infection involves the toenails, it can cause the nails to become discolored and thick. Also, if left untreated, athlete's foot can infect other parts of the body.

Doctors don't agree on exactly how athlete's foot is spread, but most believe it's passed by direct contact with an infected person or with a contaminated surface, such as the floor of a shower stall. But Shaw says the real determinants of whether or not you'll get the infection are how susceptible you are and how dry you keep your feet.

While some severe cases of athlete's foot require a doctor's care, most can be effectively treated at home. The following strategies can help you soothe and heal athlete's foot and keep it from cropping up in the future.

MOVE AWAY FROM MOISTURE.
When you think about athlete's foot fungus, remember that it likes moist, warm, dark environments. All of your treatment and prevention strategies should center around keeping your feet as dry as possible.

DRY BETWEEN YOUR TOES.
"Don't just use your damp bath towel to dry between your toes," says Schink. "Use a thin, dry hand towel and thoroughly dry between each toe." If you can't get your feet dry enough with a towel, try drying them with a hand-held hair dryer on the "warm" setting.

HELLO, DOCTOR?

While most cases of athlete's foot can be effectively treated with home remedies, you should see a doctor if:

• You develop cracks in the webs between your toes. Studies have shown that cracking in the webs between the toes may indicate cellulitis, an inflammation of the connective tissue, which must be treated by a doctor, says Margaret Robertson, M.D.

• Your athlete's foot infection doesn't respond to home remedies within two to three weeks. If your condition isn't responding to treatment, it may indicate that you have some other problem, says James Shaw, M.D. "There are a whole host of things that can mimic a fungal infection," he says. Robertson agrees. "Often, fungal infections mimic other problems, like eczema and psoriasis," she says. Your doctor can perform a simple test to determine if athlete's foot is really the problem, she adds.

WASH THOSE FEET.
Twice a day, wash your feet in soap and water, and dry them thoroughly, says Shaw.

KICK OFF YOUR SHOES.
Go barefoot or wear open-toed sandals whenever you can. "Going barefoot is good for the feet and great for treating and preventing athlete's foot," says Schink. Of course, it's not always possible to go barefoot, especially

• Your infection is getting worse despite treatment. Some strains are hardier and are able to resist over-the-counter medication. Robertson says the antifungal medications available by prescription, such as ketoconazole and griseofulvin, are stronger and can knock out more persistent infections.

• One or both feet swell.

• Pus appears in the lesions.

• The fungus spreads to your hands. Robertson says that when athlete's foot travels to the hands, it's called "two-foot, one-hand disease" because it often affects only one hand. Treatment may require prescription oral medication.

• The toenails appear thick and discolored. This indicates the toenails have become infected with the fungus. "Fungal infections of the toenails are very difficult to treat," says Robertson. "Most of the over-the-counter topical medications that are supposed to treat fungus of the toenails don't work, because the nail is so thick."

when you're at work. But you may be able to sneak off those shoes during lunch, at break time, or when you're sitting at your desk.

MEDICATE 'EM.
Over-the-counter antifungal preparations are very effective for most cases of athlete's foot, says Parker. These products come in creams, sprays, or solutions and contain tolnaftate (Tinactin), miconazole (Micatin), or

undecylenic acid (Desenex). Creams seem to be more effective, but powders can help absorb moisture. Parker recommends washing and drying the feet, then applying the medication thoroughly twice a day.

Experiment. If one product doesn't work, try another. "Different products seem to work better for different people," says Margaret Robertson, M.D., a board-certified dermatologist in private practice and a staff physician at St. Vincent Hospital and Medical Center in Portland, Oregon.

BE PERSISTENT.

Too often, people stop using the antifungal preparations as soon as the symptoms of athlete's foot infection go away. The fungus, however, may still be present. "Fungus is slow-dividing," Robertson explains. "You have to be persistent and use the medication for three to six weeks to see improvement." Once the infection has cleared, keep using the antifungal cream, powder, or lotion once a day or once a week—whatever will keep your feet fungus-free.

MAKE TEA FOR TOES.

To help dry out the infection and ease the itching that accompanies athlete's foot, Schink advises soaking your feet in a quart of warm water containing six black tea bags. "The tannic acid in the tea is very soothing and helps kill the fungus," he says.

SOAK THEM IN BETADINE.

If the infection has caused redness and cracks between the toes, the fungal infection may be compounded by a bacterial infection. Robertson suggests soaking your feet once a day for 20 minutes in two capfuls of Betadine (available over-the-counter at pharmacies) to one quart of warm water. After the Betadine soak, dry your feet well, and apply antifungal medication.

DON'T BLEACH.

While the idea is to dry out the infection, avoid home remedies that involve strong chemicals and solvents, such as bleach, alcohol, and floor cleaners. "Many people are tempted to use what's at hand to treat their problem," says Shaw. "But harsh chemicals won't necessarily kill the fungus, and they can really damage your skin."

TAN YOUR TOOTSIES.

Ultraviolet light can help dry up the infection and kill active fungus on your skin. Kick off those shoes and let the sun shine on your feet for a little while. Avoid extensive sun exposure, however, since it can promote wrinkling and skin cancer. And be careful not to burn the tops of your feet.

TREAT YOUR SHOES.

If you have fungus on your feet, you've got fungus in your shoes. To keep from reinfecting yourself every time you put your shoes on, Schink recommends treating your shoes with Lysol spray or an antifungal spray or powder every time you take off your shoes.

AIR 'EM OUT.

On sunny days, Schink advises taking the laces out of your shoes, pulling up their tongues, and setting them in a sunny, well-ventilated place. The sun will help dry out the shoes, eliminate odors, and kill the fungus.

HOW CONTAGIOUS IS IT?

We've all heard stories about someone picking up athlete's foot in public showers and locker rooms. While it's true that such moist places probably do harbor fungus, your bathroom probably does, too. Relax and forget about trying to scrub all of the fungus from your life. It's everywhere, and you're not going to avoid it no matter how much you scrub and clean.

Does it mean you have to suffer with athlete's foot? Not necessarily, says Margaret Robertson, M.D. "It's a matter of genetics and exposure," she explains. "Some people are more susceptible to the fungus, and some strains of fungus are more infectious than others."

Robertson says that the type of athlete's foot fungus that causes red, weepy lesions is more infectious than the type that creates a white scale. Being exposed to the more

ALTERNATE SHOES.

Switch every other day, says Schink. Treat the pair not being worn with sun and an antifungal medicine.

Some people's feet are simply more prone to sweating, according to Robertson. If you're one of those "sweaty feet types," you may have to change your shoes a couple of times a day to keep your feet dry.

CHOOSE SHOES WITH CARE.

When you have to wear shoes, opt for sandals or other opened-toed shoes, if possible. "Choose shoes that don't infectious type doesn't mean you're going to get it, however. "My husband has battled chronic athlete's foot for 20 years," confesses Robertson, "and I've never been infected."

"It's not really all that contagious, like many of the other skin infections," says James Shaw, M.D. "If you have it, you don't have to worry too much about infecting others." Follow these simple tips to reduce the risk of infecting others:

• After bathing, wash out the tub or shower with an antiseptic cleaner like Lysol.

• Don't share your towel.

• Wash your socks twice in extra-hot water to kill fungal spores.

• Wear thongs in public showers.

• Keep your feet dry, and use the over-the-counter medications and treatments already discussed to clear your infection up quickly.

make your feet sweat," says Robertson. Avoid shoes made of plastic or rubber or shoes that are watertight. These shoes trap perspiration and create the warm, moist conditions perfect for growing a new crop of fungus. When you must wear closed-toed shoes, opt for natural, "breathable" materials like leather.

EXERCISE YOUR SOCK OPTIONS.
Socks made of natural fibers, such as cotton and wool, help to absorb perspiration and keep the feet dry. However, recent research suggests that acrylic socks

may do an even better job of keeping the feet dry by wicking moisture away from the feet. So what kind of sock should you choose? Try a pair of natural-fiber socks and a pair of acrylic, and see which one keeps your feet drier and more comfortable.

If your feet naturally sweat a lot or if you're participating in activities like sports that make your feet sweat more than usual, change your socks two or three times a day.

WEAR THONGS.
When you're in a public place likely to harbor athlete's foot fungus, like the locker room of your favorite gym, wear thongs to limit your exposure to fungus, says Shaw. Although this technique isn't foolproof, it will decrease your risk of athlete's foot, and it may prevent you from picking up other nasty foot maladies, such as plantar warts.

Back pain

19 Ways to Keep Back Pain at Bay

Maybe you lifted something heavy or swung a golf club a little too enthusiastically. Or maybe you've been sitting in an uncomfortable desk chair for two weeks, sweating over a deadline. Whatever the reason, now you're flat on your back, wishing for something—anything—that will put an end to the agony.

Take heart—you're not alone. Almost every American suffers from back pain at some point in his or her life. The bad news is that unless you have a major injury or disc problem, your doctor may not be able to do much for you other than prescribe some pain medication and advise you to rest. The good news is that by following some simple steps, you can be on your feet again in just a few days. Even better, you can avoid having to endure similar discomfort in the future.

EASING THE PAIN

The following remedies are appropriate for anyone who is suffering from back pain that is the result of tight, aching muscles or a strain. However, if you are experiencing pain, weakness, or numbness in the legs or a loss of bowel or bladder control, be sure to see a doctor without delay.

GO TO BED.

"Bed rest is a way of removing the strain from the muscles," says Daniel S. J. Choy, M.D., director of the Laser Laboratory at St. Luke's–Roosevelt Hospital Center and an assistant clinical professor of medicine at Columbia University College of Physicians and Surgeons in New York. "The back muscles' job is to hold you erect. If you lie down, it takes the stress off of the muscles." The best way to lie is flat on your back with two pillows underneath your knees. Never lie facedown, Choy says, since this position forces you to twist your head to breathe and may cause neck pain. Make an effort to get up and start moving around after three days, since longer periods of bed rest may make the muscles weaker and more prone to strain, he adds.

ICE IT.

Applying an ice pack to the painful area within 24 hours of the injury can help keep inflammation and discomfort to a minimum, according to Willibald Nagler, M.D., Anne and Jerome Fisher Physiatrist-in-Chief and chairman of the Department of Rehabilitation Medicine at The New York Hospital–Cornell Medical Center in New York. "Ice does one thing—it decreases the nerve's ability to conduct a painful stimulus," he says. Nagler suggests wrapping ice cubes in a plastic bag, then applying the bag on top of a thin towel that has been placed on the skin. Leave the ice pack on for 20 minutes, take it off for 30 minutes, then replace it for another 20 minutes, he says.

TAKE A HOT BATH.

If more than 24 hours have passed since the injury occurred, ice will not help reduce pain or inflammation. After that time, heat may help increase the elasticity of the muscles by about ten percent, Nagler says. Jerold Lancourt, M.D., an orthopedic surgeon at North Dallas Orthopedics & Rehabilitation, P.A., in Dallas, tells his patients to soak in a hot bath for 20 minutes or more. Pregnant women, however, should not sit in a hot bath for too long, since raising the body temperature over 100 degrees Fahrenheit for long periods may cause birth defects or miscarriage.

INVEST IN A NEW MATTRESS.

A soft, sagging mattress may contribute to the development of back problems or worsen an existing problem, according to Henry J. Bienert, Jr., M.D., an orthopedic surgeon at Tulane University School of Medicine in New

Orleans. If a new mattress is not in your budget, how-ever, a three-quarter-inch-thick piece of plywood placed between the mattress and box spring may help some-what. "The verdict's not back yet on water beds," he adds. In any case, try to sleep on your back with two pil-lows underneath your knees.

GET A MASSAGE.

If you're lucky enough to have an accommodating spouse, friend, or roommate, ask him or her to give you a rubdown. "Lie facedown and have someone knead the muscles," Choy says. Local massage therapists may also make house calls. You can check the yellow pages for listings or ask a friend for a referral.

RELAX.

Much back pain is the result of muscles made tight by emotional tension, Lancourt says. He recommends that his patients practice relaxation and deep-breathing ex-ercises, such as closing their eyes, breathing deeply, and counting backward from 100.

TAKE TWO ASPIRIN.

Taking an over-the-counter analgesic such as aspirin, ac-etaminophen, or ibuprofen may help relieve your pain. However, be aware that not all medications—not even nonprescription ones—are for everyone. Pregnant women, for example, should not take any medication without first checking with their doctor. And people with ulcers should stay away from analgesics containing as-pirin, according to Lancourt. "Any medicine should be taken with knowledge of its side effects," he says. "Make sure to get the advice of your doctor."

PREVENTING FUTURE PAIN

Many daily activities—sitting, lifting, bending, carrying—can put a strain on your back. By learning new ways of going about these activities, you can help prevent back pain and ensure the health of your back for years to come. The tips that follow can help.

USE A CUSHION.

"The seats of most cars and trucks are not well designed," Choy says. "They should support the small of your back." If your seat doesn't, Choy suggests that you buy a small cushion that can be fitted to provide the missing support. He adds that the most desirable sitting position is not one in which your back is straight up and down. It's better to be leaning back at an angle of about 110 degrees. If you sit for long hours, Choy also recommends that you periodically get up and walk around.

PUT YOUR ARM BEHIND YOUR BACK.

If you have to sit for long periods in a chair that doesn't support your lower back and you don't have a cushion, try rolling up a towel or sweater so that it has about the same circumference as your forearm. Then slide the rolled-up cloth between your lower back and the chair, recommends Billy Glisan, M.S., an exercise physiologist and the director of injury prevention programs for the Texas Back Institute in Dallas. In a pinch, you can simply slide your forearm between your lower back and the back of the chair to ease the strain on your back. Even with the best back support, however, sitting is still stressful on your back, so try to make small adjustments in the curvature of your lower back every few minutes or so, advises Glisan.

SWIM.

Swimming is the best aerobic exercise for a bad back, according to Choy. Doing laps in the pool can help tone and tighten the muscles of the back and abdomen. Walking is second best, he says. You can also try the "Back-Saving Exercises."

LIFT WITH YOUR KNEES BENT.

The large muscles of your legs and buttocks are better equipped to bear heavy weights than your back muscles are, according to Bienert. "Pretend you have a goldfish bowl filled with water on the top of your head," he says. "When you squat down to pick something up, don't spill a drop." Bienert also recommends strengthening leg and buttock muscles to facilitate squatting.

CARRY OBJECTS CLOSE TO YOUR BODY.

When picking up and carrying heavy objects, pull in your elbows and hold the object close to your body, Choy recommends. "If you have to reach something on a shelf, get right under it and rest it on your head," he says. "Then, the weight is carried by the erect spine, and you don't ask as much of your muscles."

STAY ALERT.

Careless activity is the number-one cause of back injury, according to Lancourt. "If you have had previous back pain, be very careful," he says. "Avoid bending and twisting and lifting. Avoid being caught off guard. Sometimes it's better to hire somebody to do things, such as yard work or carrying heavy suitcases, than to hurt yourself and miss three months of work."

(Continued on page 70)

....

BACK-SAVING EXERCISES

The following back exercises were provided by exercise physiologist Billy Glisan, M.S. For best results, do the exercises daily, and don't discontinue them, even after the pain gets better, since strength and flexibility can only be maintained through consistent exercise. Stretches may be done twice a day. Although these exercises are safe and effective for most back pain caused by muscle strain or spasm, Glisan cautions that people with disc or other structural problems should not engage in any type of exercise without advice from their doctor.

Single Knee-to-Chest: Lie on your back with your knees bent and your feet on the floor. Grasp the back of one thigh with both hands; gently and slowly pull toward your chest until you feel mild tension—not to the point of pain. Hold to the count of ten, without bouncing, then release. Repeat four to five times with the same leg, then switch sides. This exercise stretches muscles in the hips, buttocks, and lower back—all muscles that become shortened and tight after a long day of sitting or standing. It is a good warm-up to the other exercises.

Double Knee-to-Chest: Lie on your back with your knees bent and your feet on the floor. Grasp both thighs, and gently and slowly pull them as close to your chest as you can. Pull only to the point of slight tension, and don't bounce. Hold to the count of ten, then release. Repeat four or five times before doing the next exercise.

Lumbar Rotation: Lie on your back with your hips and knees bent, your feet flat on the floor, and your heels touching your buttocks. Keeping your knees together and your shoulders on the floor, slowly allow your knees to rotate to the right, until you reach a point of mild tension. Hold for a count of ten, then return to the starting position. Repeat four to five times on the right side, then switch to the left.

Partial Sit-Up: Lie on your back with your knees bent, your feet flat on the floor, and your hands gently supporting your head. Slowly curl up just to the point where your shoulders come off the floor. Avoid bending your neck. Hold for a few counts, then roll slowly back down. Remember to breathe as you do the exercise. Repeat 10 to 15 times. This exercise strengthens the abdominal muscles; strong abdominal muscles help you maintain good posture and reduce the possibility of back injury.

Active Back Extension: Lie on your chest on the floor. You can put a pillow under your stomach (not under your hips) if that feels comfortable. Put your arms at your sides, with your hands next to your buttocks. Slowly extend your head and neck and raise your upper body slowly off the floor. Hold for five to ten counts. Slowly lower yourself back to the starting position. Remember to breathe as you do the exercise. Repeat five to ten times.

Office exercises: Poor sitting posture puts stress on the ligaments and other tissues. To give your lower back a break, periodically get up to a standing position, with your feet shoulder-width apart and your hands on your hips. Slowly lean back to a point of mild tension and hold for a count of ten. Repeat four to five times.

WATCH YOUR WEIGHT.

Maintaining your ideal weight may help take the strain off the back muscles, according to Bienert. "The less you have to carry, the less load you have," he says. "Secondly, when you gain weight in your abdomen, you may become sway-backed, which can accentuate back pain."

Bad breath

6 Refreshing Fixes

"**H**alitosis is better than no breath at all," jokes one dentist. But the problem of halitosis, or bad breath, has plagued mankind for centuries, leaving few people laughing about it. To conquer bad breath, the ancient Greeks reputedly rinsed with white wine, anise seed, and myrrh, while the Italians mixed up a mouthwash of sage, cinnamon, juniper seeds, root of cypress, and rosemary leaves, according to the Academy of General Dentistry.

Today, Americans spend more than half a billion dollars each year for mouthwashes that often contain little more than alcohol and flavoring. But people worry about their breath. Indeed, *New York Times* health columnist Jane E. Brody has written that she receives more questions about bad breath than she does about any other common medical problem.

Maybe one explanation is the simple fact that you can't really tell whether you've got bad breath. This is a time when you have to depend on the honesty and kindness of friends to let you know. "We're immune to our own breath," says Linda Niessen, D.M.D., M.P.H., associate professor and chair of geriatric oral medicine in the Department of Community Health and Preventive Dentistry at Baylor College of Dentistry in Dallas.

What if you're on your way to that important meeting and you simply *must* know if your breath will precede you through the door? You can try breathing into a handkerchief or running floss between your teeth, suggests Erwin Barrington, D.D.S., professor of periodontics at the University of Illinois at Chicago.

Fixing bad breath depends on what's causing it. Most often, bad breath is the result of nothing more serious than a dirty mouth. Plaque, the nearly invisible film of bacteria that's constantly forming in your mouth, is often responsible. Other dental culprits include cavities and gum disease. "Tooth decay by itself doesn't smell bad, but the trapped food does," explains Niessen.

Occasionally, bad breath is due to something in the lungs or gastrointestinal tract or to a systemic (body-wide) condition. "Eating a garlicky meal is one of the most common causes," says Niessen. The strong odors of foods like garlic, onions, and alcohol are carried through the bloodstream and exhaled by the lungs. Another big loser when it comes to turning your breath sour—and harming your health—is tobacco.

In addition, some health problems, such as sinus infections or diabetes (which may give the breath a chemical smell), can cause bad breath, points out Barrington.

Figuring out the cause of bad breath is the first step, obviously, in doing something about it. Here's what you can do to keep your breath as fresh as possible:

WHAT ABOUT MOUTHWASH?

Madison Avenue has played to our fears of bad breath in advertising claims for mouthwashes. But do they really work?

"Mouthwashes will cover odors," says Linda Niessen, D.M.D., M.P.H. The effects, however, are short-lived: Dental researchers agree that commercial mouthwashes mask odors only temporarily (from about 20 minutes to about 2 hours). These products don't prevent bad breath, either, says Erwin Barrington, D.D.S. While they may be able to kill bacteria that contribute to bad breath, a new batch of bacteria crops up fairly quickly.

If you do decide to use a mouthwash, Niessen recommends choosing a product with fluoride for its cavity-fighting potential or one that is accepted by the American Dental Association for removing plaque.

KEEP YOUR MOUTH CLEAN.
"That's the key thing," stresses Sebastian G. Ciancio, D.D.S., professor and chairman of the Department of Periodontology and clinical professor of pharmacology at the School of Dental Medicine at the State University of New York at Buffalo. That means a thorough brushing twice a day. It also means flossing regularly. Food and bacteria trapped between teeth and at the gum line can only be removed with floss; if it's left to linger, it's not going to smell nice.

HELLO, DOCTOR?

Persistent bad breath may be due to a treatable cause, such as an undiagnosed cavity or periodontal (gum) disease. Sometimes, a broken filling can trap food particles. If you visit the dentist and are given a clean bill of health, you may want to investigate further and talk to your physician about other possible causes.

CLEAN YOUR TONGUE, TOO.
Bacteria left on your tongue can certainly contribute to less-than-fresh breath, so be sure to brush your tongue after you've polished your pearly whites.

WET YOUR WHISTLE.
A dry mouth can equal smelly breath. Saliva helps clean your mouth; it has a natural antibacterial action and it washes away food particles, says Ciancio. (Reduced saliva flow at night explains morning breath.) Sugarless gum or sucking on mints can stimulate saliva production.

RINSE.
If nothing else, at least rinse your mouth with plain water after eating, recommends Virginia L. Woodward, R.D.H., past president of the American Dental Hygienists' Association. Swishing the water around in your mouth may help to remove some of the food particles left in the mouth after a meal.

MUNCH ON PARSLEY.

That green sprig of parsley that came with your meal can do more than decorate your plate. While munching on parsley or spearmint won't cure bad breath, the scent of the herb itself can help temporarily cover up offending oral odor. (You're basically trading an offensive odor for a more acceptable one.)

EAT TO SMELL SWEET.

Foods that help fight plaque may also help fight mouth odor, says Woodward. Opt for celery, carrots, peanuts, or a bit of low-fat cheese if you want something to snack on. "A healthy diet will help your teeth as well," Barrington points out.

Belching

8 Ways to Squelch the Belch

In certain cultures, a belch after dinner is traditionally considered a compliment to the cook. In the Western world, if an adult belches after dinner—or at any time, for that matter—it is considered a breach of manners.

Babies burp, and it is certainly a satisfying sound to the mother or father who has been patting or rubbing the baby's back. Children belch, too, because they think it's a funny game, and sometimes the competition gets noisily intense. Over the years, however, such child's play can turn into a habit of frequently and unconsciously swallowing air—a habit that can result in belching.

If you suffer from aerophagia—the medical name for repetitive belching—you have probably endured the embarrassment of an unexpected outburst at precisely the most inelegant moment. But your habit can easily be broken if you just become aware of when and how you swallow air and stop doing it. Here's how:

STIFLE IT.

"Chronic belchers may force themselves to belch because it provides temporary relief," says Lawrence S. Friedman, M.D., associate professor of medicine at Jefferson Medical College in Philadelphia. In fact, it has been demonstrated that repeated belching produces more of the same. On a fluoroscope (a special type of X ray used to visualize a body part in motion), a belching person can be seen forcing air into the mouth and esophagus. So if you're a chronic belcher, you need to make a concious effort to squelch that belch.

DON'T SMOKE.

Here is yet another reason to give up smoking. "By inhaling on cigarettes, cigars, or pipes, you are swallowing excessive amounts of air—much more than the belch can let out," says Gayle Randall, M.D., assistant professor of medicine in the Department of Medicine at the University of California at Los Angeles School of Medicine. And if you are counting on chewing gum or sucking on hard candy to help you kick the habit, think again; these activities stimulate air swallowing.

MIND YOUR MANNERS.

Mom was right again when she told you not to talk with your mouth full. "This habit allows air into the mouth, which is then swallowed with the food," says Thomas Stahl, M.D., assistant professor of general surgery at Georgetown University Medical Center in Washington, D.C. Anyway, he adds, it's an unappealing form of behavior.

EAT SLOWLY.
People who gulp down food and beverages are, for one thing, swallowing excessive amounts of air. They're also crowding the stomach with too much to digest, which causes a gaseous buildup. "Once you take a mouthful, put down your fork and chew your food well before taking another bite," advises Randall.

RELAX.
Anxiety and stress can cause you to swallow more often, which increases the amount of air taken in. "You'll have to make a conscious effort to minimize air swallowing even though you may feel that your mouth is dry, because you'll only complicate your stress with stomach gas," says Stahl.

DON'T CATCH COLD.
One sure thing about a cold is that it brings along postnasal drip, which will probably make you swallow much more frequently. So try to blow your nose to clear your nasal passages. Better yet, you should try to protect yourself from exposure to cold viruses.

AVOID BUBBLY BEVERAGES.
Drinking carbonated beverages, including beer, creates air in the stomach. "Stay away from these drinks," advises Randall.

GO STRAWLESS.
Drinking through a straw will only increase the amount
of air you swallow.

Bites

19 Ways to Fight Bites

B ites can range from itchy to painful to life threatening. And you needn't live out in the wilderness to
run the risk of getting one. In fact, one of the most dangerous kinds of bites can be inflicted in your very own
home—a bite from a fellow human being! (Doctors agree
that humans have more bacteria in their mouths than
most wild animals, no matter how often we brush our
teeth.)

Many bites can be treated at home, although others,
like a bite from a human, require an immediate visit to
the doctor or the emergency room. The trick is distin-
guishing those bites that are dangerous from those that
are benign.

The following is a guide to treating the most common
types of bites, as well as a few tips on how to avoid getting bitten in the first place. Of course, if you have had a
run-in with a creature that you suspect is dangerous,
whether or not it is discussed here, don't attempt self-
treatment. See a doctor without delay. The same advice
holds true if you experience any signs of illness (such
as fever, loss of consciousness, nausea, dizziness, or
vomiting) following a bite.

ICE AN ITCH.

Itchy mosquito bites may benefit from an ice-cold compress, according to Karl Singer, M.D., F.P., I.M., a physician in Exeter, New Hampshire. He recommends icing the bite for 20 minutes at a time every few hours. Treat nonpoisonous spider bites the same.

TRY AN OLD FAIL-SAFE.

When you had a mosquito bite as a child, your mother probably used calamine lotion—a thin, chalky, pink liquid—to stop the itch. Sold over the counter (and quite economical, too, compared with alternatives such as hydrocortisone), it is just as effective today, says Michael R. Stefan, M.D., a physician specializing in internal medicine in Los Angeles.

GIVE AN ANTIHISTAMINE A TRY.

Over-the-counter antihistamines can also help an itchy bite, since the itch is really a mild allergic reaction, says Singer. Of course, antihistamines should not be used by sensitive individuals, pregnant women, people with allergies to ingredients in the products, or those who are taking conflicting medications. Check with your doctor or pharmacist if you are in doubt.

RECOGNIZE THE SIGNS OF A SEVERE REACTION.

The bite from a venomous spider can cause a severe allergic reaction. It is important, therefore, to recognize the signs of an allergic reaction before it is too late, according to Lawrence H. Bernstein, M.D., a family physician in Storrs, Connecticut. Symptoms of anaphylaxis, or severe allergic reaction, include difficulty breathing, hives all over the body, and loss of consciousness.

Anyone experiencing these warning signals should be rushed to the nearest emergency room, he says. Hospital physicians usually treat anaphylaxis with steroids, adrenaline, and antihistamines.

DON'T PANIC IF YOU'VE BEEN BITTEN BY A TICK.

Lyme disease, a tick-borne illness that can cause chills, fever, headache, and other complications, has received lots of play in the media of late. But not all ticks carry the disease, and not every Lyme-carrying tick will transmit it to you if you happen to be bitten. Generally, a tick must remain on the skin for 24 to 48 hours in order to transmit the organism that causes Lyme disease, according to Bernstein. "The best thing to do, if you're in a place where there might be ticks, is to check yourself on a daily basis," he says. If you remove a tick from your skin (using the directions that follow), Bernstein recommends saving it in a small jar of alcohol, so that if a suspicious infection develops, the tick can be analyzed for Lyme disease. There is no need to see a doctor unless you notice any signs of swelling or redness around the bite (a sign of infection), a bull's-eye-shaped rash (often a symptom of Lyme disease), a fever, or a skin rash, Bernstein says.

REMOVE TICKS WITH CARE.

To remove a tick from your skin, grasp the insect's mouthparts with tweezers as close as possible to your skin and slowly pull straight upward. Do not attempt to pull the tick's body or head, as it may break off, leaving the mouthparts underneath your skin, Bernstein says. Use the tweezers to remove any remaining parts of the tick. Next, apply a local antiseptic, such as alcohol or an antibiotic ointment, to the bite.

STOP THE BLEEDING.

If an animal bite has caused severe bleeding, apply pressure to the area with the palm of your hand, says Michael O. Fleming, M.D., F.A.A.F.P., a family physician in Shreveport, Louisiana. If the wound is large, tie a scarf, towel, or T-shirt tightly around the site to create pressure over a larger area (not tightly enough to cut off circulation). Immobilize the area. If the bite is on a limb, elevate the limb above the level of the heart. See a physician pronto.

DON'T TREAT A PUNCTURE LIKE A SCRATCH.

A bite that leaves a scratch but doesn't really break the skin may simply be washed with soap and water, then covered with an antibacterial cream or ointment. Not so for a bite that breaks or punctures the skin, according to Bernstein. The latter needs the expertise of a doctor, he says. "You need to establish whether the animal is rabid or not," he advises. "Observe the animal carefully. With wild animals, if the animal is particularly placid—for example, if you can walk up to a squirrel and feed it—there's something wrong with that animal. It's sick." He suggests calling a doctor or veterinarian to find out if there have been any reported outbreaks of rabies in wild or domestic animals in your area.

GET A TETANUS BOOSTER.

If you've been bitten by a wild or domestic animal and the bite has broken the skin, it's probably wise to contact your doctor to see if you need a tetanus booster shot (whether or not you need one depends, in part, on the type of wound and the timing of your last tetanus shot). "Animal bites and human bites are easily infected," Fleming says. "All animals have a very large number of bacteria that live in their mouths." He also advises watching the wound for signs of infection, such as redness and swelling. If you should notice any such signs, consult your doctor as soon as possible.

REPORT AN ANIMAL TO THE AUTHORITIES.

If you've been bitten by an animal in your community, call your local Society for the Prevention of Cruelty to Animals (SPCA) or animal catcher (check your local phone directory for the number) to report the incident. If the animal was wild or a stray, the proper agency may want to track it down and capture it for observation, especially if rabies is suspected. If the animal belongs to a neighbor, report it to the pet's owner, and, if you choose, to the authorities (many communities have laws concerning pet bites).

DON'T GET BITTEN IN THE FIRST PLACE.

Perhaps the most sensible way to treat a bite is in advance—before you get bitten—Stefan says. Stay away from wild animals, even if they let you approach, and don't pester snakes, spiders, bees, or anything else that looks threatening. "Most animals and insects will not attack you unless you are bothering them," he says. Even animals that do not look threatening, such as ground squirrels, may be trouble, Stefan adds, since they may carry fleas that can transmit diseases. Insect and tick repellents may also help you avoid bites when spending long periods of time outdoors.

HANDLING SNAKEBITES

If you've been bitten by a snake that you suspect is poisonous, the best thing to do is to hightail it to the nearest emergency room. Some snakebites, most notably those from rattlesnakes such as the Eastern diamondback, can be fatal. However, hospital emergency units stock very effective antivenoms that will have you feeling better in no time, says Michael R. Stefan, M.D.

One fact that may make you less nervous is that snakes only envenomate, or inject their venom, between 25 percent and 75 percent of the time, according to Richard E. Hannigan, M.D. The rest of the time they leave nothing more than fang holes and a frightened victim.

If you are far from medical attention, Hannigan recommends taking the following steps while help is being sought or while you are on the way to the hospital:

• Have someone catch the snake and kill it—if the capture can be accomplished without excessive danger. Put the corpse in a bag, and take it to the hospital with you (but don't delay treatment for this reason). This way, hospital staff can accurately identify the snake and will be sure to administer the correct antivenom.

KNOW YOUR LOCAL FAUNA.
It's best to keep abreast of the insects and animals in your area, so that you know what to watch out for. For example, you may live in an area where there has been an outbreak of rabies among domestic animals or a large

• Stay quiet, still, and warm. Do your best not to panic. Getting upset stimulates the heart to pump more blood, which means that more venom will be circulated throughout your system. Taking a couple long, slow, deep breaths may help.

• If you have been bitten on a limb, remove any rings, bracelets, shoes, or socks, since the extremity may swell. If possible, immobilize the limb and let it rest at a level below the heart.

• You may tie a scarf, tie, belt, or piece of fabric above the level of the fang mark, but do not make it tight enough to cut off circulation. A good guideline is to make sure that you can slide at least one finger underneath the band.

• If you have a venom-extractor kit with you, apply the suction device for 30 to 40 minutes, or until you get to the hospital.

• Do not apply ice, cut the snakebite with a knife, or attempt to suck venom from the wound. These are outdated methods of treatment that may actually cause more harm than good.

• Ask for help. If you have been envenomated, you may begin to feel dizzy or ill. Do not attempt to drive yourself to the hospital.

number of Lyme-carrying ticks, according to Richard E. Hannigan, M.D., an internist in private practice in Helotes, Texas. Likewise, you should know if rattlesnakes, poisonous spiders, or scorpions are likely to take up residence around your neighborhood. If you live in an area, such as the Southwest, that is home to poisonous snakes and scorpions, learn how to recognize them and avoid them like the plague, Hannigan says.

Bladder infection

15 Self-Care Techniques

You have to *go*, and you have to go *now*. Come to think of it, it seems like you've had to go every 15 minutes today. And each time, it's been the same story. Not much comes out, but it burns like crazy.

If you have pain or burning on urination, the frequent urge to urinate, and/or blood in your urine, chances are you have a bladder infection (also called cystitis, urinary tract infection, or UTI). These symptoms may also be accompanied by lower abdominal pain, fever and chills, and an all-over ill feeling.

Bladder infections are caused by a bacterial invasion of the bladder and urinary tract. "The urine in the bladder is normally sterile," explains Amanda Clark, M.D., assistant professor of obstetrics and gynecology at Oregon Health Sciences University in Portland. "However, if it becomes contaminated with bacteria, a bladder infection can develop."

If you're a woman who suffers from bladder infections, you're not alone. "Women tend to suffer more bladder infections than men because the female urethra, the tube leading from the bladder to the outside of the body, is only about one-and-a-half inches long—a short distance for bacteria to travel," says Sadja Greenwood, M.D., a women's health specialist and assistant clinical professor in the Department of Obstetrics, Gynecology, and Reproductive Sciences at the University of California at San Francisco. (A man's urethra is about eight inches long.) Frequently, the urinary tract becomes contaminated with *Escherichia coli*, bacteria that are normally present in the bowel and anal area. In 10 to 15 percent of cases, bladder infections are caused by another organism, such as *Chlamydia trachomatis*.

Women also suffer more bladder infections because sexual intercourse can irritate the urethra and contribute to the transport of bacteria from the anal area and vagina into the bladder. "We don't really know exactly why intercourse increases the risk of bladder infections," says Clark. "We think it might make the bladder tissues a little more receptive to having an infection or it may cause more bacteria to move up the urethra."

Women who use the diaphragm for birth control have a greater risk of bladder infections, too, says Clark. The diaphragm presses against the neck of the bladder, which inhibits normal urination, she says. As urine flow decreases, pressure within the bladder increases, and the bladder is unable to completely empty itself. The pooled urine then acts as a growth medium for bacteria.

Pregnant women are also more likely to suffer from bladder infections. The changing hormones of pregnancy and the pressure exerted by the enlarged uterus on the bladder and ureters (the tubes that carry urine from the kidneys to the bladder) put pregnant women at risk.

Men can also suffer from this malady. In men, bladder infections are almost always secondary to an infection of the prostate gland (prostatitis), according to Theodore Lehman, M.D., a urologist in private practice and director of The Oregon Impotence Center in Portland. "Primary infection of the bladder in men just doesn't happen, because the bladder is well protected," explains Lehman. "But the prostate sits right in front of the bladder, and bacteria can get into it—through sexual intercourse, trauma like bouncing on a bicycle seat, or some kind of blockage—and it stirs up an infection in the prostate. Then the prostate infection can 'move upstream,' if you will, and infect the bladder."

In men, prostate infection usually feels like "you're sitting on a brick," says Lehman. When the infection extends to the bladder, the symptoms of irritation, urinary frequency, and pain and burning on urination join the achy-bottom feeling.

Bladder infections can often be treated at home with the self-care tips that follow. However, if your symptoms persist for more than 24 hours, if they don't respond to home remedies, or if you suspect that your symptoms may be due to a sexually transmitted disease or other infection, see your physician.

LOAD UP ON FLUIDS.

At the first sign of bladder infection, start drinking water and don't stop. During the first 24 hours, Greenwood recommends drinking at least one eight-ounce glass of water every hour. People who suffer from recurrent bladder infections usually don't drink enough liquids. So even when you don't have an active infection, you should drink eight glasses of water every day.

According to Lehman, drinking lots of fluid not only dilutes the urine, giving bacteria less to feed on, it also has a "washout" effect on bacteria. "The more bacteria you can wash out," says Lehman, "the less there will be to reproduce."

Clark warns, however, that people who suffer from urinary leakage (incontinence) probably shouldn't increase their fluids. She says it can make the bladder infection and the incontinence worse.

HAVE A CRANBERRY COCKTAIL.

If you've never developed a taste for the sweet tanginess of cranberry juice, now's the time. Cranberry juice (without added sugar) may make urine more acidic and less hospitable for bacterial growth, says Clark. Drinking cranberry juice is also a way to increase your fluid intake.

GO, GO, GO.

Lehman advises both men and women to avoid what he calls "L.A.-freeway-driver bladder." "Many people don't urinate when they first get the urge because it's inconvenient or there isn't the time or place," he says. "Take a guy who gets off work, has a couple of cups of coffee or a couple of beers, and gets on the freeway in rush-hour traffic. He feels the urge to urinate, but he can't get off the freeway. When he finally gets home and urinates, it's difficult and it burns. By the next day, he's calling his doctor with a prostate infection."

Holding urine allows it to concentrate in the bladder, creating a perfect medium for bacterial growth. In older men, holding urine can cause congestion, inflammation, and obstruction of the prostate and can eventually lead to a prostate infection or sometimes even to a bladder infection.

Not urinating at the first urge also causes the bladder to distend and stretch. "Essentially, the bladder is a hollow muscle," says Lehman. "If you repeatedly stretch it, then it won't void completely and creates a place for bacteria to grow."

HEAT IT UP.

For lower abdominal pain, use a heating pad or hot-water bottle or take a hot bath, advises Greenwood. Lehman says that heat not only relieves the symptoms, it also brings more blood with white blood cells and other infection-fighting blood products to the affected area. (Pregnant women, however, should not sit in a hot bath or hot tub for too long, since raising the body temperature above 100 degrees Fahrenheit for long periods may cause birth defects or miscarriage.)

TAKE A BATH.

If you have a lot of burning, a warm "sitz" bath (sitting three to four inches of water) can help to ease the pain.

TAKE A BREAK.

Rest in bed, especially if you have a fever. You'll conserve energy and speed healing.

WEAR COTTON UNDERWEAR.

Cotton underwear, cotton-lined panty hose, and loose clothing will allow the genital area to breathe and stay dry. For men, boxer-type shorts rather than jockey-style shorts are better if prostate and bladder infections are a problem.

HELLO, DOCTOR?

In many cases, bladder infections can be successfully treated at home with the remedies described here. However, call your doctor if you:

• Have a personal history of kidney disease

• Are diabetic

• Are pregnant or may be pregnant

• Have shaking spells or have vomited within the last 12 hours (may indicate kidney infection or septicemia, a bacterial infection in the blood that can be fatal)

• Have symptoms and fever that increase after 48 hours of home treatment

• Have blood in your urine

• Have had an abdominal or back injury within two weeks prior to the onset of your symptoms (may indicate kidney injury)

• Have high blood pressure

• Are male and over age 50

• Have or suspect that you have a sexually transmitted disease

AVOID ALCOHOL.

Alcohol is a urinary tract irritant for both men and women and should be avoided during a bladder infection.

What about spicy foods, tea, and coffee? Clark says, "They really shouldn't hurt a bladder infection." However, the caffeine in coffee, tea, and colas does stimulate the kidneys to produce more urine and makes the bladder fill up faster during a time when urination is painful. If caffeine seems to make your symptoms worse, avoid it until the infection goes away.

TAKE A PAIN RELIEVER.
Bladder infections can be painful. Acetaminophen, ibuprofen, or aspirin, especially at bedtime, can help.

WASH UP, LOVERS.
Both partners should wash up before intercourse.

URINATE AFTER LOVEMAKING.
If you have recurrent bladder infections, urinate just before and after intercourse, advises Clark. This can help flush out bacteria in the urinary tract.

SWITCH BIRTH-CONTROL METHODS.
Women who use a diaphragm and suffer from recurrent infections should try switching to condoms or a cervical cap. "If you have recurrent bladder infections, see your doctor to have your diaphragm's fit rechecked," says Clark. "You may do better with a smaller diaphragm or a cervical cap."

KEEP A BLADDER-INFECTION DIARY.
If you suffer from recurrent bladder infections, keep a diary to discover what patterns precede an attack. Some people find that their infections are related to stress, menstruation, lovemaking, or other factors. Once you discover what precipitates your infections, you can make changes to alter those patterns.

WIPE FROM FRONT TO BACK.

Most women wipe from back to front, which moves bacteria from the rectum dangerously close to the urethra.

USE CONDOMS.

Prostate infection, which can lead to bladder infection, is more common among men with multiple sex partners. Practice safe sex, and always use condoms with partners.

Blisters

18 Ways to Treat—and Beat—Them

You just couldn't resist a bargain. Those shoes looked great with your new outfit, even if they didn't feel so great on your feet. "They'll stretch out," you told yourself, and then patted yourself on the back for getting such a good deal. Unfortunately, you got more than you bargained for—namely, painful blisters to go with your new shoes.

Blisters are tender spots that fill up with fluid released by tiny blood vessels in an area where delicate skin tissues have been burned, pinched, or just plain irritated. Virtually everyone has experienced friction blisters, the kind caused by hot, sweaty, or ill-fitting shoes. If you have one now, read on to find out how to take care of it. Then continue reading to learn how you can help protect your tender tootsies in the future.

TREATING YOUR BLISTER

A blister is your body's way of telling you that skin and tissues are being injured. So while you take steps to relieve the discomfort, protect the injured area.

MAKE A TENT.

Instead of simply placing an adhesive bandage right on top of the blister, "tent" the bandage by bringing in its the padding in the middle raises up a bit. "This will not only protect the blister but allow air to circulate, which will aid in healing," says Nelson Lee Novick, M.D., associate clinical professor of dermatology at Mount Sinai School of Medicine in New York.

USE A DOUBLE-DUTY BANDAGE.

Another type of bandage, available in pharmacies, contains a gel and antiseptic to cushion and "clean" the blister, says Wilma Bergfeld, M.D., head of clinical research in the Department of Dermatology at the Cleveland Clinic Foundation in Ohio. Ask your pharmacist about it.

LET IT BREATHE.

Some physicians believe that a blister should not be covered at all for maximum aeration. Jerome Z. Litt, M.D., assistant clinical professor of dermatology at Case Western Reserve University School of Medicine in Cleveland, is one such doctor. He even suggests slipping your shoe off while you sit at your desk at work in order to give your blister some air.

SMEAR ON AN OINTMENT.

Whether you decide to cover your blister or not, you should apply an antibacterial/antibiotic ointment to it.

Doctors generally recommend Bacitracin or Polysporin, which may be less likely to cause an allergic reaction or sensitivity than other over-the-counter ointments.

PAD IT.

When a blister is in a particularly annoying spot, like the bottom of the foot, padding might provide more of a cushion than just a bandage would, advises Bergfeld. She suggests using the circular pads made of foam adhesive found in the foot-care aisle of drug- and beauty-aid stores. "Pharmacies also carry sheets of padding that you can cut to size for a more exact fit," says Bergfeld. Cut the padding in the shape of a donut, and place it on the skin surrounding the blister so that the blister fits in the hole in the opening of the donut. Then gently cover the blister with an antibacterial ointment and bandage.

PUT IT UP.

Elevating the blistered area can help relieve the pressure, advises Bergfeld.

BE PATIENT.

Expect it to take about a week to ten days for the blister's fluid to be reabsorbed by the body.

DRAIN IT.

While some doctors believe that a blister should never be popped because of the risk of infection, most agree that a blister causing extreme pressure—such as one on a finger or toe or under a nail—is a candidate for draining. If you should decide to pop it, first wipe the blister and a sewing needle with alcohol. "Never sterilize a needle over a flame," says Novick. "It can create soot on the

tip of the needle, which can 'tattoo,' or dirty, the blister."
Prick the blister once or twice near its edging; then
slowly and gently press out the fluid.

KEEP THE ROOF ON IT.
Once you have popped the blister and drained the fluid,
do not remove the deflated top skin. This skin, called
the blister's roof, protects the blister from infection and
forms a "bridge" for new cells to migrate across on their
journey to heal the site.

SOAK FIRST.
To drain a blister on a tough-skinned area, such as the
sole of the foot, Litt suggests first soaking the blister in
Burow's solution, available from pharmacies in packets
or tablets (follow the directions on the package). He recommends soaking the blister for 15 minutes, three to
four times a day. A day or two of this will soften the blister and make draining easier.

WATCH FOR SIGNS OF INFECTION.
Redness, red streaks, or pus in an intact or a "popped"
blister should be treated by a doctor.

PREVENTING BLISTERS
Here are ways to prevent friction blisters, according
to Glenn B. Gastwirth, D.P.M., Deputy Executive Director
of the American Podiatric Medical Association in
Bethesda, Maryland:

BUY SHOES IN THE AFTERNOON.
"Over the course of the day, your feet may swell by as
much as half a shoe size," says Gastwirth. When trying

on shoes, wear the same type of socks that you plan to use with the shoes.

LOOK FOR LEATHER.

Unlike nonporous vinyl and plastic materials, leather has microscopic pores that allow air to circulate, keeping the foot drier. In the same way, so do the clusters of perforated holes primarily found on many styles of sports footwear. A dry foot is less likely to develop blisters.

DON'T EXERCISE AT MIDDAY.

The heat of midday, especially in the summer, can make the feet perspire more, making them more blister-prone.

NEVER WEAR WET SHOES.

The wetness can cause more "dragging" between the foot and shoe and can result in blisters. If you jog twice a day, for instance, you may want to buy a second pair of running shoes for your second run each day.

PROTECT "HOT SPOTS."

If you have a chronic "hot spot," or place where blisters tend to develop, apply petroleum jelly to it, then slip on your sock. Foam or felt pads, used alone, can also absorb the friction and protect a hot spot. For best results, make sure the padding covers more area than you think a blister would take up, since the neighboring areas can become irritated, too.

WEAR THE RIGHT SOCKS.

Specially made sport socks with extra padding in hot spots can help prevent blisters. Natural fibers such as cotton and wool tend to keep the feet dry by absorbing moisture. However, according to Gastwirth, recent research suggests that acrylic fibers may, through a wicking action, actually move moisture away from the foot, keeping it drier and making it less prone to blistering. Your best bet? Try them both and see which type of fiber keeps your feet drier and more comfortable. In addition, make sure the sock fits your foot, so there is less chance of it bunching up inside the shoe and causing a blister.

TRY A SPRINKLE.
Foot powders may aid in keeping the foot dry and preventing painful blisters from forming.

Body odor
6 Steps to Sweet-Smelling Success

L et's face it, in the United States, a pungent body aroma is simply not going to make you the life of the party. So powerful is our cultural distaste for body odor that every day, some 95 percent of all Americans over the age of 12 reach for one product or another that will enable them to feel safe and secure in the company of others.

Body odor begins with sweat. The body has two types of sweat glands, and both types produce sweat that is made up largely of water. The eccrine glands, which are located on almost every part of the body, produce the sweat that cools the body. The apocrine glands, which are located in the armpits, around the nipples, and in the groin, produce sweat whose function, at least in modern times, is not clear. One thing is obvious, however. The sweat from the apocrine glands can make you stink, because it contains a substantial amount of oil, which provides food for bacteria. It's this bacterial feeding frenzy that causes the offensive odor. Here's what the experts recommend you do to come up smelling like roses:

KEEP IT CLEAN.

"The best way to prevent body odor is to wash away the sweat that forms on the skin in the area of the apocrine glands and reduce the number of bacteria waiting there to feed upon it," says Donald Rudikoff, M.D., assistant clinical professor of dermatology at Mount Sinai School of Medicine in New York. So, clean the underarm and groin area with soap, preferably a deodorant soap, and water at least once a day.

BATHE YOUR BRITCHES.

Sweat that seeps into your clothing may remind you of its presence at very inopportune times. What's more, dried, bacteria-containing sweat can damage the fibers of your clothing. "You should wash your washable clothing each time you wear it," advises Rudikoff.

TRY A DEODORANT.

For milder cases of body odor, a deodorant may help. Deodorants are considered cosmetics. Most contain a substance that helps kill the bacteria that are waiting to feed on your sweat. They may also help mask body odor by substituting a more acceptable scent.

GET TOUGH WITH AN ANTIPERSPIRANT.

Since body odor begins with sweat, one of the best ways to control it is to reduce the amount of sweat. "You can probably reduce perspiration by as much as 50 percent with an antiperspirant," says Allan L. Lorincz, M.D., professor of dermatology at the University of Chicago Medical Center.

Antiperspirants are classified as over-the-counter drugs because they are intended to alter a natural body function—they decrease production of eccrine sweat. (While apocrine sweat contains the oil upon which bacteria feed, neither an antiperspirant nor a deodorant can decrease apocrine sweat.) By decreasing production of eccrine sweat, antiperspirants help keep you drier, thus reducing the moisture that creates a breeding ground for bacteria. Antiperspirants usually also contain an antibacterial agent that fights odors. (For tips on choosing an antiperspirant, see EXCESSIVE PERSPIRATION.)

BEAT IRRITATION AND ODOR.

If you've tried antiperspirants and deodorants and found that they irritate your skin, you might instead try an antibacterial soap such as chlorhexidine (Hibiclens) or an over-the-counter antibiotic ointment. Talcum powder or baking soda can also be used.

QUIET YOUR DIET.

Certain foods, such as hot peppers, can affect the amount of sweat an individual produces. And the aroma of other pungent foods, such as garlic, can be carried in your sweat. "If your aim is to prevent body odor, cut out foods like onions, garlic, hot spices, and beer," suggests Rudikoff.

Breast discomfort

6 Soothing Strategies

For many women, breasts are a source of sensual pleasure. For breast-feeding mothers, they are a part of the bonding between mother and baby and a way of nurturing a new life. But at certain times in a woman's life, breasts can be uncomfortable or downright painful. They may even become the focus of worry and anxiety.

Breast discomfort is a normal part of being a woman. It is almost always not a sign of breast cancer. Breasts are mammary glands that are responsive to natural hormonal changes, especially fluctuations in estrogen, that occur at menstruation, menopause, and pregnancy. Hormonal changes can cause breasts to become hot, swollen, tender, and painful to the touch. "Breast discomfort is really common for women," says Amanda Clark, M.D., assistant professor of obstetrics and gynecology at Oregon Health Sciences University in Portland. "We see it a great deal during early pregnancy, with menstruation, and during early hormone therapy at menopause."

All of the hormonal changes that occur just before menstruation and during pregnancy prepare the woman's breasts for breast-feeding. With the onset of menstruation, estrogen declines and the breasts return to normal.

With pregnancy, the hormonal changes continue, and the breasts begin producing milk for the baby. Lactating breasts present their own special problems and challenges. Sometimes, a mother's milk comes in too early or too heavily and causes a painful condition called engorgement. Nursing nipples can become sore. Milk ducts may become backed up and can lead to a painful infection called mastitis. (For more information on preventing and treating discomfort associated with breast-feeding, see BREAST-FEEDING DISCOMFORT.)

During menopause, many women opt for hormone therapy to reduce menopausal symptoms such as hot flashes and to reduce their risk of developing the bone-thinning disease osteoporosis. However, it often takes a while to find just the right combination and dosage of hormones for each woman. During this period, many women experience breast discomfort.

Some women also suffer from a noncancerous breast condition called fibrocystic breasts that can cause the breasts to feel lumpy, painful, and tender. The condition is related to monthly hormonal fluctuations. As many as 30 percent of all women suffer from fibrocystic breasts, according to Sadja Greenwood, M.D., assistant clinical professor in the Department of Obstetrics, Gynecology, and Reproductive Sciences at the University of California at San Francisco. "Fibrocystic breasts were once considered a disease," she says. "But it's very common and is considered a normal—although somewhat painful—condition."

Even young girls who are just beginning to develop breasts are subject to hormonal fluctuations and can therefore experience breast tenderness. "Breast discomfort in prepubescent young women with breast bud-

HELLO, DOCTOR?

While some causes of breast discomfort can be effectively treated at home, see a doctor if you have any of the following symptoms:
- A lump or firmness
- Soreness in only one breast
- A change in your breast self-exam
- Nipple discharge on one side (Lactating breasts may secrete white/yellow discharge for up to a year after nursing is discontinued.)

In addition, be sure to examine your breasts monthly, regardless of whether you are having any discomfort or not. Self-examination of the breasts is an effective way to detect cancerous changes early. The best time to perform the examination is during the week following your menstrual period. If you do not know how to do a breast self-examination or are not sure if you are doing it properly, talk to your doctor.

ding is normal," says Deborah Purcell, M.D., a pediatrician in private practice and past chairperson of the Department of Pediatrics at St. Vincent Hospital and Medical Center in Portland, Oregon. "Even young boys can experience some enlargement of the breasts and discomfort during this growth spurt," says Purcell.

While you can't escape hormonal fluctuations, you can make yourself and your breasts more comfortable.

WEAR A SUPPORTIVE BRA.

Breasts often swell with fluid during periods of hormonal fluctuation. Susan Woodruff, B.S.N., childbirth and parenting education coordinator at Tuality Community Hospital in Hillsboro, Oregon, advises women to wear a supportive bra, especially if their breasts are large. "You may have to wear it 24 hours a day when the breasts are tender," she says. "Try one of those soft athletic bras that provide comfort and good support."

TRY CUTTING BACK ON CAFFEINE.

Greenwood says that the scientific evidence is mixed about whether or not eliminating caffeine helps lumpy, fibrocystic breasts. One study, reported by the National Institutes of Health, which included more than 3,000 women, found no relationship between caffeine consumption and fibrocystic disease. On the other hand, some women have reported good results from cutting back or eliminating caffeinated coffees, teas, colas, and chocolate. Try reducing your consumption of caffeine to see if your breast discomfort decreases.

CUT SALT.

Many women retain fluid, particularly near their menstrual periods, says Clark. "Avoiding salt around this time can help minimize fluid retention," she says.

APPLY HEAT/COLD PACKS.

Woodruff says that some women find relief by alternating a warm heating pad and ice packs. Try the heating pad for 30 minutes, then the ice packs for 10 minutes, then the heating pad for 30 minutes, and so on.

TRY A NONPRESCRIPTION PAIN RELIEVER.

Aspirin, ibuprofen, or acetaminophen can ease the pain of premenstrual breasts, says Clark. For fibrocystic breasts, Purcell recommends ibuprofen.

CHECK OUT YOUR COSMETICS.

Some herbal cosmetics and remedies, such as those made with ginseng, can have steroidal effects similar to estrogen. If you suspect that a product that you use may have such an effect, try avoiding the product temporarily to see if your condition improves.

Breast-feeding discomfort
15 Ways to Beat the Breast-feeding Blues

Throughout your pregnancy, you probably fantasized about the wonderful experience breast-feeding would be for both you and your baby. All you could think about was looking down into that tiny, trusting face and feeling the closeness between you and this new little being. So naturally, when it finally came time to put baby to breast, you were excited. But now, you're in agony. Your nipples are sore, cracked, and bleeding. If your milk has already come in, your breasts may be painfully swollen.

The milk may not flow when you need it to and may seem to flow uncontrollably when you most wish it wouldn't (like when you're standing in line at the grocery store or sitting at a dinner party). So where are those tender, happy moments you've seen in the magazine and television advertisements?

Well, hang in there. Those moments do actually exist, just not right off the bat. The problem is, many mothers give up breast-feeding in frustration because they don't realize that things will get better with time. They also don't realize that there are things they can do to decrease breast-feeding discomfort.

Breast-feeding pain can occur in different parts of the breast. Nipple pain is often caused by the baby latching onto the nipple incorrectly. "If the baby doesn't latch on in a way that allows the nipple to get adjusted correctly in his palate, it can be very traumatic for the breast," says Phyllis Frey, A.R.N.P., a nurse practitioner with Bellegrove OB-GYN, Inc., in Bellevue, Washington. In addition, she notes, "American women tend to experience more nipple discomfort than foreign women because we always wear bras to protect that sensitive skin. Foreign women, however, go braless more often and sunbathe topless, which toughens the nipples." Preexisting conditions, such as inverted nipples or nipple sensitivity that developed during pregnancy, can also cause problems.

Pain in the fleshy part of the breast is most often caused by engorgement of the breast with milk when the milk first comes in. Engorgement may also make the breasts feel sore between feedings.

While you can't escape all initial breast-feeding discomfort, there are some tips to lessen the pain.

MAKE SURE THE BABY LATCHES ON CORRECTLY.

Despite what you may have been told, breast-feeding is a learned skill, and it takes time and practice to perfect. "If the baby is latching on at the very end of the nipple, he is really mashing his gums against that tender skin," says Raven Fox, R.N., I.B.C.L.C., a registered nurse and lactation consultant/educator at Evergreen Hospital Medical Center in Kirkland, Washington. "If this motion persists, the nipples can start to crack, bleed, and blister, all of which leaves them more vulnerable to infection," she continues. The key is to get the baby's mouth open wide, lift your breast from underneath, and pull the baby in close as quickly as possible. "You want to get the baby to close down on the areola (the darkened area around the nipple), rather than on the nipple itself. And if you bring him in too slowly, he will clamp down as soon as his lips touch the nipple," Fox explains. When the baby does close directly on the nipple, you'll know it. "You may feel a general tenderness when the baby first latches on, or you may experience a real sharp pain, almost as if someone had pinched you," she warns.

USE A PROP.

Place the baby on a pillow on your lap when breast-feeding. "Doing so lifts the baby up a little higher so that once on, he isn't further irritating the nipple area by tugging down on it," says Frey.

GO EASY AT FIRST.

"It's so exciting initially to breast-feed your baby, and you often feel you don't want to interrupt him when he's

(Continued on page 108)

TREATING BREAST INFECTIONS

Cracked and bleeding nipples brought on by those first few days of breast-feeding can leave you vulnerable to infection of the breast, which is referred to as mastitis. While it is rarely serious, mastitis can be quite painful and cannot be cured without the use of an antibiotic.

According to Raven Fox, R.N., I.B.C.L.C., signs that you may have mastitis include a reddened area on the fleshy part of the breast that is painful to the touch and ranges from the size of a quarter to the whole side of the breast, a fever of up to 102 degrees Fahrenheit, general achiness, and chills. You may have one or two of these symptoms, or you may have all of them at once. They tend to come on very rapidly. "You may be feeling a little off at 7:30 in the morning and an hour later feel as if a truck ran over you," says Fox.

While you will need to see a doctor if you suspect a breast infection, there are a few things you should do on your own during the course of an infection.

Continue nursing, starting with the infected breast each time. This may sound like sheer lunacy when you are in so much pain, but it helps clear the infection and will not hurt the baby. "The milk is absolutely not infected. It is the area around the milk duct that is infected," stresses Fox. She recommends nursing at least every two to three hours, and more frequently if the baby is willing.

Prior to nursing, pack the breast in heat. Again, use a warm towel with a plastic bag over it to maintain the heat. "Then massage and stroke the breast from the fleshy part down to the nipple, focusing especially on that sore spot," says Phyllis Frey, A.R.N.P.

Get in bed. You need to go on full bed rest. This is your time to take care of yourself and let everyone else nurture you while you get over the infection. Usually, it takes only about 24 to 36 hours for the pain to pass. But Fox stresses the importance of continuing the antibiotics throughout their full 10- to 14-day course, despite the fact that you're feeling better.

Other problems causing discomfort include yeast infections in the nipple and clogged milk ducts. "Yeast infections can cause ongoing discomfort in the nipple and need to be diagnosed and treated by your doctor," says Frey.

Clogged ducts, on the other hand, usually resolve themselves within 24 hours. They are characterized by a hard, uncomfortable lump in the fleshy part of the breast. It can be very tender to the touch but isn't usually accompanied by a fever. To relieve the pain of a clogged duct, pack the breast in heat before feedings, get the baby to nurse on the infected breast first, and massage the hard spot the whole time the baby is nursing in order to loosen up the milk and unclog the duct.

"If the milk is locked in the duct for more than 24 hours, it can start leaking into the breast tissue and leave a moist breeding ground for bacteria," cautions Frey. "And once it becomes infected, it is a hot spot that hurts all of the time." Fox adds, the pattern tends to be sore nipples, engorgement, clogged ducts, and mastitis. Solving the first two problems usually prevents the latter.

finally latched on and gulping away," says Frey. "But you will pay later," she warns. Limit the breast-feeding time for the first five days. Try five minutes on each breast at first. If you don't notice yourself getting tender, you can increase that time rather quickly.

TAKING THE PAIN OUT OF WEANING

Once you get through the initial discomfort of breast-feeding, nursing becomes easy and relatively painless until that fateful day when you decide it is time to wean your baby off of the breast. In addition to producing some emotional discomfort, weaning can cause physical pain. As you decrease feedings, it takes a little time for the body to catch on and produce less milk in response, so the engorgement of those early days often returns.

"Every expert is a little different in terms of their advice on how to best wean a baby," says Harold Zimmer, M.D. "Some advise you to go 'cold turkey' and some advise you to truly wean," he continues. For Mom, it is a little more comfortable to do it gradually, but some babies will decide to wean themselves and will abruptly reject the breast for good. "Generally, trying to drop one feeding about every two days is what I recommend," says Zimmer. "And the last feedings to be dropped should be the first one in the morning and the last one at night because the baby tends to be most attached to breast-feeding at these times," he

THEN, NURSE, NURSE, NURSE.

Once your milk comes in, let the baby nurse as long as he or she wants to. "Babies go through a marathon nursing period right as their mother's milk is coming in, and we recommend letting the baby nurse constantly during this

explains. It is also important to never drop two feedings in a row. In other words, if you typically breast-feed your baby twice in the morning, twice in the afternoon, and twice in the evening, avoid dropping one morning feeding one day and another morning feeding two days later. Instead, try dropping one morning feeding, then an afternoon feeding, then an evening feeding.

As far as the pain of engorgement that can result, there are a few things you can do. "Tying a towel or Ace bandage around your breasts can help decrease your milk supply, because the extra pressure collapses the glands so that they can't hold as much milk," says Zimmer. "Applying ice packs to the breasts decreases circulation and further reduces the degree of engorgement and swelling," he continues. And once you have started to wean, he gives his OK to taking aspirin. "Aspirin is a good anti-inflammatory and can relieve some of the discomfort of engorgement," he says.

Whatever you do, avoid any extra stimulation to the breasts during the weaning process. "Anything that stimulates the breasts will promote more milk production," according to Zimmer.

12- to 24-hour period. Just get it into your head that this will be your sole job for the next 24 hours," advises Fox. "We're finding that women who resign themselves to doing this are totally missing that initial engorgement period because the baby is helping to siphon off all of the excess milk the body initially produces." After all, the body automatically makes enough milk for twins; it then gradually lowers its milk production to meet one baby's needs if there is no twin. Fox goes on to say that if you trap yourself into feeding the baby every three to four hours and letting the baby sleep for as long as he or she wants, your milk will come in and it will make your breasts look and feel as though they're going to explode. "The engorgement period should only last 36 to 48 hours, but the pain makes it seem like 5 years," she says.

DON'T REACH FOR THE PUMP.

If you do get engorged, resist the urge to express milk with a manual or electric breast pump. Unfortunately, the body doesn't know the difference between a pump and a baby's mouth. Whenever milk is drawn from the breast, the body thinks it's being used by the baby and makes more to compensate for that loss. So the more you pump, the more milk your body produces. "In essence, using a breast pump introduces a twin to your body," says Fox. The only time this advice wouldn't apply is when you are on a trip away from your baby and want to continue nursing regularly when you return, or when your baby is ill and his or her appetite is temporarily down. In these instances, you would want to pump at the baby's normal feeding times to keep up your milk supply.

AIR THEM OUT.

Try to expose your nipples to air whenever possible to help toughen them up. "If you finish nursing and immediately put your bra back on with a nursing pad in it, you're likely to get some milk leakage that will wet the pad and keep moisture against the nipple," says Frey. "This further softens the nipple, which is not what you want." Instead, she suggests keeping your bra flaps open (on a nursing bra) or going braless under a light T-shirt for at least 15 minutes after feeding. If you were planning to nap after a feeding, you might consider napping braless, as well.

STAND IN A WARM SHOWER.

This causes some milk to drip from the breasts, which can relieve some of the pressure, according to Frey. But unlike pumping the breast, this technique doesn't cause the body to produce more milk. It just provides relief as long as the water is directly hitting the breasts. "Another way to get similar relief is to fill the sink with warm water, take your bra off, lean over the sink, and splash the water up over your breasts," says Fox.

TRY "COLD STORAGE."

Between feedings, pack your breasts in ice, and wear a bra to hold the ice in place. "My favorite way to do this is to freeze four Ziploc bags of unpopped popcorn. The popcorn holds the cold much longer than the frozen peas and carrots many people use, and it doesn't get mushy. It also molds to the shape of your breasts so that you don't have big, bulky ice cubes lying on you," says Fox. "Usually, engorgement in between feedings lasts no more than seven to ten days after the baby's birth. This is because the mother's milk production and the baby's milk consumption are still balancing out," explains Harold Zimmer, M.D., an obstetrician and gynecologist in private practice in Bellevue, Washington.

WARM UP FOR FEEDINGS.

Fifteen minutes before feeding your baby, warm up your breasts. "Soak a bath towel in hot water, wring it out, and place it across your breasts with a plastic garbage bag over it to maintain the heat a little longer," advises Fox. Then take it off and massage the breast from the fleshy part down to the nipple to encourage the release of milk into the nipple. "Latching your baby onto an empty nipple can hurt so much more than if there is milk in the nipple," says Frey.

TRY THE "BURP AND SWITCH" STRATEGY.

Always begin a feeding on the sorest breast or the one that seems fullest. "Once the baby is latched on, let him nurse for five minutes, and then burp him and switch him to the other side for five minutes. Continue switching him every five minutes until he is finished eating," recommends Fox. This method ensures that the baby drains both breasts sufficiently, rather than tanking up on one and leaving the other ready to explode.

TRY SOME TEA.

Placing warm tea bags on your nipples a few times a day is one of the best home remedies around for nipple discomfort, according to Zimmer. Fox stresses that it has to be black tea, as opposed to chamomile or yellow tea, because black tea contains tannin, and the tannic acid is what soothes and toughens up the nipples. Soak the

HELLO, DOCTOR?

If none of these tips seems to help much, it's time to see your doctor to rule out the possibility of a breast infection. In addition, your local chapter of the La Leche League and most hospital maternity wards can offer over-the-phone answers to your breast-feeding questions.

tea bags in warm water for a few minutes, squeeze them out, and place them on the nipples for ten minutes.

MASSAGE THE NIPPLES WITH AN ICE CUBE.

"This will numb the painful area and give you some temporary relief," says Zimmer. But he goes on to say that once the numbness wears off, the nipples will be just as painful as before. "It is not a healing remedy as much as it is a relief mechanism," he explains.

WEAR A WELL-SUPPORTING BRA.

"You want to avoid as much additional trauma to the breasts as possible, and this is one way to protect them somewhat," says Zimmer.

TAKE ACETAMINOPHEN IF YOU DEVELOP A FEVER.

It is very common to develop a low-grade fever as high as 100.2 to 100.6 degrees Fahrenheit, according to Fox.

Acetaminophen should help to lower it and make you feel a little better. Be sure to check with your doctor, however, before taking any medication while you are nursing.

TAKE IBUPROFEN IF YOU FEEL ACHY.
"It is also not uncommon to feel as if a truck has run over you," warns Fox. If this is the case, ibuprofen should help relieve some of the aches and discomfort. Once again, however, check with your doctor before taking any medications.

Bruises
14 Tips for Coping with the Color Purple

When something goes bump in the night, and it's you, you may end up with the most common type of injury known to man. Bruises, those purplish blue testimonies to our physical foibles, occur when blood seeps from damaged blood vessels into the surrounding tissue. Known medically as contusions, bruises are usually caused by what doctors call direct trauma. Whether from hitting the coffee table or being kicked in the shin, the result is a painful reminder of our not-so-best moments.

Thankfully, bruises generally heal in about 10 to 14 days. Along the way, their coloring changes and fades from a dark purple to a yellowish blue. The changing colors indicate that "scavenger" white blood cells have moved into the area to break down ruptured red blood cells (called corpuscles) into iron by-products. These by-products can then be whisked away by the blood. When a greenish maroon color appears, healing is almost complete.

While your body is taking care of healing the injury, there are some things you can do to minimize discoloration, maximize pain relief, and prevent bruises from "hitting" you in the future.

COOL IT DOWN.

To stop the bleeding from the damaged blood vessels, use a cold compress. "The sooner you apply ice, the better," says Wilma Bergfeld, M.D., head of clinical research in the Department of Dermatology at the Cleveland Clinic Foundation in Ohio. The cold also helps prevent swelling. Wrap the ice in a damp cloth and apply it for about 10 to 15 minutes. If your fingers or toes are bruised, plunge them into ice-cold water for quick results. Never place ice directly on the skin, however, or keep a compress on for prolonged periods of time, because an ice burn can result.

TAKE A LOAD OFF.

No matter where the injury occurred, it's important to rest the affected area.

GIVE IT A LIFT.

Elevation is helpful for bruises to the arms or legs, because less blood is pumped into the injured site when gravity lends a hand. Try supporting your arm on the

UNEXPLAINED BRUISING

If you find a bruise or multiple bruises that seem to have appeared spontaneously or from the slightest touch, you should consult your family physician or dermatologist. These types of bruises may be the result of other problems or factors, such as the following:

Senile purpura. Many older people suffer from this condition, which loosely means "bruises of the elderly." As people age, the collagen (elastic fiber) that gives the skin and blood vessels their suppleness becomes thinner and frayed, allowing blood to seep through the vessel walls. The result: oversized bruises that can cover the entire length of an arm or leg. While the appearance of these colossal bruises may be frightening, the condition is an unfortunate part of the aging process and not life threatening. "It's fairly common," says Nelson Lee Novick, M.D. "I see patients with senile purpura all the time in my practice." The home-treatment procedure for senile purpura is the

back of a chair or propping your leg up on a few pillows for 30 minutes each hour for the first few hours after the injury.

SWITCH TO HEAT.
About 24 hours after the injury, once the bleeding has stopped and the healing process has begun, use heat to help reduce the muscle spasms that can accompany

same as that for common bruises; however, a physician should be consulted for a proper diagnosis, since large-scale bruising may indicate other diseases.

Drugs. Besides aspirin and acetaminophen, hundreds of over-the-counter and prescription medications can cause adverse reactions, which can lead to or aggravate bruising. Among the culprits: cortisone-like medications, often used to treat inflammation; some antibiotics; and certain heart medications. Check with your doctor or pharmacist if you suspect that your bruises may be related to a medication you are taking.

Blood disorders. Hematological, or blood-related, problems, such as a low platelet count, may show up first as bruising. (Platelets are the blood cells that aid in blood clotting.) Leukemia, or cancer of the blood, may also be indicated by bruises.

Vitamin K deficiency. Vitamin K is essential for proper blood clotting. A lack of the vitamin may reveal itself as bruising.

bruising. "The muscles contract to 'splint' an injury, especially near a joint," explains Nelson Lee Novick, M.D., associate clinical professor of dermatology at Mount Sinai School of Medicine in New York. Apply lukewarm compresses for half an hour to an hour, three to four times a day, to relax the muscles around the bruise.

While either moist or dry heat can be used—whichever is most comfortable for you—many physicians say that for reasons unknown, moist heat seems to be more effective in treating bruises. "But no matter which heating method you use, the heat should never be too high," warns Bergfeld. If you use a heating pad, for example, it should be set on the lowest temperature.

KEEP YOUR ASPIRIN IN THE CABINET.

You may be tempted to reach for aspirin to dull the pain of the injury, but don't do it. "Both aspirin and acetaminophen contain anticoagulants, commonly known as 'blood thinning' agents, which can aggravate the bruise," says Jerome Z. Litt, M.D., an assistant clinical professor of dermatology at Case Western Reserve University School of Medicine in Cleveland. Instead, you can help ease the pain of the injury with ibuprofen, the other major nonprescription painkiller, which does not contain anticoagulant factors.

PUT YOUR MOISTURIZER IN THE FRIDGE.

If you decide to treat the bruise with dry heat and the area becomes dry, use an emollient, preferably a hypoallergenic one, to help smooth and soothe the affected area. Gently pat—do not rub—it on, a few times a day. "By keeping the lotion in the refrigerator, it will feel pleasantly cool on your hot, tender skin when you use it," says Bergfeld.

BE A TEETOTALER.

Alcoholic beverages, whether wine coolers, beer, or hard liquor, can dilate (open up) blood vessels, which in turn can aggravate the bruising, warns Novick. Alcohol consumption is also a major contributor to accidents in the home.

WEAR LOOSE CLOTHING.

Tight, restrictive clothes will only increase the bruise's tenderness. For bruises on the legs, for example, try going without panty hose or socks for a day if you can.

WATCH THE WAY YOU DECORATE.

Furniture that is more rounded or that has softer edges—such as Queen Anne-style coffee tables—may be less hazardous to your legs and hips than squared-off styles, especially in small rooms where space is tight.

CONSIDER PUTTING DOWN CARPETING.

You might be less likely to slip on carpeting than on linoleum or tile, and if you do happen to fall, the carpet may help to prevent more serious injury by acting as a cushion.

TACK DOWN AREA RUGS.

Those small throw rugs, often found in entry halls, bathrooms, and kitchens, frequently slide around or bunch up, leaving you open to an unexpected trip and a potentially bruising fall. To remedy the problem, use adhesive tape or specially made tacking to adhere them to the floor.

LIGHT THE WAY TO SAFETY.

Night lights or lights set on timers are a relatively low-cost way to illuminate your path for late-night trips to the kitchen or bathroom. You might also try keeping a small flashlight on your nightstand so you can take it along when navigating dark hallways or stairways. Motion sensor fixtures, which turn on when movement is detected nearby, are great for outdoor use because they will instantly light up your driveway or sidewalk as you approach.

IMPROVE YOUR FOOTING IN THE TUB.

Put a rubber mat in your bathtub or shower stall to help prevent slipping. You might even consider installing a handrail to decrease your risk of slipping while getting in or out of the tub.

PUT EVERYTHING IN ITS PLACE.

Clutter can be hazardous to your health. Just think about the times you found a missing item by literally tripping over it.

Burns

27 Skin-Saving Strategies

It can take just an instant: A harried cook grabs the pan of burning food out of the oven; a cup of hot coffee comes tumbling down over the side of the table onto a curious child; a toddler manages to turn on the hot-water faucet during bath time.

Many burns are minor and can be treated at home. The injured skin turns red; that's known as a first-degree burn. Sometimes, tiny blood vessels may be damaged and may leak fluid, causing swelling and a weepy appearance. If blisters appear, the burn is classified as second degree. In third-degree burns, blisters do not form, and the skin turns white instead of red. "Usually, the deeper the burn, the less the pain," says Mick Crowley, R.N., B.S.N., department manager of the Burn Care Center/Neurosurgical Unit at the University of Missouri Hospital and Clinics in Columbia.

TREATING A BURN

Here's what to do when a burn occurs:

PUT OUT THE FIRE FIRST.

If your clothes are on fire, your first concern is to put out the flame. "Drop and roll," says Crowley. If a hot object is responsible, remove it.

KNOW WHEN TO SEEK MEDICAL HELP.

There are times when first-aid methods at home just won't be enough. Get medical attention immediately if you have burns on your hands or face or over a joint, like the elbow; if your burns blister or you suspect that you have a third-degree burn; or if you've suffered chemical or electrical burns. Electrical burns can be "very, very tricky" says Crowley, because the damage often occurs out of sight, below the surface of the skin. In addition, consult your doctor before applying any products to burned skin.

COOL THE BURN.

For minor burns, gently run cool water over the burned area, use cool compresses, or place the area in a bowl of cool water. "Don't turn the faucet on full force," warns Patricia Fosarelli, M.D., assistant professor of pediatrics at Johns Hopkins School of Medicine in Baltimore. You risk further injury to the skin. "And use cool, but not ice-cold, water." The coolness will actually stop the burn from spreading by eliminating the thermal energy, says Terry L. Hankey, M.D., clinical associate professor of family practice at the University of Wisconsin School of Medicine in Madison.

LEAVE THE ICE IN THE FREEZER.

Just because cool water is good for a burn doesn't mean ice is better. "Putting ice on the burn will restrict the blood flow," says Crowley.

SKIP THE BUTTER.

Putting butter on a burn is an old folk remedy that can be downright dangerous. Butter isn't sterile. "It will also insulate the area and hold the heat in," says Crowley. And the salted kind will irritate broken skin.

DON'T WORRY ABOUT DIRT.

Most first-degree burns aren't dirty, Fosarelli says. If, for some reason, yours is, gently clean it with soap and water. "Gently is the operative word," she says. "Don't rub."

BANDAGE THE BURN FOR A CHILD.

If the burn occurs in an area that could be injured again or where a child might pick at it, you may want to cover the burn with some gauze or a bandage. Forgo any covering if it's an open, weeping wound, however, because the bandage will stick to the wound, says Crowley.

DON'T POP ANY BLISTERS.

If a blister does develop, keep your hands off of it. "It's the body's way of keeping the burn sterile," explains Fosarelli. "Don't rub, poke, or break it."

PROTECT YOURSELF

Some common-sense advice for adults:
• Don't spray lighter fluid on charcoal that's already lit.
• Don't smoke in bed.
• Let the engine cool before you open the radiator cap.
• Don't prime the carburetor with gasoline.
• Keep oven mitts and pot holders handy when cooking.
• When opening a package of microwaved popcorn, keep the package directed away from your face.

PREVENTING BURNS IN CHILDREN

Even the best remedy can't beat prevention. Take the following steps and you will help protect your child from burns:

TURN HANDLES IN ON THE STOVE.

Probably the most common cause of indoor accidents that burn children is a pan of something hot falling (or being pulled) off the stove.

PUT COFFEE OUT OF REACH.

You're sitting on the couch, relaxing, your cup of steaming hot coffee nearby on the aptly named coffee table. Before you know what's happening, your toddling little boy or girl grabs the cup and dumps it on himself or herself.

LOWER THE THERMOSTAT ON THE HOT-WATER HEATER.

Set it for under 120 degrees Fahrenheit, recommends Fosarelli. "A second-degree burn can happen in seconds in water over 120 degrees."

KEEP A WATCHFUL EYE.

Never, ever leave a child unattended in a room with a fireplace (even if it has a screen in front of it), a wood-burning stove, a kerosene heater, or any kind of space heater. "Not even for a minute," warns Fosarelli. Don't leave a young child alone in the bathroom, either.

PLUG ELECTRICAL OUTLETS.

Cover all electrical outlets with specially made caps.

DON'T RUN ELECTRICAL CORDS ACROSS THE FLOOR.

"A child reaches down and bites the cord and that spells tragedy," says Fosarelli.

KEEP MATCHES AWAY FROM YOUNG CHILDREN.

That goes for lighters, too. And don't leave them in your purse, where children can find them, either.

HAVE FIRE DRILLS.

That means you need to establish escape routes in your house and demonstrate to your child how to follow them.

TELL YOUR CHILD ABOUT "911."

"Even a four-year-old can learn to dial this, especially if you have it programmed on your phone," says Fosarelli.

GET FIRE EXTINGUISHERS.

Keep them accessible and in good repair. Explain to your children that a fire extinguisher, not water, should be used on a grease fire in the kitchen.

MAKE THE STOVE OFF-LIMITS.

Keep younger children away from the stove, especially when you're cooking, and discourage older kids from cooking when you're not around.

KEEP SMOKE ALARMS IN WORKING ORDER.

Check them monthly, if not more often.

PROTECT AGAINST SUNBURN.

See SUNBURN PAIN for tips on preventing this type of burn.

Canker sores

9 Soothing Strategies

It may only be the size of a pencil eraser, but a canker sore can be hard to ignore. It hurts like the dickens, especially whenever you eat or drink something.

Fortunately, a canker sore is usually a fairly short-lived misery, and there are a few things you can do to find some temporary relief.

First, however, you need to be able to tell the difference between a canker sore and what's called a cold sore, or fever blister, which is caused by the herpes virus. A cold sore often begins as several tiny blisters that eventually form one larger sore. They appear most often on the lips and face.

In contrast, canker sores usually travel alone. And unlike a sore caused by the herpes virus, a canker sore is not contagious. A canker sore has a yellow or white-gray center with a well-defined red border. It generally measures three to five millimeters in diameter (approximately the size of a pencil eraser) and is usually located on the inside of the lip or cheek or, less commonly, on the tongue.

What causes canker sores? No one knows for sure, says Robert P. Langlais, D.D.S., M.S., professor in the Department of Dental Diagnostic Science at the University of Texas Health Science Center at San Antonio. "Being run down or tired, or suffering from stress or poor nutrition may contribute."

"You see them in students around finals," says Alan S. Levy, D.D.S., clinical instructor at the University of Southern California School of Dentistry in Los Angeles. He points out that they may also occur as a result of a minor injury in the mouth, such as from a slip of the toothbrush or a jab from a taco shell. Certain foods, such as spicy dishes and citrus fruits, have also taken some of the blame.

About 20 percent of the population gets canker sores occasionally, and women are more likely than men to suffer from them. Some women tend to get canker sores at certain times during their menstrual cycle.

Here's what you can do to help relieve the discomfort of a canker sore. Keep in mind, though, that "a canker sore will last seven days with treatment and one week without treatment," Levy says. A canker sore can take up to two weeks to heal; if one sticks around longer than that, see your dentist.

GET OUT THE STYPTIC PENCIL.

Many a barber has used a styptic pencil to stem bleeding from minor nicks and cuts. Used on a canker sore, it will numb the nerve endings, temporarily reducing the pain.

MAKE YOUR OWN REMEDY.

It may sound like a strange combination, but several dentists swear by this homemade remedy. Mix together equal amounts of Milk of Magnesia or Kaopectate and Benylin or Benadryl. Milk of Magnesia and Kaopectate both contain ingredients that coat wet tissues, such as those in the mouth. Benylin and Benadryl contain ingredients that act as mild topical anesthetics and antihistamines (which reduce inflammation). Apply the mixture to the canker sore using a cotton swab. Be careful not to swallow the stuff; you could end up anesthetizing (numbing) the reflex that keeps the windpipe closed when you swallow, warns Langlais.

GO OVER THE COUNTER.

Use an over-the-counter product like Orabase with Benzocaine. "It's like an oral bandage," says Becky DeSpain, R.D.H., M.Ed., director of the Caruth School of Dental Hygiene at Baylor College of Dentistry in Dallas. "It covers up the surface." If you use something that keeps the sore coated, you'll help prevent a secondary infection, says Levy. Products with xylocaine, a local anesthetic, can also dull the pain.

HELLO, DOCTOR?

If you are suffering from frequent canker sores, talk to your dentist about them. Same goes if you have a canker sore that is an inch in diameter or leaves a scar when it heals. And definitely get to your dentist or physician if you develop a fever; a fever may indicate that the canker sore has become infected (from poor oral hygiene, dirty fingers in the mouth, or chewing tobacco), in which case you would likely need an antibiotic.

If you've got a sore that doesn't go away or has been around indefinitely, see your dentist. "Don't think that because it doesn't hurt, it's not serious," says Alan S. Levy, D.D.S. Ironically, while a canker sore hurts and stings, "lesions that are oral cancer rarely cause pain." And while a canker sore will usually disappear in seven to ten days, a cancerous lesion will not. More than 30,000 cases of oral cancer are diagnosed each year, says Levy.

Other conditions can also cause mouth ulcers that resemble canker sores, says Robert P. Langlais, D.D.S., M.S. These include iron deficiency anemia, pernicious (vitamin B_{12} deficiency) anemia, folic acid deficiency, gluten intolerance, celiac disease, and Crohn's disease.

TAKE TWO ASPIRIN.
You can take aspirin, acetaminophen, or ibuprofen to help relieve the pain, especially before meals if the canker sore interferes with eating, says Langlais.

STICK TO COOL FOODS.

Stay away from foods that are hot—in terms of temperature and spiciness. They'll burn and sting tender canker sores, says DeSpain.

BE GENTLE.

Wield that toothbrush extra carefully to avoid irritating a canker sore. You may want to avoid rough, scratchy foods such as chips for the time being as well.

STOP BAD HABITS.

Alcohol and smoking can irritate a canker sore, says Richard Price, D.M.D., consumer advisor/spokesperson for the American Dental Association. A little abstinence may provide a lot of relief.

CHECK OUT YOUR DIET.

One old wives' tale blames canker sores on tomatoes. Experts admit some sort of allergic reaction to foods may be to blame, but others point out that food allergies can cause lesions that resemble canker sores. If you're plagued with frequent canker sores, pay attention to your diet and notice whether an outbreak seems to be linked with any particular food. Likely offenders: nuts, shellfish, chocolate, and tomatoes. What to do if you discover a connection? You guessed it—avoid eating the offending food.

LEARN TO HANDLE STRESS.

That's the best advice for preventing canker sores. Try to find some method of relieving or coping with stress. Examples that you might try include engaging in a hobby, an exercise program, yoga, or meditation.

Carpal tunnel syndrome

24 Tips for Protecting Your Wrists

If, for you, working nine to five means tapping a computer keyboard, punching cash-register keys, working a jackhammer, or doing any other repetitive motion with your hands, you may be at risk for a painful condition called carpal tunnel syndrome (CTS). CTS is a collection of symptoms that can include tingling, numbness, burning, and pain from the wrist to the fingers. By far the most common cause of CTS is repetitive motion with the hands. For this reason, CTS is considered a "cumulative trauma disorder." However, medical conditions such as rheumatoid arthritis, hypothyroidism (low levels of thyroid hormone), pregnancy, and overweight can also cause symptoms of CTS.

If you suffer from CTS, you're not alone. According to the United States Bureau of Labor Statistics, cumulative trauma disorders, including CTS, currently account for more than half of all occupational illnesses reported in the United States today. To understand why CTS occurs, it helps to take a look inside the wrist. The carpal tunnel is a narrow passageway that runs through the wrist. It is only about the size of a postage stamp, but it is crowded with nerves, blood vessels, and nine different tendons, packed in like strands of spaghetti, that control finger movement. Repetitive motions or medical conditions can cause the tendons to swell, decreasing blood flow and compressing the median nerve, which supplies the thumb, index finger, and middle finger. This compression can cause the numbness, pain, tingling, and burning we call carpal tunnel syndrome. If left unchecked, muscle wasting and permanent damage to nerves can result.

For most people, the key to beating this syndrome is prevention—making changes before CTS becomes a problem. If you're already experiencing the tingling, numbness, and pain associated with CTS, you may be able to prevent further damage and promote healing by making a few simple changes in your lifestyle. The tips that follow can help you keep your hands and wrists healthy and help reduce symptoms of CTS. If your symptoms are severe or if they don't resolve after two weeks of self-care, however, see your doctor.

STAY IN SHAPE.

You'll be less likely to suffer injury if your body's circulation and repair systems work well, says Mark Tager, M.D., president of Great Performance, Inc., a company in Beaverton, Oregon, specializing in occupational health. He suggests practicing good nutrition, getting adequate sleep, taking frequent exercise breaks, and avoiding smoking, which cuts down circulation.

TAKE MINIBREAKS.

Fatigue in the joints or muscles is a warning, says Michael Martindale, L.P.T., a physical therapist at the Sports Medicine Center at Portland Adventist Medical Center in Oregon. "The body is trying to tell you something," he says. "It's up to you to listen and take a break."

STAY LOOSE

"A lot of times, initial problems with the wrist are actually tendon problems that don't yet involve the nerve," says David Rempel, M.D. "Exercises may help."

Rempel says that in many work settings today, the problem is that workers don't move around enough. "You're seated in front of a computer for hours in the same position," he says. "It's bound to cause problems. Exercises can help promote blood flow and strengthen the muscles and tendons."

The National Safety Council suggests performing the following four exercises twice a day or whenever you need a break. Stop doing any exercise, however, if it makes your symptoms worse.

Wrist Circles: With your palms down and your hands out, rotate both wrists five times in each direction.

Thumb Stretch: Hold out your right hand, and grasp your right thumb with your left hand. Pull the thumb out and back until you feel a gentle stretch. Hold for five to ten seconds, and release. Repeat three to five times on each thumb.

Five-Finger Stretch: Spread the fingers of both hands far apart and hold for five to ten seconds. Repeat three to five times.

David Rempel, M.D., assistant professor of medicine and director of the Ergonomics Laboratory at the University of California at San Francisco, advises you to

Finger-Thumb Squeeze: Squeeze a small rubber ball tightly in one hand five to ten times. Afterward, stretch the fingers. Repeat with the other hand.

In addition to doing the exercises from the National Safety Council, Rempel suggests strengthening the wrist tendons by doing the following exercises using small hand-held weights. Once again, however, stop any exercise if it seems to make any of your symptoms worse.

Palm-Up Wrist Curls: Rest your forearms on a table, with your palms facing upward and your hands held straight out over the edge of the table. With a light weight (one to two pounds) in each hand, flex your wrists up ten times. Over the course of several weeks, gradually build up to 40 repetitions. Increase the weight of the dumbbells each week by one pound to a maximum of five pounds. Don't exceed five pounds with this exercise, however, or you may traumatize the wrist.

Palm-Down Wrist Curls: Adopt the same position as in the previous exercise, but have your palms facing downward. Flex your wrists up ten times. Gradually increase the number of repetitions over several weeks.

Arm Curls: Stand and hold the weights at your sides, palms facing forward. Slowly curl your arms up, keeping your wrists straight. Do 10 curls, and over several weeks, build up to 40 curls.

give your wrists an occasional rest: "A 1- to 2-minute break every 20 or 30 minutes is a good idea. Then take a longer break every hour."

DON'T SNOOZE AND LOSE.

Some people are bothered more by CTS symptoms at night. Many doctors believe this is because the fluid in the body is redistributed when you lie down, so more of it accumulates in the wrist. In addition, many people unwittingly cause wrist-nerve compression by sleeping with one hand tucked under their head, says Tager. He suggests altering your sleep position to keep your wrist from being bent or compressed.

TAKE SOME WEIGHT OFF.

Excess weight can compress the nerves in the wrist, says Tager. He advises keeping your weight within five to ten pounds of your ideal weight by eating a low-fat diet and getting plenty of exercise.

ROTATE JOBS.

Experts at the National Safety Council suggest that you rotate between jobs that use different muscles and avoid doing the same task for more than a few hours at a time.

Rempel offers the following example: "If your job is to tie a knot in a rope, and the guy down the line cuts the rope, see if you can modify your job so that either you switch tasks frequently or you combine tasks so you're not just doing the same thing over and over."

If your job doesn't allow rotation, talk with your supervisor or union about a change. Rotation reduces job stresses and minimizes production losses.

KEEP IT IN "NEUTRAL."

"Work with your body and your wrists in a comfortable, neutral position," advises Rempel. For wrists, a "neutral" position is straight, not cocked. Check the height of your computer screen (it should be at eye level). Rearrange the level of your keyboard or workstation so that you don't have to strain, reach, or bend your wrists. Your wrists should always be in a straight line with your forearms. And be sure your work is within your "comfort zone" (not too close or too far away).

GET THE RIGHT GRIP ON IT.

Most of us have a tendency to grip with only the thumb, index, and middle fingers, which can increase pressure on the wrist. If you have to grip or twist something, such as the lid of a jar, Tager suggests you use your whole hand.

ALTERNATE HANDS.

Whenever possible, Martindale suggests, give your dominant hand a break.

WATCH THOSE PRESSURE POINTS.

Too often, typists rest their wrists on the sharp edge of a desk or table as they work, which can cause excess pressure on the wrists, says Rempel. Adjust your workstation, if necessary, to keep your wrists off the edge.

SOFTEN UP AND SLOW DOWN.

It's often powerful movements done at high speed that cause carpal tunnel problems. Martindale suggests slowing down and applying only the force needed.

DECREASE BAD VIBES.

People who use vibrating tools, such as sanders and jackhammers, for extended periods are at risk for wrist problems. If you are one of these folks, take frequent breaks and, when possible, operate the tool at the speed that causes the least vibration.

GO "ERGO."

Often, CTS can be prevented or treated by adopting tools and workstations that have been "ergonomically" redesigned to cause less stress on the body. Some tools have been designed to work with less force, while others now feature better grips and handles. Some knife manufacturers, for example, have redesigned knives for meat packers that require less wrist bending. Other companies have created special aids such as wrist rests for computer users that can prevent or reduce the problems of CTS.

Look for items that can ease the strain on your wrists and hands, but be wary of miracle machines and gadgets. "Some of the ergonomic aids can be really helpful," says Rempel. "But I tell people to be careful about devices that make medical claims that say they'll cure CTS."

WATCH FOR SYMPTOMS, AND TAKE ACTION.

Pay attention to early warning signs of CTS, such as morning stiffness in the hands or arms, clumsiness, inability to make a fist, or thumb weakness, and take preventive and self-care action immediately, says Tager.

ICE IT.

If you're having CTS symptoms, use ice to reduce swelling and inflammation. Place an ice pack on the wrist and forearm for 5 to 15 minutes two or three times a day, advises Rempel. At the same time, however, be sure to take steps to eliminate the cause of the trauma to your wrist.

TAKE THE HEAT OFF.

Heat can worsen CTS. "Heat may be good for loosening sore muscles, but you should never use heat with a nerve problem," says Rempel. "Heat causes the tissue to swell, which can make the problem worse."

NIX FLIMSY SPLINTS.

Wrist splints that are prescribed by physicians can help CTS; too often, however, people who develop CTS symptoms rush to the pharmacy for a wrist splint as a home remedy. Rempel says these splints can do more harm than good. "The wrist splints you buy at the pharmacies are pretty flimsy," he says. "They often allow the wrist to move. If people put them on and don't take them off for long periods of time, they can cause muscle shrinking (atrophy)."

REACH FOR OVER-THE-COUNTER RELIEF.

For minor pain and swelling, take aspirin or ibuprofen.

Chafing

13 Ways to Snub the Rub

D oes your skin—or your clothing—rub you the wrong way? If so, you're probably suffering from a condition called chafing. While chafing is rarely a serious problem, nothing can take the spring out of your step like sore, irritated, chafed skin.

Chafing is a condition in which the skin's normal balancing act is disturbed. Normally, the body constantly sheds skin cells, a few at a time, and replaces them with new skin. "During chafing, persistent friction against the skin rubs off more of the skin's outer layer than the skin is able to replenish," says Rodney Basler, M.D., dermatologist and assistant professor of internal medicine at the University of Nebraska Medical Center in Omaha.

Redness and irritation are the first telltale signs of chafing. As the problem worsens, so does the pain and aggravation to the skin. "Left untreated, or if the area becomes wet through constant sweat or wetting, the skin may split and ooze or even bleed," says William Dvorine, M.D., dermatologist and chief of dermatology at St. Agnes Hospital in Baltimore. Ultimately, infection may set in. Fortunately, chafing rarely gets that bad.

Those most prone to this bothersome condition are overweight people and athletes. "If there are greater areas of skin touching skin [as with heavy or very muscular people], then it's more likely that friction injuries will develop," says Basler, who is also chairman of the Task Force on Sports Medicine for the American Academy of Dermatology. When athletes are in motion, the movement of skin against skin is increased. Also, they may wear rough fabrics that irritate the skin.

Target zones for chafing include the upper, inner thighs; under the arms; beneath the breasts in women; and, surprisingly, men's nipples (see "Joggers Beware"). Joggers often experience chafing between the thighs, but Basler says it's largely a male problem. He chalks up this difference between the sexes to the angle of the hips.

Whether you're a man or a woman, chafing doesn't have to cramp your style. Here are several simple tips:

JOGGERS BEWARE

Despite its rather odd-sounding name, "joggers' nipple" is actually a common chafing condition among runners, especially those who go long distances. "At the end of a marathon, you will see a number of people running with bloodstains on the front of their jogging shirts," says Rodney Basler, M.D. Caused by rough fabric, you see it "ten to one in men over women, who are protected by bras," says Basler.

The following tips from Basler should help you avoid joggers' nipple.

For Women:

• When running, wear a soft, supportive, well-fitting bra.

For Men:

• If weather permits, run without a shirt.

• Choose shirts of soft, natural material, such as cotton, rather than more irritating synthetic fabrics.

• Before running, put a thick cream on your nipples for lubrication.

• If all else fails, apply an adhesive strip, cut so it just covers the nipple and areola (the dark area surrounding the nipple). Scaling down the size of the bandage in this way will help prevent tape burn and painful hair pulling.

KEEP YOUR CLOTHES CLEAN.
This is especially important for the outfits you jog or exercise in. "Dirt and sweat can accumulate in fabric and

act as an irritant," says Dvorine. Choose a mild cleanser, and wash clothes frequently.

GO EASY ON THE BLEACH.

Bleach can irritate chafed skin. "I've seen this particularly in people who do martial arts," says Dvorine. "They will often wash their uniforms in bleach and may not wash the bleach out thoroughly enough." Avoid bleaching your clothes, or at least make sure the bleach is thoroughly rinsed out.

RINSE YOUR SUIT.

The chlorine used in swimming pools can also irritate chafed skin, so after a swim in a chlorinated pool, be sure to rinse off your suit and your skin.

SPRINKLE WITH POWDER.

Powder, applied to chafed areas during the day or before a workout, can act as a buffer and cut down on friction. "Using powder may prevent a mild case of chafing from progressing into a more serious one," says Dvorine.

Most any powder will do, but you may be wise to look for one with talc or cornstarch, suggests Hillard H. Pearlstein, M.D., assistant clinical professor of dermatology at Mount Sinai School of Medicine in New York. "They are excellent drying agents that absorb water and moisture," says Pearlstein.

If you're chafed in the groin area and you've had a fungal infection such as jock itch in the past, an over-the-counter antifungal powder may be in order. "That gives you the added benefit of not only cutting down on the friction but killing any fungus that might be present," says Dvorine.

HELLO, DOCTOR?

Chafing can usually be taken care of at home, but in some cases it requires professional help. According to William Dvorine, M.D., here are some red flags that should send you to the doctor:

• Your chafing gets worse despite using the powder/cream treatment for a week.

• Your skin is oozing and cracking.

• You have fever or chills and a feeling of heat on the skin.

DAB ON SOME CREAM.

Applying 0.5 percent or 1 percent hydrocortisone cream (available without a prescription) to the chafed area can provide soothing relief. "Cortisone quiets down the inflammatory response in the skin and allows the skin to heal itself, which it will do if just given half a chance," says Dvorine. You can apply the cream during the day or only at night. If you apply it at night, Dvorine suggests removing it with mineral or baby oil in the morning and using the powder by day. Avoid soap and water to wash off the cream, as that can further irritate chafed skin.

GIVE YOUR UNDERARMS A BREAK.

Hold off on deodorants or antiperspirants—or at least use them sparingly—if your underarms are chafed. Until the condition clears, don't shave or trim the hair in your armpits, either, says Dvorine. These practices will only further aggravate the skin.

WEAR "BUN HUGGERS."
"The advent of the bun huggers in the last five years has been wonderful for eliminating chafing," says Basler. These sports briefs with tight-fitting legs that end about midthigh are great for runners.

CUT BACK.
While most cases of chafing don't get this bad, you may find it is simply too painful to do whatever activity caused the chafing. In that case, Basler suggests you take a few days off from the activity and let the skin heal. Then, when you're ready to begin again, protect your skin: Before each workout, smooth thick cream on areas where you usually get chafed.

Chapped lips

7 Tips for Smoother Lips

If puckering is painful and pursing is too much to bear, you're probably suffering from chapped lips. Harsh winter weather, dry indoor heat, a habit of constantly licking your lips—all of these factors can help dry out the skin of your lips by causing the moisture in the skin to evaporate. The result: Rough, cracked, sensitive lips that leave you little to smile about.

Protecting your lips from chapping is not only important for appearance and comfort, but for health. Cold sores, bacterial infections, and other problems are more likely to strike lips that are already damaged by chapping. Here's what you can do to keep your lips soft and moist:

DON'T LICK YOUR LIPS.

The repeated exposure to water actually robs moisture from the lips, causing them to become dry. "People feel better if they lick their lips, but it just aggravates the problem," says Paul Lazar, M.D., professor of clinical dermatology at Northwestern University School of Medicine in Chicago.

USE A LIP BALM.

Numerous products are available over the counter. Pick one that you like so you'll use it frequently. Most lip balm products are waxy or greasy and work by sealing in moisture with a protective barrier.

TRY PETROLATUM.

Plain old petrolatum is good, too, says Jerome Z. Litt, M.D., assistant clinical professor of dermatology at Case Western Reserve University School of Medicine in Cleveland.

WEAR LIPSTICK.

"If you look at old men and old women, you'll see a difference in their lips, especially the lower," says Albert M. Kligman, M.D., Ph.D., emeritus professor of dermatology at the University of Pennsylvania School of Medicine in Philadelphia. He attributes that difference to the "moderately helpful" properties of lipstick in moisturizing and protecting against the sun's ultraviolet rays. Be careful of cosmetics made outside of the United States, however, since the purity of such products may vary.

SCREEN OUT THE SUN.

The sun's ultraviolet rays can damage and dry the sensitive skin on your lips. Indeed, the lips are a common site for skin cancer. "Your lips don't contain melanin [the pigment, or coloring, that can help protect skin from the sun] and they sunburn easier," points out Ruby Ghadially, M.D., assistant clinical professor in the Department of Dermatology at the University of California at San Francisco. Certain skin cancers that appear on the lips may be more serious and more likely to spread, she says. So if you'll be out in the sun, use a lip balm that contains sunscreen. Choose a product that has a sun protection factor (SPF) of 15 or higher.

CHECK OUT YOUR TOOTHPASTE.

An allergy—to your toothpaste or mouthwash—could be to blame for the rough, red skin on your lips, says Litt. Try switching brands of toothpaste and going without the mouthwash for a few days to see if the problem clears. Rinse well after brushing.

WATCH WHAT PASSES BETWEEN THEM.

When your lips are chapped, they're more sensitive, and certain foods can irritate them. Lazar recommends holding off on pepper, mustard, barbecue sauce, orange juice, and alcoholic beverages to give your lips a break as they heal.

Colds

11 Tips for Fighting the "Cold" War

Headache. Stuffy nose. Cough. Fever. Itchy eyes. Sore throat. Muscle aches. If you're like most people, you know the symptoms of the common cold all too well. Although Americans spend more than $5 billion annually on doctor visits and cold remedies—everything from tissues and vitamin C to over-the-counter decongestants and herb teas—there is no cure for the common cold.

Colds, also called upper respiratory infections, are caused by hundreds of different viruses, according to David N. Gilbert, M.D., director of the Department of Medical Education at Providence Medical Center in Portland, Oregon. "But we don't have any drugs that can kill or inhibit these viruses," he says. "We have to depend on the body's natural defenses."

During a cold, virus particles penetrate the mucous layer of the nose and throat and attach themselves to cells there. The viruses punch holes in the cell membranes, allowing viral genetic material to enter the cells. Within a short time, the virus takes over and forces the cells to produce thousands of new virus particles.

In response to this viral invasion, the body marshals its defenses: The nose and throat release chemicals that spark the immune system; injured cells produce chemicals called prostaglandins, which trigger inflammation and attract infection-fighting white blood cells; tiny blood vessels stretch, allowing spaces to open up to allow

145

DON'T PASS IT ON

Unfortunately, there is no cold vaccine that will protect us from the hundreds of cold viruses just waiting for an opportunity to take up residence and multiply. As a result, getting at least one cold a year is "pretty inevitable," says Stephen R. Jones, M.D. But if you get a cold, you don't have to pass it on. By learning some simple techniques, you can keep your cold to yourself.

Most authorities on the common cold are now convinced that cold viruses are passed in two ways—by direct contact and by viral-filled droplets from the nose being inhaled by others (the so-called "aerosol method"). The direct-contact method works something like this, says David N. Gilbert, M.D.: "You get a virus in your nose, then blow your nose, which contaminates your fingers with the virus, and then you shake hands with someone. They touch their noses and get the cold."

blood fluid (plasma) and specialized white cells to enter the infected area; the body temperature rises, enhancing the immune response; and histamine is released, increasing the production of nasal mucus in an effort to trap viral particles and remove them from the body.

As the battle against the cold virus rages on, the body counterattacks with its heavy artillery—specialized white blood cells called monocytes and lymphocytes; interferon, often called the "body's own antiviral drug"; and 20 or more proteins that circulate in the blood plasma and

Viruses can also live on inanimate objects such as telephones, doorknobs, and cloth handkerchiefs. But no one is really sure just how long they live. To avoid spreading your cold to others by direct contact, Gilbert advises washing your hands frequently and using paper tissues instead of a cloth handkerchief. Be sure to dispose of the tissues promptly after use.

People can also get your cold by directly inhaling viral particles. While most of us feel uncomfortable around someone who is sneezing and coughing, the truth is that those symptoms are late-stage and usually come on when the person is least infectious. Most people spread their colds to others during the first few days when their throat feels sore and they're just coming down with a cold. To avoid giving your cold to others, you may want to stay away from coworkers and friends for a day or two during the onset of a cold. "Avoid crowded places if you can, and cover your nose when you cough or sneeze," says Jones.

coat the viruses and infected cells, making it easier for the white blood cells to identify and destroy them.

The symptoms you experience as a cold are actually the body's natural immune response. In fact, says Michael Castleman, author of *Cold Cures*, by the time you feel like you're coming down with a cold, you've likely already had it for a day and a half.

Many people believe the old adage, "Do nothing and your cold will last seven days. Do everything and it will last a week." While we may not be able to cure the common cold, the simple self-care techniques that follow can help you feel more comfortable and speed healing.

DRINK PLENTY OF FLUIDS.

"Fluids keep the mucus thin," says Gilbert. Donald Girard, M.D., head of the Division of General Internal Medicine at Oregon Health Sciences University in Portland, agrees. "Colds can make you somewhat dehydrated and you don't even know it," says Girard. Drink at least eight ounces of fluid every two hours.

COOK UP SOME CHICKEN SOUP.

One of the most beneficial hot fluids you can consume when you have a cold is chicken soup. It was first prescribed for the common cold by rabbi/physician Moses Maimonides in twelfth-century Egypt and has been a favorite folk remedy ever since. In 1978, Marvin Sackner, M.D., of Mount Sinai Hospital in Miami Beach, Florida, included chicken soup in a test of the effects of sipping hot and cold water on the clearance of mucus. Chicken soup placed first, hot water second, and cold water a distant third. Sackner's work has since been replicated by other researchers. While doctors aren't sure exactly why chicken soup helps clear nasal passages, they agree "it's just what the doctor ordered."

REST.

Doctors disagree about whether or not you should take a day or two off from work when you come down with a cold. However, they do agree that extra rest helps. Staying away from the work site may be a good idea from a prevention standpoint, too. Your coworkers will probably appreciate your not spreading your cold virus

HELLO, DOCTOR?

While most colds can be effectively treated at home, you should call your doctor if:

• You have a headache and stiff neck with no other cold symptoms. (Your symptoms may indicate meningitis.)

• You have a headache and sore throat with no other cold symptoms. (It may be strep throat.)

• You have cold symptoms and significant pain across your nose and face that doesn't go away. (You may have a sinus infection, which requires antibiotics.)

• You have a fever above 101 degrees Fahrenheit (adults), you've taken aspirin, and the fever isn't going down.

• Your child has a fever above 102 degrees Fahrenheit.

• Your cold symptoms seem to be going away, but you suddenly develop a fever. (It may indicate pneumonia, which is more likely to set in toward the end of a cold.)

• You have a "dry" cough—one that doesn't bring up phlegm—for more than ten days.

• You cough up blood.

around the office. If you do decide to stay home, forgo chores and take it easy, read a good book, take a nap.

Girard adds that you should skip your normal exercise routine when you've got a cold. In fact, he says, if you're feeling pretty bad, you should just head for bed.

(Continued on page 152)

WHAT ABOUT "COLD MEDICINES?"

When cold season arrives, doctors' offices fill up with people searching for a "cold cure." Unfortunately, modern medicine doesn't have any medication that is effective against viruses, including the more than 100 viruses that can cause the common cold. Antibiotics, such as penicillin, don't work against cold viruses. "The first thing you shouldn't do," says David N. Gilbert, M.D., "is go to the doctor's office and get a penicillin shot. They're ineffective, expensive, and they expose you to unnecessary side effects."

OK, if the doctor can't help, what about all those "cold remedies" touted on television and radio? Surely they must work.

Not really. Some cold experts believe that popular cold remedies may actually inhibit the body's immune responses as they suppress cold symptoms. All of your cold symptoms are part of your body's natural response in its battle against the viral invaders. To stop or suppress those responses may actually prolong your cold.

For example, cold experts say a mild fever—below 102 degrees Fahrenheit—enhances the body's ability to fight the cold virus. Gilbert, therefore, suggests forgoing aspirin and acetaminophen to lower a mild fever. (If you're over 60, have heart disease, or have any immune-compromising health condition, however, contact your physician at the first sign of a fever.)

Another example of potentially counter-productive cold remedies is antihistamines, which are common ingredients in multisymptom cold formulas. Antihistamines stop the runny nose, but they may do more harm than good. "Antihistamines dry up mucous membranes, which are already irritated," says Gilbert. "They thicken the nasal mucus so you feel like you need more decongestant, and they can cause an irritated cough."

One over-the-counter cold remedy that can bring symptomatic relief is pseudoephedrine, a decongestant ingredient found in products such as Sudafed, says Stephen R. Jones, M.D. "This ingredient effectively shuts down the swelling and fluid production and promotes drainage," he says. People who have high blood pressure or heart disease, however, should avoid this drug.

Cough syrups that contain glyceryl guaiacolate (but not dextromethorphan) can help loosen thick sputum, making it easier to cough up, according to Donald Girard, M.D.

If you think you need over-the-counter remedies to cope with your cold, most authorities recommend single-action remedies rather than the "shotgun" approach of multisymptom products. Most people get their cold symptoms serially—sore throat first, cough last. But multisymptom cold remedies say that they cure all of your cold symptoms at once, even the ones you don't have. Why take medications—and risk their side effects—when you don't need them?

"These multisymptom cold remedies don't really do anything," Jones says. "The reason people like the nighttime cold remedies is that many of them contain large amounts of alcohol. They're expensive and ineffective. I tell my patients to avoid them."

STAY WARM.

"I usually recommend people stay indoors and stay warm when they have a cold," says Girard. If nothing else, staying warm may make you feel more comfortable, especially if you have a fever.

USE A SALTWATER WASH.

The inflammation and swelling in the nose during a cold is caused by molecules called cytokines, or lymphokines, which are made by the lymphocytes, explains Stephen R. Jones, M.D., chief of medicine at Good Samaritan Hospital and Medical Center in Portland, Oregon. "Recent evidence has shown that if we can wash out those cytokines, it reduces the swelling and fluid production." Jones recommends filling a clean nasal-spray bottle with dilute salt water (one level teaspoon salt to one quart water) and spraying each nostril three or four times. Repeat five to six times per day.

GARGLE.

Girard says gargling with warm salt water (a quarter teaspoon salt in four ounces warm water) every one to two hours can soothe your sore throat. "Salt water is an astringent that is very soothing to the inflamed tissues, and it tends to loosen mucus," he says.

CONSIDER VITAMIN C.

Although studies suggest that vitamin C may boost the body's immune system, the use of this vitamin in treating colds is still controversial. Many physicians don't recommend vitamin C as a cold remedy. Others, including cold researcher Elliot Dick, Ph.D., chief of the Respiratory Virus Research Laboratory at the University of Wisconsin–Madison, have found that taking 2,000 milligrams or more of vitamin C daily can lessen the severity of cold symptoms.

If you do decide to try boosting your vitamin C intake during a cold, don't overdo it. While vitamin C has been found to be relatively safe at doses of up to 10,000 milligrams per day, some people find vitamin C causes diarrhea at or above the 10,000-milligram level. Perhaps the safest way to get more vitamin C is to choose vitamin C-rich foods more often. For example, since you'll need to increase your fluid intake while you have a cold, fill some of that requirement with orange juice.

VAPORIZE IT.
The steam from a vaporizer can loosen mucus, especially if the sputum is thick, says Girard. It may also raise the humidity in the immediate area slightly, which may make you feel more comfortable.

STOP SMOKING.
"Smokers have colds longer in duration than nonsmokers," says Gilbert. "If you chronically irritate the bronchial tubes while you have a cold, you're more likely to develop a complication like pneumonia."

In addition to irritating the throat and bronchial tubes, smoking has been shown to depress the immune system. Since you have to depend on your own immune system rather than medicine to cure a cold, you'll want it to be in the best condition possible.

STAY AWAY FROM "HOT TODDIES."
While a hot alcoholic beverage might sound good when you're feeling achy and stuffy, Gilbert says it increases

mucous membrane congestion. "If you want to minimize your discomfort," he says, "stay away from alcohol."

MAINTAIN A POSITIVE ATTITUDE.

Although mind-body science is in its infancy, some researchers suggest that a positive I-can-beat-this-cold attitude may actually stimulate the immune system. "If you give up, so does your immune system," says Castleman. "Buoyancy and self-confidence help rev up the immune system or at least keep it from collapsing while it fights your cold."

Jones isn't as convinced about the connection between the mind and the immune system. He says the evidence directly linking one's thoughts with immunity is "interesting, but inconclusive." But, he admits, "a positive attitude is always best and certainly couldn't hurt your cold."

Cold sores

6 Ways to Foil Cold Sores

It never fails. Every time you have a big meeting coming up or an important presentation to give, you develop an unsightly cold sore on your lip. You wake up with a small cluster of tiny, harmless-looking, white blisters, which quickly explode into a painful sore the size of Rhode Island (OK, so maybe it just *looks* that big).

"True cold sores, the ones that occur on the lips, are caused by the herpes simplex virus I," says Evan T. Bell,

HELLO, DOCTOR?

"Many people choose to leave cold sores alone and let them go their own way since they are usually not severe or life threatening," says Evan T. Bell, M.D. And doing so certainly won't hurt you.

On the other hand, if you have frequent or severe cold sores, see your doctor. "There is a prescription drug called acyclovir that works actively against initial outbreaks of herpes simplex viruses," says Bell. Although the drug tends to be less effective for recurrences, you and your doctor may decide that it's worth a shot.

M.D., a specialist in infectious diseases at Lenox Hill Hospital in New York. "Herpes viruses presumably lie dormant in certain nerve cells of the body lifelong, until something like stress, strain, a cold, or excessive exposure to the sun causes them to manifest. In the case of herpes simplex virus I, it happens to be on the lip," he explains. The sores last from 7 to 14 days.

Although many use the terms "cold sore" and "canker sore" interchangeably, they are different. Unlike cold sores, canker sores are oral lesions that are characterized by small, round, white areas inside the mouth surrounded by a sharp halo of red. And, while cold sores are highly contagious, canker sores are not.

Unfortunately, attempting to camouflage cold sores with makeup often produces an even worse effect. Still, while you can't do much about the way they look, you can do a few things to help decrease discomfort, speed healing, and keep them from coming back. You can even take steps to prevent passing on your cold sores to others. Here's how:

COVER IT WITH A PROTECTIVE PETROLEUM-BASED PRODUCT.

"This will protect it from infection and help it to heal a little quicker," says Marcia Kielhofner, M.D., clinical assistant professor of medicine at Baylor College of Medicine in Houston, Texas.

REACH FOR ASPIRIN, ACETAMINOPHEN, OR IBUPROFEN.

"These sores can be quite painful because they are in an area that tends to be easily and continually irritated," says Kielhofner. "An over-the-counter painkiller can greatly reduce this discomfort."

AVOID SALTY OR ACIDIC FOODS.

Things like potato chips or citrus fruits can further irritate cold sores and add to the pain, according to Kielhofner.

APPLY AN OVER-THE-COUNTER ANESTHETIC.

Putting a local anesthetic ointment containing benzocaine on the cold sore can help numb the pain temporarily.

PROTECT YOUR LIPS FROM THE SUN.

Applying sunscreen to your lips may help prevent sun-induced recurrences of cold sores, according to a study by the National Institutes of Health. Look for a sunscreen, designed especially for the lips, that has an SPF of 15 or higher. Some colored lipsticks now also contain sunscreen; check the cosmetic counter at your local department store.

KEEP IT TO YOURSELF.

One important thing to keep in mind with cold sores is that they are extremely contagious. While you have a cold sore, avoid kissing and sharing cups, towels, or other such items. And wash your hands frequently.

Colic

15 Ways to Help You and Your Baby Cope

When you brought your new baby home from the hospital, he seemed so quiet, so sweet, so well behaved. Suddenly, about two weeks after your child's arrival, Mommy's angel turned into a crying, squalling, red-faced little devil. At times, the child may have appeared to be in pain: He drew his legs up to his belly and appeared to pass gas more frequently. Perhaps you took your child to the pediatrician for a diagnosis, or maybe you were able to recognize the symptoms yourself—the demon of colic had invaded your once-peaceful home. By now, you've probably reached the end of your rope.

You feel frustrated and tired. You may have started to doubt your ability to parent your child properly. You may have even considered packing up your bags and leaving home.

The first step to take is to relax in the knowledge that your feelings are perfectly normal. Parents are often conditioned to believe that if their child is crying, something is wrong—something that they should be able to fix. Fortunately, you can take solace in the fact that your child is probably otherwise healthy. Colic does not indicate the presence of a serious medical problem. And a certain amount of crying is normal and healthy, says William B. Carey, M.D., a clinical professor of pediatrics at the University of Pennsylvania School of Medicine and director of Behavioral Pediatrics in the Division of General Pediatrics at Children's Hospital, both in Philadelphia. Still, to set your mind at ease, it may be helpful to take your child to the pediatrician to ensure that his or her crying is not a sign of a medical problem, says Carey. It can also be reassuring to keep in mind that most cases of colic go away by the time the child has reached three months of age.

The bad news is that doctors still don't know what causes colic, what the disorder really is, or how to cure it. They don't even know if colicky babies really are in pain. However, there are some tried-and-true ways to help soothe your baby and to help you keep a hold on your sanity in the process. These are included in the tips that follow.

SET THE BABY IN MOTION.
As most parents can attest, mild repetitious motion, such as that of a moving car or a rocking chair, can calm a

cranky baby. With a colicky child, that knowledge is doubly important, according to Cheston M. Berlin, Jr., M.D., a professor of pediatrics and of pharmacology at Pennsylvania State University College of Medicine's Milton S. Hershey Medical Center in Hershey. "Motion is the best thing for children who are having so much trouble," he says. If taking the child out in the car is too inconvenient, he recommends putting the child in a safety seat and placing it atop a running dryer (but don't leave the baby unattended).

There are also devices on the market that will rock or vibrate the baby's crib, Berlin says. Some of these devices even have sound sensors that will start the motion only when the baby starts crying and will stop after it senses that the baby has calmed down or gone to sleep. One device even simulates the motion of a car moving at 55 miles per hour. Some physicians find it effective, while others feel that it makes little difference.

LET THE BABY SLEEP.

Many parenting books and pediatricians would have you believe that you should pick the baby up every time he or she cries, says Carey. However, babies often cry because they are tired. If this is the case, picking up the child only stimulates him or her further. "I think some of the time you should be leaving the baby alone," Carey says. "If you pick up a tired baby, he'll cry more."

To assess whether your child is crying because of fatigue, try everything else first: feeding, burping, changing, cuddling. Then, if the baby is still crying, put him or her down to sleep, and walk out of the room. Often, according to Carey, the child will settle down within five minutes.

COLIC MEDICATIONS AND BABIES: A POOR COMBINATION

Several colic medications have been tried throughout the years, with varying degrees of success. However, recent studies out of the Southwest SIDS (Sudden Infant Death Syndrome) Research Institute in Lake Jackson, Texas, and Children's Hospital in Camperdown, New South Wales, Australia, have found that colic medications may prove dangerous and even fatal.

The Texas researchers studied eight infants who were experiencing life-threatening respiratory and gastro-intestinal symptoms. All of the babies had previously been given a premixed colic medication containing Dramamine, a popular antihistamine used to relieve motion sickness, and Donnatal, a drug prescribed for irritable bowel syndrome and other intestinal disorders. Donnatal contains, among other things, phenobarbital, a barbiturate used as a sedative. In an article published in the journal **Clinical**

STAY CALM.
"It is important to emphasize that colic is a benign disorder," according to Berlin. "It has never been known to cause or represent any serious medical problem," he adds. Keeping that knowledge in mind can help parents to understand and accept that this is just a stage in their child's development—an unpleasant stage, but one that will soon pass.

Pediatrics, the researchers wrote that the possibility that the drug can lead to respiratory and gastrointestinal problems in certain infants "requires serious consideration and further evaluation."

In the Australian study, investigators described a case where atropine—an ingredient in Donnatal and a drug that is often prescribed for diarrhea, cramping, and other intestinal ailments—caused serious side effects in an infant who received it as a colic medication. The adverse effects were caused by a faulty prescription of the drug. "In view of the potential for serious toxicity resulting from either inappropriate prescription, preparation, or administration, alternative methods of treatment should be employed," the researchers wrote in the **Journal of Paediatrics and Child Health**.

Since colic symptoms tend to go away by the time the child has reached three months of age, it's probably a good idea to avoid any colic medications and patiently wait it out.

TAKE YOUR BABY OFF COW'S MILK.

Some studies have shown an improvement in colic after dairy products have been removed from babies' diets, according to Ronald G. Barr, M.D.C.M., an associate professor of pediatrics and psychiatry at McGill University and director of the Child Development Program at Montreal Children's Hospital, both in Montreal. The culprit seems to be a protein in cow's milk, which is present in many infant formulas and is also found in the milk of breast-feeding mothers who eat dairy products, Barr says. The protein may be responsible for colic in about five to ten percent of babies who suffer from the condition. Changing the baby's formula (there are many soy-based formulas available) or staying off dairy products yourself if you are breast-feeding is worth a try. If your baby's crying does not seem to improve after two weeks, you can assume milk was not the problem.

TRY PEPPERMINT WATER.

Although it has never been definitively proven to be effective, peppermint-flavored water is a century-old remedy for colic, according to Berlin. "It was very recently discovered that the active ingredient in peppermint oil is a calcium-channel blocker, a substance that may relax the gut," he says. He recommends soaking a piece of a peppermint stick in water, then feeding a bottleful of the flavored water to the baby. Do not use straight peppermint oil, he says, as this may be too strong for the baby.

ADD FIBER TO YOUR BABY'S FORMULA.

Some studies have shown that colic seemed to improve in certain infants when fiber was added to their formula, according to William R. Treem, M.D., a pediatric gastroenterologist in the Division of Pediatric Gastroenterology and Nutrition at Hartford Hospital in Connecticut and associate professor of pediatrics at the University of Connecticut School of Medicine. "Some babies seemed to be dramatically better when we added fiber to their formula," he said. "We used Citrucel, a bulking agent that draws water into the stool. We have added anywhere from one-half teaspoon three times a day to one-half teaspoon six times a day. I think it's best to start small and build up to the higher doses." Although not the answer for every baby, adding fiber is certainly safe and is definitely worth a try, Treem says.

TAKE A SHOWER.

If your baby's crying has driven you to the point of near madness, it's time to stop and take a break, Berlin says, since an overly frustrated parent can be of no help to anyone. "I recommend 20 to 30 minutes in a warm shower," he says, adding that the sound of the water can successfully mask the baby's crying. (Be sure the baby is in a safe place, such as a crib.)

KEEP A CALENDAR.

A record of your baby's weight and the frequency and length of crying bouts may be of help in tracking his or her progress, Barr says. It can also be a handy record to take to the pediatrician's office, he says. A useful bonus of the charting is that it reminds you that your baby does cry a lot, but that there are breaks in between. "Parents tend to feel like the baby just cries all the time," Barr says.

BE REALISTIC.

"The babies that you see in magazines and books—the babies who are neat, clean, and happy—well, you can expect your baby to be like that for about 30 minutes out of every 24 hours," says Edward R. Christophersen, Ph.D., professor of pediatrics at the University of Missouri at Kansas City School of Medicine and chief of the Behavioral Pediatrics Section at Children's Mercy Hospital in Kansas City, Missouri. "Keep in mind that the

HOW MUCH DOES A NORMAL BABY CRY?

In 1962, the famous pediatrician T. Berry Brazelton, M.D., published a study of the crying patterns of 80 normal, middle-class infants. He found that their crying lasted for about two hours per day at two weeks of age, increased to a peak of almost three hours per day by the time they were six weeks of age, and then gradually decreased to about one hour per day by the time they had reached three months of age.

The generally accepted medical definition of colic is a condition in which a young infant who is otherwise healthy and well fed has bouts of irritability, fussing, or crying that can persist for a total of more than three hours a day on more than three days of the week, according to William B. Carey, M.D. Sometimes, doctors add the stipulation that the baby's excessive crying continue for a period of more than three weeks to be considered colic.

Carey emphasizes this simple point: Normal babies cry—a lot. So don't assume that just because your child is putting up a fuss for three hours a day, he or she is abnormal. More than likely, it's just your baby's way of letting you know that he or she is healthy, energetic, and alive. Lastly, try to keep in mind and take solace in the fact that by three months of age, this phase will be over and you're most likely to have a great deal more peace and quiet around the house.

only exercise babies get is crying and nursing." In other words, don't be discouraged: Your baby is not abnormal just because he or she cries a lot.

SOOTHE, DON'T STIMULATE.

Since crying, colicky babies are already overly stimulated, try soothing the baby instead of bouncing or rocking him or her, says Carey. Some time-honored tools: a hot-water bottle, filled with warm—not hot—water and placed on a towel on the child's back or stomach; a pacifier; or the use of repetitious sounds, such as the noise of a fan or humidifier.

MAINTAIN AS MUCH DIRECT CONTACT AS POSSIBLE.

Pediatricians often recommend carrying and cuddling a colicky baby as much as possible. However, studies have failed to show that carrying actually causes a reduction in crying. On the other hand, carrying the baby more frequently before colic ever sets in may prevent the condition from developing in the first place, says Barr. He mentions a study where the caretakers of 99 normal infants increased their carrying of the infants by the age of three weeks. The result? The babies cried 43 percent less than other babies of the same age. "The carrying prevented the crying peak from ever occurring in those infants," according to Barr. He also describes studies of a tribe of Botswanian hunter-gatherers, the !Kung San, whose infants cry as often as North American babies, but only for about half as long. Barr says that mothers in the tribe spend significantly more time with their babies held close to their bodies than North American mothers do.

FEED MORE OFTEN.

One reason that the !Kung San spend so much time holding their babies is that they feed them almost continuously, Barr says. "They feed very frequently—approximately four times per hour, four minutes per feed," he says. This type of feeding schedule may be partly responsible for the reduced crying of the !Kung San infants, according to Barr. "Parents do have the option to feed more frequently," he says. "I think there is lots of room for changing the frequency of feeding that is within the range of what is normal." Even if continuous feeding does not fit into your schedule, adding a few extra feedings still may help, Barr says.

PUT YOUR BABY ON A SCHEDULE.

Some children cry excessively because they don't know how to calm themselves down enough to go to sleep, says Christophersen. Since babies younger than 12 weeks often fall asleep while being fed, it is sometimes difficult for them to fall asleep without feeding, he says. He suggests starting your baby on a regular schedule of sleeping and waking and trying to get him or her to fall asleep without your assistance. "Kiss them, hug them, sing them songs, then let them fall asleep on their own," he says. "This way, they learn to make their own transition from the alert, crying state to the sleeping state."

TOUCH BASE WITH YOUR PEDIATRICIAN.

Your pediatrician can be an invaluable source of ideas, experience, and reassurance, says Christophersen. "Parents can get very discouraged with a colicky child," he says. He recommends taking advantage of all support systems that are available to you.

WAIT IT OUT.
If all else fails, take solace in the fact that colic generally stops by three months of age, Berlin says. The longest you'll have to wait is until the baby reaches six months, although colic this long-lasting is rare. Unfortunately, "there's no dramatic cure," he says.

Constipation

11 Ways to Keep Things Moving

Irregularity is one of those things that no one likes to talk about. It's personal and, well, a little embarrassing. But if you're one of the millions of people who's ever been constipated, you know it can put a real damper on your day.

The first thing to realize when you're talking about constipation is that "regularity" is a relative term. Everyone has his or her own natural rhythm. Ask four people to define regularity, and you're likely to get at least four different answers. Normal bowel habits can span anywhere from three bowel movements a day to three a week, according to Marvin Schuster, M.D., professor of medicine with a joint appointment in psychiatry at Johns Hopkins University School of Medicine and chief of the Division of Digestive Diseases at Francis Scott Key Medical Center, both in Baltimore.

"One of the most common forms of constipation is imaginary or misconceived constipation," says Schuster.

CONSTIPATION

It's based on the idea that if you don't have the "magical" one bowel movement a day, then something's wrong. Constipation has a lot to do with a person's comfort level, says Peter Banks, M.D., director of Clinical Gastroenterology Service at Brigham and Women's Hospital and lecturer on medicine at Harvard Medical School, both in Boston. People who are constipated often strain a lot in the bathroom, produce unusually hard stools, and feel gassy and bloated.

Schuster calls it "constipation" if you have fewer than three bowel movements a week or if you experience a marked change in your normal bowel patterns. A sudden change in bowel habits merits a visit to your doctor to rule out any more serious underlying problems (see "Hello, Doctor?"). But for the occasional bout of constipation, here are some tips to put you back on track:

GET MOVING.
Exercise seems not only to boost your fitness but to promote regularity as well. "The thinking is that lack of activity puts the bowels to rest," says Banks. That may partially explain why older people, who may be more sedentary, and those who are bedridden are prone to becoming constipated. "We encourage people to get up and be more active," says Banks. So gear up and get moving. You don't have to run a marathon; a simple walking workout doesn't take much time and can be very beneficial. When it comes to regularity, even a little exercise is better than none at all.

RAISE YOUR GLASS.
Drinking an adequate amount of liquids may help to alleviate constipation or prevent it from happening in the

....

HELLO, DOCTOR?

Constipation can be a symptom of a more serious problem, such as an underactive thyroid, irritable bowel syndrome, or cancer, to name a few. See your doctor if you have any of these symptoms:

- A major change in your bowel pattern
- Constipation lasting for several weeks or longer
- Blood in your stool
- Severe pain during bowel movements
- Unusual stomach distention

....

first place. The reason for this is simple. "If you dehydrate yourself or drink too little fluid, that will dry out your stool as well and make it hard to pass," says Schuster.

On the other hand, some people have the misconception that if you drink far more than you need, you can treat constipation. Schuster disagrees, saying the excess fluid will just get urinated out.

To achieve a balanced intake of liquids, a good rule of thumb is to drink eight cups of fluid a day, says Mindy Hermann, R.D., a registered dietitian and spokesperson for the American Dietetic Association. (This rule of thumb doesn't apply, however, if you have a kidney or liver problem or any other medical condition that may require restricting your intake of fluid.) Drink even more when it's hot or when you're exercising. Hermann suggests that athletes weigh themselves before and after a workout. Any weight lost during the activity reflects water loss. To replace it, they should drink two cups of liquid for every lost pound of body weight.

For those who are constipated, all liquids are not created equal. Avoid drinking coffee or caffeinated drinks, urges Elyse Sosin, R.D., a registered dietitian and the supervisor of clinical nutrition at Mount Sinai Medical Center in New York. Caffeine acts as a diuretic, taking fluid out of your body when you want to retain it. She suggests drinking water, seltzer, juice, or milk.

DON'T FIGHT THE URGE.

Often, because people are busy or have erratic schedules or because they don't want to use public bathrooms, they suppress the urge to have a bowel movement. "If they do this over a period of time, it can block the urge so it doesn't come," explains Schuster. If at all possible, heed the call when you feel it.

TAKE ADVANTAGE OF AN INBORN REFLEX.

We're all born with a reflex to defecate shortly after we're fed, says Schuster. With socialization, we learn to control our bladders and bowels and we inhibit this reflex. Schuster suggests that you try to revive this reflex by choosing one meal a day and trying to have a movement after it. "Very often, people can program the colon to respond to that meal," Schuster says. He notes that this works better with younger people than with the elderly.

KNOW YOUR MEDICATIONS.

A number of prescription and over-the-counter medications can cause constipation. If you are currently taking any medication, you might want to ask your doctor or pharmacist whether it could be causing your constipation. Among the drugs that can cause constipation are calcium-channel blockers taken for high blood pressure, beta-blockers, some antidepressants, narcotics and other pain medications, antihistamines (to a lesser degree), certain decongestants, and some antacids. Antacids that contain calcium or aluminum are binding and can cause constipation. When choosing an antacid, Schuster suggests you keep in mind that the names of most of those with aluminum start with the letter "a." Those that start with the letter "m" contain magnesium, which does not constipate. If you are unsure, ask your pharmacist.

BULK UP.

Many times, adding fiber or roughage to your diet is all that's needed to ensure regularity. Fiber, the indigestible parts of plant foods, adds mass to the stool and stimulates the colon to push things along. Fiber is found in fruits, vegetables, grains, and beans. Meats, chicken, fish, and fats come up empty-handed in the fiber category. The current recommendations for daily dietary fiber are 20 to 35 grams. "Most people eat between 10 and 15 grams," says Hermann. So there's plenty of room for improvement. Fiber supplements may be helpful, but most doctors and dietitians agree that it's preferable to get your fiber from food (see "Laxative Alert").

ADD FIBER SLOWLY.

People assimilate high-fiber foods into their diet more easily if they do it gradually. "You need to add one high-fiber food at a time, start with small amounts, and wait a couple of days before adding something else so you don't

LAXATIVE ALERT

Laxatives seem like an easy solution for constipation woes, but they can cause many more problems than they solve. Indeed, these tablets, gums, powders, suppositories, and liquids can be habit forming and produce substantial side effects if used incorrectly.

Laxatives work in many different ways, and "each one has its problems," says Marvin Schuster, M.D. Some lubricate, others soften the stools, some draw water into the bowel, and still others are bulk forming. One real danger is that people can become dependent on them, needing ever-increasing amounts to do the job. Eventually, some types of laxatives can damage the nerve cells of the colon until the person can't evacuate anymore. Some laxatives inhibit the absorption or effectiveness of drugs. Those with a mineral-oil base can prevent the absorption of vitamins A, D, K, and E. Still others can damage and inflame the lining of the intestine.

"I think laxatives ought to be avoided if at all possible and only used under a doctor's care," says Schuster. In the long run, you'll be much better off to depend on exercise, adequate fluid intake, and a high-fiber diet to keep you regular.

throw your system into chaos," says Hermann. Sosin agrees and also stresses the need to "drink an adequate amount of fluids with the fiber."

EAT AT LEAST FIVE SERVINGS OF FRUITS AND VEGETABLES DAILY.

Eat a variety of fruits and vegetables, says Hermann—some that are high in fiber and others that aren't. Potatoes (white and sweet), apples, berries, apricots, peaches, pears, oranges, prunes, corn, peas, carrots, tomatoes, broccoli, and cauliflower are good choices.

EAT 6 TO 11 SERVINGS OF GRAIN PRODUCTS DAILY.

That's in addition to the five servings of fruits and vegetables just mentioned. Grain products include cereals, breads, and starchy vegetables (such as corn, green peas, potatoes, and lima beans). "I tell people to start out the day with a high-fiber cereal because it's easy to do and it immediately knocks off a big chunk of the amount of fiber they should be getting during the day," says Hermann. Check cereal box labels; more than five or six grams of fiber per serving is high fiber. If you don't like any so-called high-fiber cereals, line up the boxes of cereal that you would be willing to eat and pick the one with the most fiber, suggests Hermann.

Read labels when choosing breads as well. "Just because a bread is brown doesn't mean it has a lot of fiber in it," says Hermann. Find a bread that has at least two grams of fiber per slice. Watch the portion size, too, when looking for high-fiber foods. "Sometimes they will give you a very large size that's unrealistic for one serving," says Sosin.

BRING HOME THE BEANS.

Dried beans and legumes—whether pinto, red, lima, navy, or garbanzo—are excellent sources of fiber. Many people don't like them because of the gassiness they may cause. Cooking beans properly can ease this problem considerably. Hermann's technique for cooking less "explosive" dried beans: Soak the beans overnight, then dump the water out. Pour new water in, and cook the beans for about 30 minutes. Throw that water out, put in new water, and cook for another 30 minutes. Drain the water out, put new water in, and finish cooking.

CUT BACK ON REFINED FOODS.

You can bump up your fiber intake by switching from refined foods to less-refined foods whenever possible. Switch from a highly processed cereal to a whole-grain cereal, move from heavily cooked vegetables to less-cooked vegetables, and choose whole-grain products over products made with white flour. A glass of orange juice provides 0.1 gram of fiber, while eating an orange gives you 2.9 grams. "As soon as you start juicing something or straining it or taking the pulp out, you're taking out the fiber," says Hermann.

Corns and calluses

22 Steps to Relief

You may refer to your feet as tootsies or dogs, but the fact remains that feet are highly sophisticated structures. The human foot is a miracle of engineering designed to stand up under a lot of wear and tear. It's a good thing, too: Your feet are the most used and abused parts of your body. According to the American Podiatric Medical Association, the average American walks 115,000 miles in a lifetime—a distance that would take you all the way around the earth four times. Your feet support the weight of your body, plus clothing and whatever extras you might be carrying. And in an average day of walking, your feet are subjected to a force equal to several hundred tons.

Despite how well designed your feet are, things can go wrong. An estimated 87 percent of American adults have some type of foot problem. Among the most common of these problems are corns and calluses.

Although both corns and calluses are patches of toughened skin that form to protect sensitive foot tissue against repeated friction and pressure, they are different in some ways. Hard corns are usually found on the tops of the toes or on the outer sides of the little toes, where the skin rubs against the shoe. Sometimes, a corn will form on the ball of the foot, beneath a callus, resulting in a sharp, localized pain with each step. Soft corns, which are moist and rubbery, form between toes, where the bones of one toe exert pressure on the bones of its neighbor. Both hard and soft corns are cone shaped, with the tip pointing into the foot (what you see is the base of the cone). When a shoe or another toe puts pressure against the corn, the tip can hit sensitive underlying tissue, causing pain.

Calluses, on the other hand, generally form over a flat surface and have no tip. They usually appear on the weight-bearing parts of the foot—the ball or the heel.

(Continued on page 178)

IF THE SHOE FITS...

"When corns and calluses form, the real underlying problem is one of mechanics—the foot inside the shoe is not functioning properly. But poor-fitting shoes may precipitate the problem," says Joseph C. D'Amico, D.P.M.

Here are some guidelines to getting a better fit the next time you shop for shoes:

• Have the salesclerk measure each foot twice before you buy any pair of shoes. Don't ask for a certain size just because it's the one you have always worn; the size of your feet changes as you grow older.

• Be sure to try on both the left and the right shoe. Stand during the fitting process, and check to see that there is adequate space (three-eighths to one-half inch) for your longest toe at the end of each shoe. Remember, your longest toe may not be your big toe; in some people, the second toe extends the farthest. Likewise, your feet may not be the exact same size. If one foot is slightly larger than the other, buy the shoes for the larger foot and use padding, if necessary, for a better fit on the smaller foot.

• Make sure that the shoe fits snugly at the heel.

• Make sure the ball of your foot fits snugly into the widest part of the shoe—called the ball pocket.

• Shop for shoes at the end of the day, when your feet are likely to be slightly swollen.

• Don't just put the shoes on and look at them in the mirror. Walk around the store in the shoes to make sure they fit and feel right as you stride along.

• Don't buy shoes that feel too tight, expecting them to stretch out with time. If the shoes that you want to purchase don't feel right in the store, they will never fit comfortably. The shoes you buy should not need to be stretched.

• If you are not sure about the fit, check into the store's refund policy. If possible, take the shoes home, wear them on a rug for an hour, and if they don't feel good, take them back.

• When buying shoes for everyday use, look for ones with fairly low heels.

• Make sure that the material of the shoe's upper is soft and pliable.

• Have several different pairs of shoes so that you do not wear the same pair day after day. Alternating your shoes is a wise move, not only for the health of your feet but for the life of your shoes.

You may discover, as most people do, that your left foot and your right foot are not exactly the same size. Or you may have a high instep, a plump foot, a very narrow foot, or especially long toes. While these characteristics may make it somewhat difficult to step into every pair of shoes you try on, they do not mean that you must resign yourself to never finding a pair of shoes that fit comfortably. All it takes is a little time and the determination to walk in comfort.

One last reminder: Like Cinderella, who was the only one in the kingdom able to fit into the glass slipper, the person who buys a pair of shoes is the only person who should wear them.

Each step presses the callus against underlying tissue and may cause aching, burning, or tenderness, but rarely sharp pain.

Try the tips that follow to relieve the discomfort associated with these two conditions. Then, if your corn or callus continues to cause discomfort, see a podiatrist. In addition, if you have diabetes or any other disorder that affects circulation, do not attempt to self-treat any foot problem; see your podiatrist right away.

PLAY DETECTIVE.

"Corns and calluses develop for a reason," says Suzanne M. Levine, D.P.M., a podiatrist in private practice in New York. "Abnormal amounts of dead, thickened skin form at certain spots on your feet to protect them from excess pressure and friction." Obviously, the real solution to corns and calluses is to track down and eliminate whatever is causing the pressure and friction. "The place to start is with your shoes," advises Levine. See "If the Shoe Fits" for tips on choosing well-fitting shoes.

TRIM THOSE TOENAILS.

Toenails are designed to protect the toes from injury. However, the pressure of a shoe on a toenail that is too long can force the joint of the toe to push up against the shoe, forming a corn. To take the pressure off, keep your toenails trimmed. Cut each toenail straight across so that it doesn't extend beyond the tip of the toe. Then, file each toenail to smooth any rough edges.

TAKE A SOAK.

While eliminating the source of the problem is essential, sometimes you need immediate relief from the sharp pain of a corn. Levine suggests soaking the affected foot in a solution of Epsom salts and warm water, then smoothing on a moisturizing cream, and wrapping the foot in a plastic bag. Keep the bag on for a couple of hours. Then remove the bag and gently rub the corn in a sideways motion with a pumice stone. "This will provide temporary relief—and I stress temporary," says Levine.

ICE A HARD CORN.

If a hard corn is so painful and swollen that you can't even think of putting a shoe on your foot, apply ice to the corn to help reduce some of the swelling and discomfort.

DON'T CUT.

There are a myriad of paring and cutting items to remove corns and calluses available in your local drugstore or variety store, but you should ignore them all, in the best interest of your feet. "Cutting corns is always dangerous," says Mary Papadopoulos, D.P.M., a podiatrist in private practice in Alexandria, Virginia. "You can expose yourself to an infection, or you may cause bleeding that is not easily stopped."

SOFT STEP IT.

"You can give yourself temporary relief from corns and calluses with shielding and padding," says Joseph C. D'Amico, D.P.M., a podiatrist in private practice in New York. What you want the padding to do is transfer the pressure of the shoe from a painful spot to one that is free of pain. Nonmedicated corn pads, for example, surround the corn with material that is higher than the corn itself, thus protecting the corn from contact with the shoe.

A similar idea applies when padding a callus. Cut a piece of moleskin (available at drugstores or camping supply stores) into two half-moon shapes and put the pieces on opposite sides of the area to protect it.

SEPARATE YOUR PIGGIES.

To relieve soft corns that form between toes, keep the toes separated with lamb's wool or cotton. A small, felt pad, like those for hard corns, may also be used for this purpose.

BABY YOUR SOFT CORN.

In addition to separating your toes, sprinkle a little corn-starch or baby powder between them to help absorb moisture.

MIX YOUR OWN CALLUS CONCOCTION.

For calluses, Levine suggests mixing up your own cal-lus softener. Make a paste using five or six aspirin tablets and a tablespoon of lemon juice, apply it to the callus, wrap your foot in a plastic bag, and wrap a warm towel around the bag. Wait ten minutes, then unwrap the foot and gently rub the callus with a pumice stone.

INVITE YOUR FEET TO TEA.

Soaking your feet in chamomile tea that has been thor-oughly diluted has a soothing effect and, according to Levine, will help dry out sweaty feet (excessive mois-ture can contribute to foot problems). The chamomile will stain your feet, but the stain can be easily removed with soap and water.

OVER-THE-COUNTER CORN AND CALLUS REMOVERS

Salicylic acid is the only over-the-counter drug that the Food and Drug Administration deems safe and effective for treating calluses and hard corns. For medicated disks, pads, or plasters, the recommended concentration is 12 percent to 40 percent; for liquid forms, it is 12 percent to 17.6 percent.

Many podiatrists, however, advise against the use of these products as home remedies, mainly because the active ingredient is an acid that can burn healthy skin as well as the dead skin of a callus or corn. If you do decide to try one of these products, follow the package directions carefully and be sure to apply the product only to the area of the corn or callus, avoiding the surrounding healthy tissue (one way to do this is to spread petrolatum in a ring shape around the corn or callus). If your corn or callus does not improve within two weeks, stop using the product and see a podiatrist. If you are diabetic or have any medical condition that hinders circulation, do not try one of these products at all; see a podiatrist at the first sign of any foot problem.

The following ingredients are not generally recognized as safe and effective for removing corns and calluses, says the FDA: iodine, ascorbic acid, acetic acid, allantoin, belladonna, chlorobutanol, diperodon hydrochloride, ichthammol, methylbenze-thonium chloride, methyl salicylate, panthenol, phenyl salicylate, and vitamin A.

COAT YOUR FEET.
If you expect to be doing an unusual amount of walking or running, coat your toes with a little petroleum jelly to reduce friction.

Cuts and scrapes

9 Ways to Care for Your "Boo-Boo"

You're hurrying along and the front of your shoe catches on a crack in the cement, sending you tumbling to the ground. When you get up, you find that not only is your ego bruised but you've managed to peel away the skin on your elbows and knees. You've got yourself a collection of painful scrapes.

You scramble home to prepare the appetizer tray for your guests. You have just one more carrot to slice when, "Ouch!"—your knife slips and slices not the carrot, but your finger. You've got a cut.

"A cut is an incision into the skin," explains Robert Matheson, M.D., a dermatologist in private practice in Portland, Oregon. "It's a vertical slice into the skin that affects only a limited number of nerves. In contrast, a scrape involves the traumatic removal of skin in a horizontal fashion. It scrapes away the skin's surface and exposes a larger number of nerves, usually making it more painful than a cut."

An amazing number of things happen when you cut or scrape yourself. When you disrupt the skin, a clear, antibody-containing fluid from the blood, called serum, leaks into the wound. The area around the cut or scrape becomes red, indicating that more blood is moving into the wound site, bringing with it nutrients and infection-fighting white blood cells. Nearby lymph nodes may swell. After a few days, pus (which contains dead white blood cells, dead bacteria, and other debris from the body's inflammatory response to infection) may form. And finally, a scab forms to protect the injury as it heals.

Even being extra careful, you can't always avoid the scrapes and cuts of life. But you can learn how to care for them and speed their healing (be sure to read "Hello, Doctor?" on the following page to determine if your injury needs a doctor's care):

STOP THE BLEEDING.

When you get a cut or scrape, the first thing to do (after admonishing yourself for being so clumsy) is to stop the bleeding. "Apply pressure with a clean cloth or tissue to stop the blood flow," says Louisa Silva, M.D., a general practitioner in Salem, Oregon, who sees plenty of cuts and scrapes in her private practice.

If possible, elevate the wound above the heart to slow the blood flow. Don't use a tourniquet.

WASH UP.

One of the most important things you can do in treating a cut or scrape is to make sure you cleanse it thoroughly. "Wash it thoroughly with soap and water," says dermatologist Paul Contorer, M.D., chief of dermatology for Kaiser Permanente in Beaverton, Oregon, and clinical professor of dermatology at Oregon Health Sciences University in Portland.

HELLO, DOCTOR?

Many cuts and scrapes can be safely treated at home, but see your doctor if:
• You notice signs of infection (redness, red streaks, swelling, pus, enlarged lymph nodes).
• The injury is located on the face.
• The cut or scrape is very deep or is too dirty to clean.
• The cut is wider than a quarter inch or is too ragged to close evenly.
• You can't stop the bleeding.
• The injury occurred in the area of tendons and nerves, and you can't feel the area or you can't move it.

Matheson says soap and water is usually sufficient, but you can also use over-the-counter cleansers like Hibiclens that don't sting. If the wound is really dirty, he recommends using hydrogen peroxide to bubble out debris. Apply it carefully, since it can damage surrounding skin.

BRING ON THE ANTIBACTERIAL OINTMENT.
Contorer says antibacterial ointments can be very helpful. Polysporin, Neosporin, and Bactine are examples of antibacterial ointments available without a prescription. Matheson says he prefers Polysporin to other ointments because it contains fewer ingredients that may cause allergic reactions.

CLOSE THE SKIN.

Properly closing the skin is important in cuts that are an eighth to a quarter inch wide. Matheson says closing makes the cut heal faster and reduces the chances of scarring. Be sure that you have thoroughly cleansed the cut before attempting to close it. Line up the edges of the cut, then apply butterfly strips or an adhesive bandage to keep the cut closed.

COVER IT.

"It's important to keep a cut or scrape covered," says Silva, "to keep the wound clean and protected." Instead of covering with plain gauze, which tends to stick to wounds, Silva recommends using Telfa, a coated, gauze-type bandage. Adhesive bandages often have Telfa on them, she says, but you can also buy larger pieces of Telfa in the pharmacy and cut them to fit. Cover the wound with the Telfa pad, and use adhesive tape to hold the pad in place.

KEEP IT CLEAN.

The initial washing isn't enough to prevent infection, says Matheson. You'll need to remove the bandage and wash the wound every day with soap and water. Then re-cover it with a clean bandage.

DON'T LET IT DRY OUT.

One of the myths about cuts and scrapes is that a thick, crusty scab is good. Not so. Says Matheson, "Don't let your wound get dry and crack. If you keep it relatively moist, you'll speed healing and minimize scarring."

If a scab forms, don't pick at it; this disrupts the skin and can introduce bacteria. Instead, Matheson recommends soaking off crusty scabs with a solution of one tablespoon of white vinegar added to one pint of water. The mildly acidic solution is soothing and kills bacteria.

Contorer advises patients to use a water/petrolatum regimen at night before retiring. "I have them wash the wound thoroughly and then cover it with a little Vaseline to seal in the moisture," he says.

Both doctors emphasize that a certain amount of air circulation is important to wound healing. You want the bandage or covering to be tight enough to protect, but not so tight that it seals out all air and causes the wound to become too moist.

DON'T GET LOCKED UP.

Silva says it's important to have a tetanus shot within 72 hours if you haven't had one in the last five years. Tetanus bacteria, which causes "lockjaw"—a condition that can involve stiffness in the jaw and other joints, paralysis, and even death—exists in our soil, she says. "It's still very much a threat in this country."

PROTECT IT FROM SUNLIGHT.

To avoid the skin darkening that often occurs when a cut or scrape heals, Contorer says to avoid sun exposure during the healing process and apply over-the-counter hydrocortisone to the wound.

Matheson suggests using a good sunscreen for several weeks on areas where you've had a wound. Look for a sunscreen with a sun protection factor (SPF) of 15 or higher. (Of course, to shield your skin from damaging ultraviolet light and protect your skin from sunburn and skin cancer, wear sunscreen on all exposed skin when you go outside, especially if you are fair skinned.)

Dandruff

11 Ways to Shake the Flakes

Don't toss out all those dark suits or that black sweater that you love. There's a better way to deal with dandruff. As a matter of fact, you may be able to simply wash it away.

If you are like most people, you have always thought of those unsightly flakes as dry skin. In reality, though, dandruff is usually a condition of oily skin and an oily scalp. The process that causes dandruff—the shedding of dead skin cells—is a natural one that goes on continually all over your body. In fact, you get a whole new suit of skin about every 27 or 28 days. The old stuff just sort of flakes away. You simply may not notice the tiny skin cells dropping off your arms and legs.

You happen to see the skin cells that make up dandruff because your hair traps them before they can float off unnoticed. Then the oil from your hair and scalp clumps up the cells until they turn into those visible flakes that decorate your shoulders. Naturally, they are even more noticeable on first dates, job interviews, and other important occasions.

According to Joseph P. Bark, M.D., chairman of dermatology at St. Joseph Hospital in Lexington, Kentucky, you should be glad your scalp flakes away. "If you didn't lose that skin progressively, everybody would be carrying their scalp around in a wheelbarrow," he says. "It would be tremendously thick."

Unfortunately, few of us are brave enough to shrug off dandruff, even if it reflects a normal and necessary process. Fortunately, you can take steps to sweep those flakes away once and for all.

SHAMPOO EACH DAY TO KEEP IT AWAY.

What easier way to get rid of dandruff than to wash it down the drain? Often, this is all that's required, says Andrew Lazar, M.D., assistant professor of clinical dermatology at Northwestern University School of Medicine in Chicago. Getting rid of excess oils and flakes through daily shampooing may be the easiest way to tame your mane.

SWITCH SHAMPOOS.

If your regular shampoo isn't doing the trick, even with daily washing, it's time to switch to an antidandruff shampoo. Check the ingredients for over-the-counter shampoos, says Fredric Haberman, M.D., author of *The Doctor's Beauty Hotline* and a member of the teaching faculty at Montefiore Medical Center—Albert Einstein School of Medicine in New York. Look for a dandruff shampoo that contains zinc pyrithione, selenium sulfide, sulfur, or salicylic acid.

SWITCH, AND SWITCH AGAIN.

Your favorite dandruff shampoo may stop working after a while. To your dismay, those little white flakes may take up residence on your shoulders again. It's not the fault of the shampoo, says Haberman. You simply may build up a resistance to the shampoo's active ingredient. Haberman recommends rotating three brands of dandruff shampoo (each with a different formulation), using each for a month. In other words, use one shampoo for a month, then switch to a second brand for a month, then to a third brand for a month, then back to the original shampoo for a month, and so on.

LATHER TWICE.

The first lathering and rinsing gets rid of the loose flakes and the oily buildup on your hair and scalp. It sort of clears the area so the second lathering can get to work. Leave the second lathering of shampoo on your hair at least five minutes before rinsing it off, advises Haberman. That gives the shampoo a chance to penetrate the skin cells and do what it's supposed to do.

TRY TAR.

If the antidandruff shampoos aren't working, it's time to try the tar shampoos. Tar shampoos have been a proven remedy for more than 200 years, says Bark. The tar decreases cell turnover quite effectively. However, there are some drawbacks. Tar shampoos have a strong odor, may stain the shaft of lighter-colored hair (it can take weeks of using a milder shampoo to get rid of the discoloration), and may irritate the skin.

RINSE.

If you decide use a tar shampoo, rinse your hair with lemon juice, a conditioner, or creme rinse to get rid of any odor from the shampoo, suggests Paul S. Russell, M.D., clinical professor of dermatology at Oregon Health Sciences University in Portland. Russell says that using a conditioner after washing with an antidandruff shampoo is a good idea anyway, because medicated shampoos tend to stiffen hair and make it less manageable.

IS IT REALLY DANDRUFF?

You may have something that's like dandruff, but isn't dandruff. Other possibilities that also involve flaking of the skin are seborrheic dermatitis and psoriasis.

Seborrheic dermatitis is a chronic disorder characterized by inflammation of the skin, along with scaling. It sometimes strikes the eyebrow area, the sides of the nose, the ears, and the central chest.

Psoriasis is characterized by red, scaly patches on the skin that are caused by unusually rapid turnover of cells in the skin.

Prescription medications are available to control both conditions. So if you still have trouble with dandruff after attempting the home remedies discussed here, see your doctor.

BE SENSITIVE TO YOUR SENSITIVITY.

There are some people who just plain shouldn't use a tar shampoo no matter how bad their dandruff problem is. Why? Because they're so sensitive. Rather, their scalp is sensitive to the ingredients in the shampoo. Bark says the tar shampoo can irritate and inflame the hair follicles in the scalp of some people and can cause a condition that dermatologists refer to as folliculitis. The cure for this type of sensitivity? Switch to a milder dandruff shampoo.

STOP THOSE ITCHY FINGERS.

Try to resist the temptation to go after those itchy patches like a dog chasing fleas. You may end up with wounds to your scalp caused by your fingernails. If you break the skin on your scalp, discontinue use of medicated shampoo for a while. Switch to a mild shampoo, such as a baby shampoo, advises Russell, and use it daily until the scratches are healed. Then you can switch back to the medicated shampoo.

SHOWER AWAY SWEAT.

After exercise or strenuous work that makes you perspire, shower and shampoo as soon as possible. Sweat irritates the scalp and speeds up the flaking of skin cells, says Lazar.

GO EASY ON THE STICKY STUFF.

Although you needn't give up the various mousses, sprays, and gels that hold your hairstyle in place, try to use them less often, says Lazar. These hair products can contribute to oily buildup, which can in turn make your dandruff problem worse.

BE KIND TO YOURSELF.

People who are under a great deal of stress seem to have more dandruff, observes Haberman. He says that stress somehow contributes to the proliferation of skin cells. Although there is no known diet connection to dandruff, "poor diet can stress you out and contribute to any dermatitis condition," says Haberman. Adopting a healthier lifestyle and finding ways to relax or let off steam can make a difference. Engaging in some form of exercise regularly can help you do both.

Denture discomfort

8 Ways to Stop Denture Discomfort

Dentures have come a long way since the wooden teeth supposedly worn by George Washington. But, as anyone who has worn them can attest, dentures can cause discomfort. There are two times when dentures often cause discomfort—during the initial "adjustment" phase, when they are new, and after several years of wearing, when dentures may stop fitting properly.

Most people become accustomed to their new dentures within a short time. However, at first, you may have difficulty talking and eating. You may find the dentures tend to "slip," or you may develop sore spots in your mouth.

Even people who have had dentures for years sometimes develop problems with them, usually problems related to fit. "When the teeth are extracted, the dentures sit on the bony ridge that's left," says Sandra Hazard, D.M.D., a managing dentist with Willamette Dental Group, Inc., in Oregon. "Without the teeth, the stimulation to the bone is gone and, over many years, the bone is reabsorbed by the body. The plastic denture, of course, stays the same but starts to fit badly."

Poor fit is probably the most common cause of denture discomfort. As the bony ridge shrinks, the dentures can slip, move around, and cause sore areas. Often, peo-

HELLO, DOCTOR?

While some denture discomforts can be handled at home, Jack W. Clinton, D.M.D., says you should see your dentist if:

• You develop soreness that doesn't improve within a week.

• You have an area on the gum that bleeds spontaneously or is filled with pus.

• There's extra tissue growing, particularly between the upper lip and the gum.

• You have a white sore for more than one week.

• You have a sore that doesn't heal completely within 10 to 14 days.

ple try to refit their dentures by using commercial denture adhesives. But using too much adhesive can change the relationship of the denture to the tissue and result in more soreness. Sometimes the body itself tries to solve the ill-fitting denture problem by causing tissue to overgrow in the mouth.

While dentures will never fit like your natural teeth, follow these tips to avoid denture discomfort:

KEEP THOSE CHOMPERS CLEAN.

When you first have your teeth extracted and your new dentures fit, it's important to keep your dentures clean, because excess bacteria can retard the gums' healing process, says Hazard.

Once you're accustomed to your dentures, it's important to clean them at least twice a day. "You can brush them with toothpaste or use a special denture cleaner," says Hazard.

Jack W. Clinton, D.M.D., associate dean of Patient Services at Oregon Health Sciences University School of Dentistry in Portland, prefers plain old soap and water to keep dentures sparkling. "Using a hand brush and soap and water works great," he says.

BRUSH THE GUMS.

Don't forget to brush your gums, too. "You can help maintain the health of the tissues that lie underneath the dentures by brushing the gums twice a day with a soft brush," says Ken Waddell, D.M.D., a dentist in private practice in Tigard, Oregon.

Brushing the gums, palate, and tongue not only stimulates the tissues and increases circulation; it also helps reduce bacteria and removes plaque.

BABY YOUR MOUTH.

At least at first, your gums will need time to adjust to the compression created by the dentures. Hazard advises patients to eat soft foods during the denture adjustment period to avoid damaging the tender tissues.

Once the gums have healed and your dentist has refit your dentures properly, you'll be able to chew more normally. But Waddell says some foods, such as apples and corn on the cob, are probably best avoided by people who wear dentures. "Advertisements show people with dentures eating all kinds of hard foods," he says. "But hard foods cause the denture to traumatize the gums and bone of the upper jaw. Cut up your apples and take the corn off the cob."

TAKE AN OVER-THE-COUNTER PAIN RELIEVER.

During the initial break-in of your dentures, your mouth is likely to feel sore. Over-the-counter pain relievers, including aspirin, ibuprofen, and acetaminophen, can take the sting out of the pain, says Hazard.

However, if you have persistent pain or if you've worn dentures for several years and pain develops, see your dentist.

TAKE THEM OUT.

When you develop a sore area in your mouth from dentures, Clinton says to do what comes naturally—take them out. "If you're uncomfortable, you probably have a soft-tissue injury," says Clinton. "Take the denture out and leave it out for an hour or so. In most cases, that takes care of it."

If you develop a red spot, go dentureless for 24 hours. If it doesn't clear up or if the soreness returns when you start using your dentures, see your dentist.

RINSE WITH SALT WATER.

If you're in the adjustment phase of wearing dentures or if you're a denture veteran who has developed a sore area in your mouth, Clinton advises rinsing the mouth with warm salt water (half a teaspoon of salt to four ounces of warm water). "Take out your dentures and rinse your mouth every three to four hours with the salt water," he says. "Not only does the salt water help clean out bacteria, it also helps toughen the tissue."

DON'T SELF-ADJUST.

Too often, people who have worn their dentures for a while and develop a fit problem try to "adjust" their dentures themselves with a pocket knife or other tool. This can cause more harm, says Clinton, because it can break down the dentures, change the dentures' "bite," and alter how the dentures fit against the gum.

Also, don't try to "fill the space" between the denture and the gum tissue with over-the-counter adhesive. If your dentures begin to slip or don't feel like they're fitting properly, see your dentist, who can reline them.

TAKE TIME OUT.

"I tell people their dentures should be out of their mouths half the time," says Clinton. "It gives the soft tissues time to recover."

Always take your dentures out at night, Clinton advises. "You don't sleep with your shoes on," he says. "It's the same with your dentures."

Dermatitis and eczema

25 Ways to Fight Them

Dermatitis, which is sometimes called eczema, can create a vicious cycle. Your skin itches, so you scratch it. It becomes red and swollen, and then tiny, red, oozing bumps appear that eventually crust over. You keep scratching because the itching is unbearable, so the rash gets even more irritated and perhaps even infected.

All too often, you don't even know what's causing the itching. It could be an allergy to the soap you use in the shower each morning. It could be irritation due to a chemical you're exposed to at work. It could be atopic eczema—a mysterious itchy rash common to people with a history of allergies and most prevalent in children.

Dermatitis is sometimes used as a catch-all term for any inflammation or swelling of the skin. The term eczema is used interchangeably with dermatitis by some experts, while others differentiate between the two as separate types of inflammation.

Regardless of what kind of dermatitis you're suffering from, however, some general rules apply when you're seeking relief. There are also some treatment and prevention tips that are specific to the type of dermatitis that you have. So first, we'll give you some basic strategies for relief—no matter which type of dermatitis has you scratching. Then we'll give you some specific helpful hints to protect your skin from some of the most common types of dermatitis.

RELIEF FROM THE ITCH

Determining what's causing your dermatitis is important in treating it, but if you can't think of *anything* but the itching at the moment, here are some steps you can take for fast relief.

COOL THE ITCH AND SWELLING.

You can do this with cool compresses. Jerome Z. Litt, M.D., assistant clinical professor of dermatology at Case Western Reserve University School of Medicine in

Cleveland, recommends using a folded handkerchief or a piece of bed linen folded eight layers thick. Dip the clean cloth into cool water or Burow's solution (available over the counter at your pharmacy) and place it on the rash for 10 to 15 minutes every hour. Wet compresses are appropriate with oozing blisters; you'll actually dry up the rash by using water on it.

Litt also says whole-milk compresses are effective. "The protein in the milk helps relieve itching."

APPLY CALAMINE LOTION.

This old standby can help relieve the itch. Apply it in a thin layer, so that the pores aren't sealed, two to three times a day. "The problem with calamine lotion is that it's visible, so it's not very elegant," says Col. Ernest Charlesworth, M.D., assistant chief of allergy and immunology at Wilford Hall U.S. Air Force Medical Center in San Antonio. At least one manufacturer, however, has come out with a version of calamine lotion that will leave you a little less "in the pink." Check your local pharmacy.

USE AN OVER-THE-COUNTER HYDROCORTISONE CREAM.

The one percent formulation is more effective, but it won't help a bacterial or fungal infection (two other common causes of rashes). "Hydrocortisone cream is the dermatologist's equivalent of 'take two aspirin and call me in the morning,'" says Litt. Hydrocortisone seems to be more effective on allergic than on irritant dermatitis, points out Alan N. Moshell, M.D., director of the Skin Disease Program at the National Institute of Arthritis and Musculoskeletal and Skin Diseases in Bethesda, Maryland.

STAY AWAY FROM PRODUCTS THAT END IN "-CAINE."

These can often cause allergies in sensitive individuals. Charlesworth tells about a pharmacist's wife who treated a bad sunburn with a product containing benzocaine and ended up with an allergic contact dermatitis on top of her burn.

DON'T TRY TOPICAL ANTIHISTAMINES.

They can cause allergic reactions. "You should swallow an antihistamine," says Litt. "Don't ever rub it on your skin. I've seen too many horror stories—you can end up with a rash squared to the second power."

TAKE AN ORAL ANTIHISTAMINE.

Try an over-the-counter product like Benadryl to relieve itching. Such products cause drowsiness, but that may help at night when itching is most severe. If you take it during the day and it makes you drowsy, avoid driving or operating heavy machinery.

DON'T SCRATCH.

By scratching the affected area, you can break the skin and cause a secondary infection, warns Alexander A. Fisher, M.D., F.A.A.D., clinical professor of dermatology at New York University Medical Center in New York. Litt recommends rubbing the itch with your fingertips instead of scratching with your nails.

TAKE A SOOTHING BATH.

Adding oatmeal or baking soda to bathwater will make it more soothing, says Litt, although it won't cure your rash. Buy an over-the-counter colloidal oatmeal bath

CONDOM DERMATITIS

More and more people are exposed to latex these days. More people are using condoms in their practice of safe sex. And physicians and dentists routinely wear latex gloves when examining patients.

As a result, more people are showing signs of allergies to latex. Around ten percent of health personnel are now allergic to rubber gloves, says Alexander A. Fisher, M.D., F.A.A.D. Between one and two percent of the general population is allergic.

That could add up to a lot of reactions, considering that 500 million condoms were sold in 1986, Fisher says. As far as condom dermatitis is concerned, you may react to a protein in the rubber itself, to some of the antioxidizing chemicals (which help keep the rubber from breaking down) contained in the rubber, or even to preservatives like paraben used in the "wet" condoms. (Most of the lubricated condoms in the United States, Fisher says, use a silicone-based lubricant that's dry.)

Symptoms of condom dermatitis include vaginal burning in women, redness and swelling in the groin area, an

treatment or add a cup of baking soda to warm, not hot, bathwater.

ALLERGIC CONTACT DERMATITIS

Some people sneeze when confronted with ragweed pollen or when exposed to dander from cats. And some eczemalike rash on the inner part of the upper thighs, or a rash around the mouth.

You may be able to switch to another brand of condom for relief. You can also try another option: Use a condom made of processed sheep's intestine. This type, however, does not protect against the AIDS virus, so Fisher suggests combining the latex condom with one of sheep's intestine. The order in which they are worn, of course, is determined by which partner suffers from the allergy.

If you're allergic to latex, you may also notice problems when you visit the doctor. "The patient goes to the gynecologist and afterwards has a vaginal itch," Fisher says, "because of the doctor's gloves during the exam. Or the rubber dam used by some dentists can cause allergies."

You can test yourself by wearing a rubber glove, or just the fingers of the glove, on your damp hand for 15 to 30 minutes and then looking for any reaction. Remember, if you react to latex on your hands, any part of your body will react to latex.

Hope for the future: the condom for women, since it's made of polyurethane instead of latex.

people break out in a rash, which is known as allergic contact dermatitis, when confronted with substances that are normally harmless to most other people. Substances that cause problems for these sensitive individuals can include the ingredients in costume jewelry or those in makeup.

EAR PIERCING ALERT

If you decide to get your ears pierced, make sure those first earring studs have stainless steel posts, warns Col. Ernest Charlesworth, M.D. Also make sure that the needle used is of stainless steel rather than nickel plated. Otherwise, they may contain nickel, and you'll risk becoming sensitized to this common allergen. The downside: It won't just be your earlobes that react the next time you're exposed to nickel. A watchband, ring, or belt buckle that touches the skin could set off an allergic reaction—and an itchy rash—in the future.

Confounding the issue: You have to be exposed at least once to become "sensitized," or allergic, to the substance in question. That means you might be able to wear your grandmother's ring for years before it brings on any symptoms or be able to try a new makeup for weeks before it causes a reaction.

Add to that the time delay in which a reaction occurs. An airborne allergen, like ragweed or animal dander, usually elicits sneezing or a runny nose within 15 minutes of exposure. But it may take up to 72 hours before a reaction shows up on your skin. That can make identifying the culprit pretty tough.

The most common allergen in allergic contact dermatitis is poison ivy, which can cause reactions in at least half of the people ever exposed to it (see POISON IVY, OAK, AND SUMAC).

The next most common allergen that causes this type of dermatitis is nickel, a metal commonly used in costume jewelry. Even 14-karat gold jewelry has some nickel in it. Up to ten percent of the population may suffer an allergic reaction to this metal, says Charlesworth. You're safest with 24-karat gold, which is pure gold, says Litt, or jewelry made of platinum or stainless steel.

Other possible causes of allergic contact dermatitis:
- Neomycin or benzocaine in topical anesthetics
- Leather
- Formaldehyde, which is used in shampoo, detergent, nail hardeners, waterless hand cleaners, and mouthwashes
- Cinnamon flavor in toothpaste and candies
- PABA, the active ingredient in some sunscreens
- Chemicals found in hair dyes
- Preservatives in cosmetics

How can you handle allergic contact dermatitis?

FERRET OUT THE CAUSE.
If the rash recurs or won't go away, you're going to have to play detective to find out what's causing it. If you're having trouble pinning down the cause, a dermatologist or allergist can help. Either can do a test using common allergens (called a patch test) and ask you the right questions to detect the culprit. "It can be difficult," Charlesworth warns. "Some of these chemicals are present in such small amounts." What's more, we use so many different products. Paul Lazar, M.D., professor of clinical dermatology at Northwestern University School of Medicine in Chicago, points out that the average

woman uses 17 different products on her scalp and head each morning.

DON'T SWEAT IT.

Wearing nickel-containing jewelry in a hot, humid environment may worsen the allergy, says Charlesworth, because perspiration leaches out some of the nickel. So before you start a workout or go out into the heat, take off any nickel-containing jewelry.

DON'T DEPEND ON THE "HYPOALLERGENIC" LABEL.

That's a "very ambiguous" term, says Charlesworth, like "low-fat" or "high-fiber" on a box of cereal. The only requirement to use the term, he says: The product has to have been tested on 200 rodent ears and not caused a reaction.

COAT NICKEL JEWELRY.

Paint the surfaces that come in contact with your skin with clear nail polish.

PROTECT YOUR SKIN.

"If you're working in the garden, wear work gloves and a long-sleeved shirt," says Lazar.

IRRITANT CONTACT DERMATITIS

Some things in this world are so harsh that prolonged exposure to them can result in a rash known as irritant contact dermatitis. Numerous chemicals in industry cause problems for workers, but the household is not without its share of hazards to your skin. Soaps, detergents, oven cleaners, bathroom cleaners, and a whole

HELLO, DOCTOR?

When should you see a doctor for your rash? "When you feel uncomfortable with what's going on," says Paul Lazar, M.D. "Patients worry they come in too soon, when many of them come in too late because a simple problem has ended up turning into a chronic disease." He adds that if you're worried about your rash, you need to seek medical attention.

multitude of products can irritate the skin by removing the skin's protective oils, explains Fisher.

What's the difference between irritant and allergic contact dermatitis? Soap, for example, can cause either one. But it's repeated exposure to soap that causes irritation, while a brief exposure to the perfume or an antibacterial agent in the soap can set off an allergic reaction, explains Moshell.

Clues to the culprit: Where is the rash on your body, and what could have touched the skin in that area?

If you suspect that an irritant has caused your red, itchy, bumpy rash, there's one very important thing you should do:

AVOID EXPOSURE TO THE IRRITANT.
Until you manage to do that, you'll keep subjecting the skin to the irritant, and the rash will continue. If expo-

sure to household cleansers is the problem and it's your hands that are suffering, wear vinyl gloves, rather than those made of rubber, when handling products such as oven cleaners or when washing dishes or doing other chores that expose your hands to water, soap, and chemicals. "No one's allergic to vinyl," Fisher points out. Wearing cotton liners with the gloves will help keep perspiration from further irritating your skin, although this can be a bulky combination.

ATOPIC DERMATITIS

This one takes its name from atopy, the term for an inherited condition that can show up as dermatitis, as allergies to airborne substances such as pollens, or as asthma. If your family members have any of these conditions, you may be at risk for atopic dermatitis.

Infants and children are most likely to be plagued, and a majority of the cases will end by adulthood. If you or your child suffers from this chronic rash, you'll need the care of a physician, most likely a dermatologist or allergist.

It's characterized by intense and miserable itching. The key to coping with this condition is to reduce irritation to the skin, says Noreen Heer Nicol, M.S., R.N., F.N.C., a dermatology clinical specialist/nurse practitioner at National Jewish Center for Immunology and Respiratory Medicine and senior clinical instructor at the University of Colorado Health Sciences Center School of Nursing, both in Denver. Here's her advice:

WASH NEW CLOTHES BEFORE WEARING.
This will help remove formaldehyde and other potentially irritating chemicals used to treat fabrics.

RINSE TWICE.
Even if you use a mild laundry detergent, it's a good idea to rinse your clothes twice to make sure that all of the soap is removed.

WEAR LOOSE, NATURAL-FABRIC CLOTHING.
You want your skin to be able to "breathe," so choose loose-fitting, open-weave, cotton or cotton-blend clothes.

KEEP TEMPERATURES CONSTANT.
Abrupt temperature changes—hot to cold or vice versa—can irritate the skin, so try to avoid them whenever possible. Try to maintain constant humidity levels in your home, too.

KEEP YOUR FINGERNAILS TRIMMED.
It's hard to scratch effectively—and therefore hard to cause further damage to your sensitive skin—if your fingernails are short.

HYDRATE YOUR SKIN WITH A BATH OR SHOWER.
Use warm, not hot, water, and soak or shower for at least 15 or 20 minutes. Nicol recommends avoiding the use of a washcloth, except for cleaning the genital area, because it's abrasive.

USE SOAP ONLY WHERE NECESSARY.
Choose a gentle soap, such as Dove, Oiltum, Alpha Keri, Neutrogena, Purpose, or Basis; a nonsoap cleanser, such as Aveeno or Emulave; or a liquid cleaner, such as Moisturel, Neutrogena, or Dove. Rinse thoroughly, gently pat away excess moisture, and then apply moistur-

izer to your still-damp skin to seal in the water. Plain petrolatum is the best after-bath sealant.

USE MOISTURIZER THROUGHOUT THE DAY.

This is extremely important in atopic dermatitis, says Moshell, to prevent excessive dryness of the skin. Nicol recommends the following products: Aquaphor ointment, Eucerin cream, Moisturel cream or lotion, D.M.L. cream or lotion, Lubriderm cream or lotion, Neutrogena emulsion, Eutra, Vaseline Intensive Care lotion, or LactiCare lotion.

PROTECT YOUR SKIN FROM THE SUN.

A sunburn is only going to irritate the skin further. Whenever you go outside during the day, use a sunscreen with a sun protection factor (SPF) of 15 or more on all exposed areas of skin.

WASH AFTER SWIMMING.

The chlorine and other chemicals found in most swimming pools can irritate the skin. So soon after you've finished your swim, take a shower or bath and use a mild soap all over. Don't forget to reapply your moisturizer as well.

CHECK OUT YOUR DIET.

Some physicians believe that food allergies may play some role in atopic dermatitis, while others say that it hasn't been proven. If you suspect that a food aggravates your rash, eliminate it from your diet for a few weeks. If your rash clears up, and then you eat the food again and the rash returns, you should probably eliminate it, suggests Fisher.

Diabetes

28 Ways to Live Well with Diabetes

Each day, some 12 million diabetics in this country walk a tightrope between too little sugar in the bloodstream and too much. Too little—which may come from a complication of medication—and they may quickly be overcome by dizziness, fatigue, headache, sweating, trembling, and, in severe cases, loss of consciousness and coma. Too much—which can happen after eating too much, especially if the person is older and overweight—and the person may experience weakness, fatigue, excessive thirst, labored breathing, and loss of consciousness. Left untreated, the picture is bleak: Blindness, kidney disease, blood vessel damage, infection, heart disease, nerve damage, high blood pressure, stroke, limb amputation, and coma may result.

Because the initial symptoms (fatigue, weakness, frequent urination) are usually mild, half of all diabetics do not realize that they have the disease. And that's a real shame, because with early diagnosis and treatment, the chances of living a long and productive life are higher than if the disease creeps along undetected until irreversible problems set in.

If you'd like some proof that diabetes is clearly a disease you can live with, take a look at these prolific diabetics: singer Ella Fitzgerald, actress Mary Tyler Moore, baseball Hall of Fame great Jim (Catfish) Hunter. Even before treatment was as sophisticated as it is today,

EARLY WARNING SIGNS

Early diagnosis and treatment is extremely important in helping diabetics live healthier, longer lives. If you notice the early warning signs listed below or suspect that you may have diabetes, see your doctor.

Some of the early warning signs of Type I diabetes are:
• Frequent urination accompanied by unusual thirst
• Extreme hunger
• Rapid weight loss with easy tiring, weakness, and fatigue
• Irritability, nausea, and vomiting

Some of the early warning signs for Type II diabetes are:
• Frequent urination accompanied by unusual thirst
• Blurred vision or any change in sight
• Tingling or numbness in the legs, feet, or fingers
• Frequent skin infection or itchy skin
• Slow healing of cuts and bruises
• Drowsiness
• Vaginitis in women
• Erectile dysfunction in men

author Ernest Hemingway and inventor Thomas Edison, both of whom suffered from diabetes, managed to leave their marks on history.

If you are one of the lucky ones whose diabetes has been diagnosed by a doctor, you have an idea of what has gone awry in your body. The disorder stems from the way your body processes carbohydrates, which you take in through food. Normally, these foods are converted into a form of sugar called glucose, which floats along in the bloodstream until the pancreas, a large gland located behind the stomach, goes into action. The pancreas produces insulin, a hormone that signals body cells to soak up the glucose. Once inside the cell, the glucose is either used to produce heat or energy or is stored as fat. A person with diabetes produces little or no insulin or else becomes resistant to the hormone's action and can't compensate. Either way, the glucose can't get into the cells; it accumulates in the blood and is later expelled in the urine. In short, blood sugar rises while cells starve.

Only about one-tenth of all diabetics have the severe form of the disease, called Type I, which usually affects children and young adults and requires daily injections of insulin. Most have what doctors refer to as Type II, or adult-onset, diabetes. While about one-third of Type II diabetics do require insulin to control blood sugar, and another one-third use medications to increase insulin production, the remaining Type II diabetics rely on nonmedical measures (such as diet, weight loss, and exercise) alone to control their disease. No matter which group you fall into, you can benefit from taking an active role in your treatment. But don't make a move without consulting your doctor first. He or she will call the shots; then it's up to you to carry through. Here's how:

DISH UP A SPECIAL DIET.

"The goal of dietary intervention for Type I diabetes is to help minimize short- and long-term complications by normalizing blood sugar levels. The goal of dietary intervention in Type II diabetes is to help the patient achieve and maintain normal body weight," says John Buse, M.D., Ph.D., assistant professor in the Department of Medicine, Section of Endocrinology, at the University of Chicago and director of the Endocrinology Clinic at the University of Chicago Medical Center.

Both Type I and Type II diabetics should follow the guidelines offered by the American Diabetes Association (ADA), which were revised in 1986 based on new research findings (see "Choose One from Column A . . .").

KNOW YOUR CARBOHYDRATES.

The traditional dogma for diabetics was this: Avoid simple carbohydrates, or simple sugars (such as table sugar), because they raise blood sugar quickly, and choose complex carbohydrates (such as the starches and fiber found in grains, potatoes, beans, and peas), because they raise blood sugar more slowly. But this dogma has given way recently to newer rules, which really aren't rules at all in the strictest sense.

"Diabetic meal planning must account for many factors," says Harold E. Lebovitz, M.D., professor of medicine, chief of the Division of Endocrinology and Diabetes, and director of the Clinical Research Center at State University of New York Health Science Center at Brooklyn. "A food eaten alone may affect blood sugar differently than when it is eaten with another food. The same variations can be noted with cooked foods versus raw foods and even with different brands of foods. And not least, different foods affect blood sugar differently in different people."

Consequently, while complex carbohydrates like lentils, soy beans, peanuts, and kidney beans are still

CHOOSE ONE FROM COLUMN A . . .

These recommendations should be considered "ground rules" for a Type II diabetic. Diets must be adjusted to meet individual needs, so be sure to discuss your diet with your doctor before making any changes.

• Raise carbohydrate intake to more than half of total calories. Every gram of carbohydrate provides four calories.

• Keep protein intake to 12 to 20 percent of total calories. A gram of protein provides four calories as well.

• Lower fat intake to less than 30 percent of total calories and make every effort to substitute polyunsaturated fat or monounsaturated fat for saturated fat. Each gram of fat provides nine calories, so go easy!

• Maintain cholesterol intake at less than 300 milligrams a day. Less saturated fat in the diet will automatically lead to reduced cholesterol.

• Include fiber in the diet; it should be part of as many meals as possible.

best for causing the slowest and lowest rise in blood sugar after a meal, present evidence suggests that sucrose (table sugar) may not be "off limits" for Type II diabetics if blood glucose levels stay normal after their ingestion. "Experimenting with 'forbidden foods' may be possible with a doctor's consent," says Lebovitz. "But before you start bingeing on bonbons, it's important to be prepared to see what happens in terms of the blood-glucose response."

GET FOND OF FIBER.

The key to the effectiveness of complex carbohydrates may lie in the fiber content. "While the cause and effect of fiber in control of Type II diabetes has yet to be established, we do know that such foods are very satiating and can help enormously toward weight loss and maintenance," says Buse.

UNDERSTAND "SWEET" TALK.

Actually, there are a number of different kinds of sugar, and each has a potentially different effect on blood sugar levels. "The most basic form of sugar is glucose, or dextrose, which will raise blood sugar levels faster than any other kind when swallowed," says Ira J. Laufer, M.D., clinical associate professor of medicine at New York University School of Medicine and medical director of The New York Eye and Ear Infirmary Diabetes Treatment Center in New York. "Sucrose also tends to raise blood sugar almost as quickly as dextrose. But fructose, sometimes called fruit sugar, generally has a very mild effect on blood sugar. If your diabetes is in good control, dietetic desserts and candies sweetened with pure fructose are not likely to raise your blood sugar levels very much," he adds. On the other hand, fructose provides as many calories as other sugars, so it may not be the wisest choice for diabetics who need to lose weight.

REDUCE YOUR RISKS.

To emphasize the fact that excess weight is a Type II diabetic's most serious problem, experts on diabetes often say that if you want to find out if there's a possibility of getting diabetes, just keep on eating and get fat. You can do other things, too, but the main thing is get fat. An estimated 80 percent of those with Type II diabetes are obese when diagnosed with the disease. Added weight can both accelerate diabetes and bring on its complications, especially cardiovascular disease and stroke.

In contrast, even a modest weight loss can have dramatic effects: High insulin levels drop, the liver begins to secrete less glucose into the blood, and peripheral muscle tissues begin to respond to insulin and take up glucose better. Just as obesity leads to insulin resistance, so weight loss reverses the condition. When persons with Type II diabetes lose weight, they frequently are no longer diabetic. "Type II diabetics may *only* need to get and stay at an ideal body weight," says Buse. "And unless they do that, nothing else will work very well." (See "Changing Your Ways" for weight-loss tips.)

DON'T "CRASH."

Too rapid weight loss rarely works in the long run and is potentially dangerous if undertaken without a doctor's advice. Sometimes, a doctor *will*, in fact, prescribe a very-low-calorie diet to initiate weight loss, but only for a very short period of time. Generally, the best approach is to lose weight gradually with a low-fat, lower-calorie, nutritionally balanced diet combined with increased activity. Avoid the use of over-the-counter appetite suppressants that contain phenylpropanolamine (PPA).

GRAZE.

Many experts believe that a Type II diabetic may more easily achieve normal blood sugar levels by not over-

CHANGING YOUR WAYS

As any dieter knows, losing weight takes more "won't" power than willpower, says John Buse, M.D., Ph.D. Sometimes, people just make it too easy for themselves to fail. Here are some tips to help you succeed:

Learn what triggers your eating. If the sight of a bakery window sets off a craving for cake, make it a habit to walk on the other side of the street. Become aware of any cues like this, and learn to control them.

Don't keep large amounts of food on hand. For some overweight people, the fact that food is within reach means that it must be eaten. Buy only enough for a few meals at a time.

Prepare your meals from scratch rather than relying on take-out. For one thing, take-out foods are likely to be high in calories because of the methods used in preparation. And you might easily order too much, which may make it easier to overeat.

loading with too much food at one time. "Three smaller meals a day—breakfast, lunch, and dinner—plus two or three snack-type meals in between is easier for the diabetic person's insulin to handle. Just be sure that you don't overshoot your calorie limit, however," advises Lebovitz.

GET A FIRM FOOTHOLD.

Neuropathy, damage to the nerves, is a common problem for diabetics. It occurs most often in the feet and legs, and its signs include repeated burning, pain, or numbness. "Neuropathy can be dangerous if it causes a loss of feeling, because then even a minor foot injury may go undiscovered—leading to serious infection, gangrene, and even amputation of the limb," says Joseph C. D'Amico, D.P.M., a podiatrist in private practice in New York. Diabetics, therefore, need to be diligent about foot care. (See "Foot Notes for Diabetics.")

BE A SPORT.

Regular exercise provides many benefits. It tones up the heart and other muscles, strengthens bones, lowers blood pressure, strengthens the respiratory system, helps raise HDL (good cholesterol), gives a sense of well-being, decreases tension, aids in weight control, enhances work capacity, and confers a sense of achievement. "For those with diabetes," says Laufer, "exercise bestows additional benefits. It promotes the movement of sugar from the bloodstream into cells, where it is burned for energy, and it improves the cells' ability to respond to insulin, thus decreasing their need for the hormone."

Not all exercises are for every diabetic person. If blood sugar is high, exercise will lower it; if it's low, exercise will lower it further. Those on medication must work with a doctor to make necessary adjustments. Because of the potential for neuropathy, diabetics need to protect the nerve endings in the feet and so may need to avoid high-impact activities such as jogging. Another consideration is that diabetics are particularly sensitive to dehydration. Also, intense exercise could endanger cap-

FOOT NOTES FOR DIABETICS

A common complaint from many people is, "My feet are killing me!" For a diabetic, the statement could be all too true. Loss of nerve function, especially on the soles of the feet, can reduce feeling and mask a sore or injury on the foot that, if left unattended, can turn into an ulcer or gangrene. "A person with diabetes must be super cautious about foot care," says Joseph C. D'Amico, D.P.M. "Remember, there's only one pair per person per lifetime."

Here's how to start at the bottom:

Look them over. Give your feet a thorough going-over every night to make sure that you haven't developed a sore, blister, cut, scrape, or any other tiny problem that could blow up into big trouble. If your vision isn't good, have someone with good eyesight check your feet for you.

Wash, rinse, and dry. A clean foot is a healthy foot, with a much lower susceptibility to infection. And clean feet feel better, too.

Avoid bathroom surgery. Under normal circumstances, there is little danger from using a pumice stone to reduce a

illaries in the eyes already weakened by diabetes, leading to rupture, vision problems, and even blindness. So you will need to choose your exercise program carefully with the aid of your doctor. And, especially if you are over 40 years old, you will need to undergo a general medical examination, including a cardiovascular screening test corn or callus. But for a diabetic, such a practice might lead to a little irritation, then a sore, then infection, and finally, a major ulcer.

Remove "removers" from reach. Caustic agents for removing corns and calluses can easily cause a serious chemical burn on a diabetic's skin. Never use them.

Take care of the little things. Any time a cut, sore, burn, scratch, or other minor injury appears on a diabetic's foot, it must be attended to immediately. "Wash the lesion with soap and water to remove all foreign matter. Cover with a protective sterile dressing. Use adhesive tape with caution, if at all, because it can weaken the skin when it is pulled off. Use paper or cloth-type tape instead," suggests D'Amico. If the sore is not healing or if you notice signs of infection, such as redness, red streaks, warmth, swelling, pain, or drainage, see a podiatrist.

Choose shoes with care. "Since a person with diabetes may not always be aware of the pain caused by shoes that are too tight, he or she must be very attentive to fit when buying new shoes," says D'Amico.

and exercise test, before proceeding with your exercise program.

Once your doctor gives you the go-ahead to begin a program of regular exercise, you need to set up realistic goals in order to avoid too-high or too-low blood sugar levels and other problems that could result from doing

....

HYPOGLYCEMIA: THE DISEASE THAT ISN'T

After eating a meal—or going too long without one—are you tired? Lightheaded? Dizzy? A little bit anxious? You may be among the thousands of people who have been told or who have convinced themselves that they have low blood sugar, or hypoglycemia—and who are wrong.

Hypoglycemia, also called "sugar blues," was a condition that appeared some years ago and was supposedly caused by eating excess sugar, which led to very high glucose levels followed by very low levels. More likely, says John Buse, M.D., Ph.D., the symptoms were caused by skipping meals, lack of sleep, or tension.

But hypoglycemia does, indeed, exist. Doctors have determined that there are two basic types. One, called fasting hypoglycemia, occurs after missing one or more meals and develops slowly as the blood sugar gradually

too much too soon. "Someone who has not spent much time engaged in physical activity who is also overweight should not be thinking in terms of running races," advises Laufer.

Swimming, bicycle riding, and brisk walking are all recommended. Indeed, walking is the one activity that all medical experts agree is ideal for a diabetic patient. "The average Type II diabetic patient is over 50, overweight, and underactive," says Laufer. Walking is a kinder, gentler activity for such individuals. Remember, drops lower and lower. It commonly produces central nervous system symptoms, and its causes can be serious underlying disorders, such as tumors that produce insulin. Type I diabetics who take too much insulin for the amount of food they eat may experience the symptoms of fasting hypoglycemia.

The second type, reactive hypoglycemia, occurs about two to four hours after eating, especially if the meals are high in carbohydrates. The usual symptoms include shakiness, weakness, sweating, rapid heartbeat, and faintness, which indicate that the body is reacting to a sudden blood sugar drop by producing adrenaline, cortisol, and glucagon—hormones that aim to bring blood sugar back to normal. People in the early stages of diabetes may rarely have this type of hypoglycemia, but it is more common after extensive abdominal surgery or other surgery.

however, that the positive effects of exercise last for only a day or two, so your goal should be to exercise at least every other day.

WATCH YOUR MOUTH.

Diabetics must be extra careful about their teeth. "Good dental hygiene is important for everyone," says Andrew Baron, D.D.S., a dentist and clinical associate professor at Lenox Hill Hospital in New York. "Because they are at increased risk for infection, diabetics should be super cautious about preventing tooth decay and periodontal disease." Keep a supply of toothbrushes so you won't have to deal with old, worn brushing aids. Brush and floss without fail after every meal and before bedtime. And see your dentist regularly for checkups and cleaning.

CHECK YOUR DENTURES.

Ill-fitting dentures or permanent bridgework cause frustration for anyone who has to live with them. For a diabetic, the consequences go far beyond annoyance. "Dentures that move around in your mouth can cause sores that don't heal," cautions Baron. "It's a shame to suffer with such problems, especially when they are so easily remedied by a dentist." If you notice sore spots in your mouth or find that your dentures are moving or slipping, see your dentist to have the problem corrected.

TAKE CHARGE.

How do you psych yourself up for a game that has no timeouts and that never ends? That's the question diabetics face every day. One way is to learn all you can about your illness so that you can better control it. "Diabetics are constantly learning and relearning lifestyle changes and behavior adjustments. It's like studying for a master's degree in diabetes—and, in this case, there is no graduation and no vacation," says Laufer.

It's a given that even in a diabetic whose disease appears to be totally under control, there will be occasional rapid and even violent swings in blood sugar levels, brought on by emotional or physical stresses, meals, medications, or even the time of day. But if they are anticipated and accepted, these episodes can be viewed as simply a bump in the road rather than a major detour.

DO SOMETHING NICE FOR YOURSELF.

While it's important to learn as much as you can about your diabetes and stay with your treatment regimen, you also need to keep things in perspective. "It is a rare individual who takes time to 'stop and smell the roses,' as it were," notes Laufer. "This is especially true for diabetics, who often get so caught up in their disease that it is difficult for them to focus on other, more positive aspects of life." Make a list of all the things you would like to do if you had the time—and then *make* the time to do at least some of them. While staring into space may be an ideal uplifter for one person, and napping the afternoon away does the same for another, straightening out a messy closet may do the trick for a third.

DO SOMETHING NICE FOR SOMEONE ELSE.

It's hard to think of your own problems when you are engaged in making another person's life more pleasant, especially someone with more severe problems than yours. "You can call your local hospital or library to inquire about volunteers," says Laufer. "Or you can knock on the door of an elderly, housebound neighbor who might appreciate a visit."

Diaper rash

10 Ways to Get Rid of It—for Good

Diaper rash. It's not a pretty sight for you, and your baby probably doesn't enjoy it much, either. While

HELLO, DOCTOR?

If all else fails, call the doctor. Diaper rash, if left untreated, can worsen, leaving your baby's bottom raw and painful. A good rule of thumb is to wait two to five days and, if the condition doesn't improve, head for the doctor's office, says James E. Bridges, M.D.

far from being a serious medical problem, diaper rash is just another of life's little discomforts.

There's not too much to say about how to recognize diaper rash—if your baby's got a red, sore bottom underneath his or her diaper, that's a pretty conclusive diagnosis. The good news is, you can cure that rash within a matter of days. And with some conscientious care, you can say goodbye to it forever.

The following are sure cures for diaper rash. Luckily, the same principles apply to the prevention side of the coin. In other words, the very things that make the rash go away are also what keep it away, so keep on doing them. Good riddance!

GET RID OF THE DIAPER.

As its name implies, diaper rash is caused by a diaper. Say goodbye to the diaper, and—voila!—no more rash, says Gregory F. Hayden, M.D., a professor of pediatrics and an attending pediatrician at the University of Virginia Health Sciences Center in Charlottesville. "If the baby has a rash, take his diaper off whenever practical," says Hayden. "This way, stool and urine won't touch the skin." To keep any mess to a minimum, you can put the baby on a rubber mat covered with a washable cloth while you air out his or her bottom.

CHANGE THE BABY OFTEN.

The best way to avoid diaper rash or to cure an existing rash is to make sure that the baby is always clean and dry, says Jeannette M. Pergam, M.D., a pediatrician and assistant professor of pediatrics at the University of Nebraska Medical Center in Omaha. "The moist, warm environment under the diaper is one that is very conducive to causing skin infections," she says.

AVOID COMMERCIAL BABY WIPES.

Many brands of store-bought baby wipes contain alcohol and other chemicals that can dry and irritate your child's skin, says Pergam. Wet, soapy washcloths are best for cleaning baby's bottom, she says. Be sure to rinse thoroughly with a clean, wet cloth or plain water to remove any soap.

DRY THAT BOTTOM.

When you change baby's diapers, dry the area thoroughly with a towel, says Pergam. She also advises leaving the area exposed to air for a few minutes just before putting on a new diaper. An old-fashioned way to keep baby's bottom dry is to brown a little cornstarch in a frying pan and apply it to the child's bottom, according to James E. Bridges, M.D., a specialist in family medicine in Fremont, Nebraska. He adds that commercial cornstarch baby powders probably work just as well.

THE GREAT DIAPER DEBATE

Are cloth diapers or disposable diapers better at preventing diaper rash? The issue is far from clear-cut, but do take into account the results of the following studies when making your decision: A 1990 study conducted at the Department of Design at Colorado State University in Fort Collins found that diapers labeled "super absorbent" kept the skin drier and retained more moisture than cloth or conventional disposable brands. In most cases, the regular disposables were less effective than cloth diapers at keeping the skin dry. Among cloth diapers, the most effective were those that contained an inner layer of nonwoven fabric, the researchers wrote.

Another study conducted at the Department of Dermatology at the University of Rochester in New York found that babies who wore diapers containing substances to absorb urine and make it "gel" had significantly less diaper rash than babies who wore regular disposables.

CHOOSE AN OINTMENT AND USE IT.

Many pediatricians recommend using a diaper-rash cream or ointment, such as A and D or Desitin, every time you change your baby. These heavy creams create a block so that stool and urine won't irritate the skin, says Hayden. "Some people worry that the ointments will keep moisture in," he says, "but they work pretty well for most skin." A cotton ball dipped in baby oil will usually take the creams off without scrubbing.

TRY BABY POWDER, BUT BE CAREFUL WHERE YOU SHAKE IT.
Dusting the baby's bottom with baby talcum powder may be another way to protect your child's skin against irritants, according to Hayden. However, studies have shown that if babies inhale the powder, it can be dangerous, even fatal. Cornstarch-based powders may pose less of a threat, Hayden adds. When using any powder, try shaking some into your hand—away from baby's face—and then sprinkling it onto the diaper area.

HANG THE DIAPERS OUT TO DRY.
"There's an old wives' tale that if you hang your baby's diapers out to dry instead of putting them in the dryer, they won't cause diaper rash," Pergam says. Although she has no explanation for the efficacy of this tip, she swears that it worked for her own children. If you have a place to hang them, you may want to give this a try to see if it helps.

FIGHT BACK AGAINST YEAST.
Sometimes, what appears to be an innocuous diaper rash can really be an infection of yeast, also called *Candida albicans*. It may be hard to tell the difference between the two, Hayden says, although a yeast infection may appear as little white specks dotting an area of red irritation. To cure a yeast infection, try using an over-the-counter antiyeast medication, such as Lotrimin, or see your pediatrician for a prescription.

TRY VINEGAR SOLUTION.

Urine is an extremely alkaline solution, says Bridges. It can burn the skin the same way that acid can. To balance out the equation, try adding half a cup of white vinegar to your rinse water when you wash the baby's diapers, he suggests. "That neutralizes the ammonia," he says. Pergam recommends wiping baby's bottom with a solution of eight parts water to one part vinegar—the theory is the same.

AVOID PLASTIC PANTS.

Plastic pants worn over a diaper keep moisture in and may cause irritation or worsen an existing infection, Hayden says. "It's better to let things evaporate and dry out."

Diarrhea

15 Ways to Go with the Flow

You may blame it on a 24-hour bug or something you ate, but if you're like the average American, you'll suffer once or twice this year from diarrhea—frequent, watery bowel movements that may be accompanied by painful cramps or nausea and vomiting.

Gastroenteritis—the catch-all medical term for intestinal flu, viral infection, and food poisoning—is the second leading cause of missed work time (the common cold beats it).

Diarrhea is uncomfortable and unpleasant, but generally no big deal in otherwise healthy adults. However, if diarrhea becomes a chronic condition, the situation changes. If it affects the very young, the elderly, or the chronically ill, it can be dangerous. And if you're not careful to drink enough fluids, you could find yourself complicating what should have been a simple situation.

What causes diarrhea? Because the condition generally lasts only a few days, doctors don't usually culture the stool to diagnose what started it in the first place. It's most often due to a viral infection, which antibiotics can't fight. You just have to tough it out for a couple of days. The virus has invaded the bowel, causing it to absorb excessive fluid, which leads to the watery stools. You may also experience cramping, nausea, vomiting, headache, fever, malaise, and even upper-respiratory-tract symptoms, such as a runny nose. One clue: If members of your family all get sick, but at different times, it's likely a virus that got passed around. Bacteria, which often cause traveler's diarrhea in certain parts of the world, can also be responsible for diarrhea as the result of food poisoning. "When the whole family goes on a picnic and six hours later, they're all sick, that's a classic sign of food poisoning," says Rosemarie L. Fisher, M.D., professor of medicine in the Division of Digestive Diseases at Yale University School of Medicine in New Haven, Connecticut.

Much rarer are microbes like amoebae and giardia that try to set up permanent housekeeping in your bowel, causing diarrhea that lasts for weeks or months. You can get these from contaminated food or water, public swimming pools, and communal hot tubs.

(Continued on page 232)

THE YOUNG AND THE OLD

For most people, diarrhea is nothing more than a minor inconvenience. But for the very young and the elderly, it can be life threatening, even fatal.

Why is it so dangerous for these groups? "Young children have a much smaller blood volume," explains Harry S. Dweck, M.D., director of the Regional Neonatal Intensive Care Unit at Westchester Medical Center in Valhalla, New York. What constitutes "a small fluid loss in an adult can make a big difference in an infant."

Dehydration can take days to occur in an adult, hours to days for a child, and seconds to minutes in a newborn, Dweck emphasizes. That's why diarrhea has been such a killer of children in many countries around the world.

If your child has diarrhea, "call the doctor right away, with the first loose stool," Dweck stresses.

Diarrhea may be harder to recognize in infants. "Newborns may have up to 6 to 9 bowel movements a day," Dweck says. "And if they're breast-fed, it's a more liquid stool." But parents generally learn fast what their baby's normal stool looks like. If it becomes more liquid, if it's explosive, or if the odor changes, it's probably diarrhea. "The best way by far to prevent diarrhea in infants is to breast-feed," Dweck points out. The colostrum, the special kind of milk produced during the first few days of the baby's life, "is loaded with antibodies and white blood cells" that are absorbed directly into the baby's gastrointestinal tract, which will help prevent gastrointestinal infections down the road.

There's also less chance of contamination with breast-feeding, since there are no bottles. And formula itself can cause allergic reactions that include diarrhea.

Diarrhea is less serious in children over 18 months of age, but diarrhea still warrants a call to the doctor. Your physician will tell you how to treat your baby and what to give him or her to prevent dehydration and electrolyte imbalance. Once kids reach the age of eight or so, you can follow the same recommendations for treating diarrhea as you would for adults.

The elderly can't stand to lose much fluid, either, but that's because their circulatory system has changed with aging. Hardening of the arteries occurs throughout the blood vessels in the body; lowered blood pressure that occurs when fluid is lost means there's not enough pressure to force blood to circulate.

"That puts them at a high risk for stroke, heart attack, or kidney failure," explains Richard Bennett, M.D.

But when the elderly have diarrhea, it's often difficult to know when they're becoming dehydrated. "They don't recognize thirst as well," says Bennett. "Or maybe they can't get around well enough to get a drink when they are thirsty." Changes in the skin that signal dehydration also aren't apparent in aged skin. The best clue: Are they still passing urine every hour or two?

If you're older and in good health but have a history of congestive heart failure and/or are taking diuretics, you should call your physician as soon as the diarrhea starts. "The doctor may want to change your dosage of diuretics, since these drugs cause you to lose fluid," says Bennett.

Certain drugs, especially antibiotics, can have diarrhea as a side effect. Magnesium-containing antacids and artificial sweeteners such as sorbitol are often overlooked culprits.

Unless diarrhea persists, you usually don't find out its cause. Treatment is aimed at relieving the symptoms and at preventing dehydration, the most serious consequence of diarrhea.

So what can you do?

RIDE IT OUT.

If you're not very young or old or suffering from any chronic illness, it may be safe just to put up with it for a couple of days. "Although there's no definite proof that diarrhea is a cleansing action, it probably serves some purpose," explains Richard Bennett, M.D., assistant professor of medicine at Johns Hopkins University School of Medicine in Baltimore.

KEEP HYDRATED.

In the meantime, make sure you "maintain your fluid and electrolyte balance," as the doctors say. Obviously, you can lose a lot of liquid in diarrhea, but you also lose electrolytes, which are minerals like sodium and potassium, that are critical in the running of your body. Here's how to replace what you're losing:

• **Drink plenty of fluids.** No one agrees on which fluid is best—again, because of the electrolyte problem. The experts do agree you need at least two quarts of fluid a day, three if you're running a fever. Plain water lacks electrolytes, although you may want to drink this part of the time. Weak tea with a little sugar is a popular choice. Some vote for Gatorade, although Fisher points

WHEN DIARRHEA LASTS AND LASTS AND LASTS

Sometimes diarrhea goes on . . . for weeks. That's when a more serious problem is probably responsible. Your doctor can ferret out the cause. Here are some of the possibilities:

Lactose intolerance. "If you get diarrhea every time you drink a glass of milk, you may suffer from this condition that involves an inability to digest lactose, the sugar in milk and dairy products. It's the most common reason for chronic diarrhea," says Rosemarie L. Fisher, M.D. Avoid milk, but take a calcium supplement, she suggests.

Celiac disease. In this case, you can't digest gluten, which is part of wheat.

Irritable bowel syndrome. Emotions play a big role in this one, which can include alternating constipation and diarrhea. "The classic picture is the young adult with diarrhea on the morning of a big exam," says Fisher.

Parasitic infections. These may last indefinitely.

Crohn's disease or ulcerative colitis. Both these conditions have inflammation of the bowel and diarrhea, often accompanied by pain.

Systemic illnesses. Chronic diarrhea may be a complication of diseases such as diabetes, scleroderma, and hyperthyroidism.

Cancer. It's not a pleasant thought, but one of the warning signs of tumors in the bowel is diarrhea, especially if blood is present.

out it's constituted to replace fluids lost through sweating, not for diarrhea, a whole different ball game. Defizzed, nondiet soda pop is recommended by some, although anything with a lot of sugar can increase diarrhea. So can caffeine. Fruit juices, particularly apple and prune, have a laxative effect, but others may be OK.

• **Buy an over-the-counter electrolyte replacement formula.** Pedialyte, Rehydralyte, and Ricelyte are available over the counter at local drugstores. These formulas contain fluids and minerals in the proper proportion.

KEEP YOUR LIQUIDS COOL BUT NOT ICE-COLD.

Whatever you choose to drink, keep it cool, suggests Peter A. Banks, M.D., director of Clinical Gastroenterology Service at Brigham and Women's Hospital and lecturer on medicine at Harvard Medical School, both in Boston. It will be less irritating that way. Sip, don't guzzle; it will be easier on your insides.

SIP SOME CHICKEN BROTH.

Or any broth, says Banks. But have it lukewarm, not hot, and add some salt.

REST IN BED.

Give your body a chance to fight the bug that's causing this.

PUT A HEATING PAD ON YOUR BELLY.

Banks says it will help relieve abdominal cramps.

TRY YOGURT.

You'll want to make sure you get a product that contains *live* lactobacillus cultures, which are friendly bugs that

HELLO, DOCTOR?

"If you see blood in your stool, that should immediately ring a bell to see your doctor," according to Rosemarie L. Fisher, M.D.

If you feel like you're getting dehydrated, get medical attention. The signs: Dizziness when you stand up, scanty and deeply yellow urine, increased thirst, dry skin. Children may cry without tears as well.

If you've got a fever or shaking chills, or the diarrhea persists past 48 to 72 hours, see the doctor.

If diarrhea occurs in the very young, the elderly (see "The Young and the Old"), or the chronically ill, a doctor should be consulted immediately.

---

normally live in the gut. "There are anecdotal reports but no good studies that yogurt works," says Bennett. "But there's no harm in trying."

EAT LIGHT.

Foods gentle on the digestive system include soups, gelatin, rice, noodles, bananas, potatoes, toast, cooked carrots, and skinless, defatted chicken.

TAKE THE PINK STUFF.

Stopping the diarrhea with an over-the-counter medication may not be the best thing for your body. Diarrhea probably reflects your body's attempt to get rid of a troublesome bug. If you do feel it's necessary, however, Pepto-Bismol is probably the safest over-the-counter antidiarrheal medicine, says Bennett. And studies show it may have a mild antibacterial effect, which would be most useful in traveler's diarrhea, since this condition is usually bacteria related (see TRAVELER'S DIARRHEA).

TAKE KAOPECTATE OR IMODIUM A-D.

Again, you're probably better off going without antidiarrheal medication. If you absolutely need some relief, however, you can try one of these over-the-counter medications. Imodium A-D slows down the motility, or movement, of the gut; Kaopectate absorbs fluid. Bennett does not recommend these for elderly patients because decreased motility can be dangerous in an infection and can lead to worse problems.

DON'T DO DAIRY.

Avoid milk or other dairy products like cheese during the time that you're having diarrhea as well as for one to three weeks afterward. The small intestine, where milk is digested, is affected by diarrhea and simply won't work as well for a while. "Milk may sound soothing," says Fisher. "But it could actually make the diarrhea worse."

CUT OUT CAFFEINE.

Just as they stimulate your nervous system, coffee and other caffeinated drinks jump-start your intestines. And that's the last thing you need to do when you have a case of diarrhea.

SAY NO TO SWEET TREATS.

High concentrations of sugar can increase diarrhea. The sugar in fruit can do the same.

STEER CLEAR OF GREASY OR HIGH-FIBER FOODS.

These are harder for your gut to handle right now. It needs foods that are kinder and gentler.

Dry hair

11 Tips for Taming It

Your hair feels like straw—dry, fly-away, unmanageable. How could you have been cursed with such a mane? You probably weren't, according to Frank Parker, M.D., professor and chairman of the Department of Dermatology at Oregon Health Sciences University in Portland. "While some people are born with hair that tends to be more dry, most dry hair problems aren't organic or genetic problems at all. They're instead due to what you're doing to your hair," he says.

That's right. Those dry locks are most likely your own fault. Exposing your hair to harsh chemicals such as hair dyes, permanent-wave solutions, and the chlorine in swimming pools and hot tubs dries out the hair. So does shampooing too often and using styling tools such as hot combs, hot rollers, and blow dryers. Even too much sun and wind can dry out your tresses.

You can learn to treat your dry hair with T.L.C. and teach it to be more manageable. Here's how:

DON'T OVERDO THE SHAMPOO.

Overshampooing is one of the most common causes of dry hair, according to Parker. "Too often, people think they have to shampoo their hair every day with harsh shampoos," he says. "It just strips away the natural oils."

On the other hand, you shouldn't go too long without a good lather. "Shampoo at least every three days," says barber, cosmetologist, and hair-care instructor Rose Dygart, owner of Le Rose Salon of Beauty in Lake Oswego, Oregon. "Gentle shampooing stimulates the oil glands."

BE KIND TO YOUR HAIR.

Dygart says dry hair is the most fragile type of hair and is subject to breakage, so it must be handled with care. "Learn to shampoo your hair very gently," she says. "Try not to pull the hair or put any tension on the hair shafts."

When lathering, avoid scrubbing with your fingernails, which can not only break the hair but can irritate your scalp. Work up a lather using your fingertips; they're great for the job.

USE A GENTLE SHAMPOO.

Dry hair needs a gentle, acidic cleanser, says Dygart. "Use a shampoo with a pH of between 4.5 and 6.7 for dry hair. Use a gentle cleanser you wouldn't be afraid to put on your face," she says. Some people recommend baby shampoos, but Dygart says their pH is far too high, and alkaline shampoos dry out the hair. Instead, she recommends acidic shampoos.

POUR ON THE CONDITIONER.

Dry hair needs conditioning, says Nelson Lee Novick, M.D., associate clinical professor of dermatology at Mount Sinai School of Medicine in New York. "Find a conditioner that has as little alcohol as possible in it, because alcohol is drying," he says. "Products that have little or no fragrance usually have less alcohol. For really dry hair, try an overnight conditioner that you put on and wear a shower cap over and rinse off the next day."

For severely dry hair, Novick recommends Moisturel body lotion, instead of a conditioner. Apply it to damp hair, and leave it on overnight beneath a shower cap. Rinse thoroughly in the morning.

POUR THE HOT OIL.

"Hot oil treatments are excellent for restoring dry hair," says Dygart. She recommends using over-the-counter hot oil products that you heat and place on the hair for 5 to 20 minutes (according to package instructions). Wear a plastic bag or shower cap over your hair while the hot oil is on. Then, wash the hair with a gentle shampoo.

SLATHER ON THE MAYO.

Mayonnaise is another excellent moisturizing treatment for dry hair, says Dygart. "Use old-fashioned mayonnaise, not diet or low-cholesterol types," she says. "First, shampoo your hair, then apply about a tablespoon of mayonnaise. Wrap the hair in a plastic bag for 20 to 30 minutes. Then shampoo and rinse thoroughly."

NIX THE 100 STROKES.

Novick says that because dry hair is so fragile, too much brushing can actually fracture the hair, causing hair fall.

He suggests brushing gently, never when hair is wet. Dygart says the type of hairbrush you use is important. She recommends boar-bristle brushes or "vent" brushes, ones with rubberized tips, that don't pull the hair excessively.

GIVE YOURSELF A SCALP MASSAGE.

One way to stimulate the oil glands on the scalp is to gently massage the scalp during shampoos, says Dygart. "Use the tips of your fingers to very gently massage all over your scalp," she says. "It not only stimulates the oil glands, it also feels great."

BE AN EGGHEAD.

Dygart suggests beating an egg in a cup and, with tepid water (not hot—it cooks the egg!), lathering the egg into the hair and then rinsing it out with tepid water. There's no need to shampoo afterward. The egg not only cleans the hair but gives it a lovely shine.

PACE YOUR HAIR TREATMENTS.

If you perm on Tuesday, dye your hair on Thursday, and put it in hot rollers on Saturday, your hair is destined to be dry and damaged. "Think about your hair like a sweater," says Novick. "How many times can you dye it repeatedly before it begins to look terrible?" Novick says people with dry hair don't have to abandon dyes, permanent waves, or hair straightening, but he says it's important to space those treatments out.

HOLD THE HEAT.

Using hot combs, hot rollers, and blow dryers is asking for dry hair trouble, says Paul Contorer, M.D., chief of dermatology for Kaiser Permanente in Beaverton, Oregon, and clinical professor of dermatology at Oregon Health Sciences University in Portland. Hot rollers are the worst because they stretch the hair while the heat shrinks it. Hot combs also tend to stretch the hair and expose hair to heat for long periods of time.

If you must use artificial heat on your hair, Dygart suggests that you use a blow dryer on a low setting and avoid pulling or stretching the hair while drying.

Dry skin

12 Ways to Fight Moisture Loss

Everyone occasionally suffers from dry skin, according to dermatologist James Shaw, M.D., chief of the Division of Dermatology at Good Samaritan Hospital and Medical Center and associate clinical professor of medicine at Oregon Health Sciences University, both in Portland. "Dry skin is largely influenced by genetics and by climate and other drying factors like taking hot showers," he says.

When there's not enough water in the skin's top layer (called the stratum corneum), the skin becomes flaky, itchy, and unsightly. In extreme cases, this layer can become rough, cracked, and scaly, and chronic dermatitis (skin irritation) can develop.

Normally, the outer layer of the skin is kept moist by fluid from the sweat glands and from underlying tissues.

Oil, produced by the sebaceous glands in the skin, helps to seal in that fluid. But lots of things rob moisture from the skin's outer layer. Some people simply have an outer skin layer that doesn't hold water well. Others may have less active sweat glands. Age is also a factor in dry skin. The older you get, the less oil the sebaceous glands produce, and the drier your skin is likely to be.

One of the greatest skin-moisture robbers is low humidity. Cold, dry air, common in many areas during the winter months, sucks water from the skin. Add the drying effects of sun or high altitude to low humidity, and the parching is compounded. Heated or air-conditioned air in your home or office may also be dry and cause your skin to lose moisture.

Water can actually take moisture from your skin. Overbathing or bathing long in hot water causes a repeated wetting and drying of the tissue that holds the outer layer of skin together and, over time, can make it less able to hold and retain water. "People who bathe several times a day or take lots of hot tubs are actually leaching important proteins from their skin that normally keep the skin moist," explains Frank Parker, M.D., professor and chairman of the Department of Dermatology at Oregon Health Sciences University in Portland.

Harsh soaps, detergents, household cleansers, and chemical solvents can also take their toll on the skin. These products can damage the skin's outer layer. People who must frequently wash and dry their hands, such as nurses and hairstylists, often complain of red, chapped hands, so-called "dishpan hands."

While you can't keep skin away from all of the external moisture robbers, here are some tips to keep your skin moist and youthful-looking for years to come:

SUN AND YOUR DRY SKIN

If you're a sun worshipper who is always "working on your tan," you're also drying out your skin and increasing your risk of developing wrinkles, age spots, and skin cancer (melanoma), warns Frank Parker, M.D. "Just as the sun dries wet clothes hanging on a clothesline, it dries out the outer layer of the skin," he says. "Over time, the damage the sun does to the skin causes it to wrinkle and develop pigmentation spots."

Even more sobering is the increased risk of developing skin cancer from excessive sun exposure. People who are fair-skinned are at greater risk of developing such cancers than are darker-skinned individuals. To avoid the dry skin, wrinkles, and increased cancer risk from sun exposure, Parker suggests these tips:

Wear sunscreen. Sunscreens are rated by their sun protection factor, or SPF. The higher the SPF number, the greater the sun protection.

Cover up. Wear a lightweight, long-sleeved shirt and a hat when you're in the sun.

Avoid the sun between 10:00 A.M. and 3:00 P.M. This is the time of day when the sun's burning rays are at their strongest, so try to plan outdoor activities for earlier or later in the day.

Use lotions. If you must sunbathe, apply cream-type lotions and occasionally "spritz" your skin with mineral water to keep it moist. Keep your tanning sessions as short as possible, and moisturize afterward.

MOISTURIZE, MOISTURIZE, MOISTURIZE.

Always keep a lotion or cream on your skin, especially if you tend toward dry skin, says Parker. "Apply moisturizer right after you bathe, while you're still damp," he says. *Pat*, don't rub, yourself dry-damp with a soft towel. Apply moisturizers throughout the day whenever your skin feels dry and before retiring to bed.

Which moisturizers should you use? "The more oil a product has in it, the more protection it offers, and the thicker the product, the more it seals in moisture," says Shaw. "Thin lotions are mostly water. Cold creams are thicker and have more oil and less water. And products like Vaseline [petrolatum] are all oil."

Dermatologist Margaret Robertson, M.D., a staff physician at St. Vincent Hospital and Medical Center in Portland, Oregon, advises using a thick, unscented moisturizer that doesn't automatically disappear on the skin. She says you can mix water with petrolatum to form a cream that provides good moisture protection.

TAKE SHORT, COOL SHOWERS AND BATHS.

Hot water actually draws out oil, the skin's natural barrier to moisture loss, and can make itching worse, says Shaw. Bathe or shower only as often as *really* necessary and no more than once a day. If you take long, hot soaks, apply a moisturizer immediately after bathing.

USE SOAP SPARINGLY.

Shaw advises decreasing soap and water washing. "People wash too much," he says. "Overwashing with soap and water harms the skin's outer layer."

People who suffer from chronically dry skin should take brief baths or showers and lather up only the groin, armpits, and bottoms of the feet, says Robertson. When you use soap, opt for milder, oilated or superfatted soaps such as Dove, Basis, or Aveenobar. For super-dry skin, try a soap substitute to cleanse your skin.

DON'T BE ABRASIVE.

Scrubbing your skin with washcloths, loofah sponges, or other scrubbing products dries your skin out even more, says Robertson. "Often, when people have dry skin, they develop scale and try to scrub it off with washcloths or sponges," she says. "But they're doing more harm than good."

OIL THAT BATH.

"Bath oils can help," says Shaw. But, he warns, if you put the bath oil in the water before you get in and get wet, the oil can coat your skin and prevent it from becoming saturated with water. Instead, he recommends adding the oil to the bath after you've been in the water for a while or applying it directly to your wet skin after bathing. (If you do add the oil to your bathwater, be sure to use extra care when getting in or out of the tub, since the oil will make the tub slippery.)

Robertson says that mineral oil makes an excellent bath oil. However, she warns not to soak, even in an oil bath, for longer than 20 minutes.

RAISE THE HUMIDITY.

The higher the humidity, the less dry the skin. "In the tropics, where the humidity is around 90 percent, no one suffers from dry skin," says Shaw. He says once the temperature drops below 50 degrees Fahrenheit, the humidity tends to drop off, too.

Sixty percent humidity is perfect for the skin. It's the point at which the skin and the air are in perfect balance and moisture isn't being drawn from the skin into the air. If you live in a dry climate or if the humidity in your office or home is less than 60 percent, consider using a home humidifier. Even a vaporizer can help somewhat.

AVOID DETERGENTS, CLEANSERS, AND SOLVENTS.

Common household products, such as cleansers, window cleaners, ammonia, turpentine, lighter fluid, and mineral spirits can dry and damage the skin's outer layer. Wear vinyl gloves and use less harsh alternatives (for example, vinegar and water make a great window cleaner) whenever possible.

NIX ALCOHOL-BASED PRODUCTS.

Some people like to cleanse their faces with alcohol wipes or astringents. They leave the skin feeling clean and tingling, but there's a price. "Alcohol-based products have a drying effect," says Shaw.

USE CREAM- OR OIL-BASED MAKEUP.

If you wear foundation and blusher, choose oil-based types that help retain moisture rather than water-based products, says Robertson. In the evening, wash off makeup with mild soap. Then, rinse thoroughly, blot dry with a soft towel, and moisturize well.

COOL IT OFF.

Wood stoves and forced air heating systems dry the skin. Shaw recommends keeping house temperatures lower for moist skin.

TOSS OFF THE ELECTRIC BLANKET, PILE ON THE COMFORTER.

The heat from electric blankets can dry out your skin, too. Shaw says that for people who have chronically dry skin, opting for an extra blanket instead of an electric one is a good idea.

AVOID TOO MUCH ALCOHOL.

The effects of excessive alcohol consumption usually don't show up on the skin for several years. "We don't really know if there's a cause-and-effect relationship between drinking alcohol and dry skin," says Robertson. "But we do know that alcoholics tend to have drier, more wrinkled skin."

Each time you drink alcohol, your skin loses moisture needed to keep it young looking. When alcohol enters the bloodstream, it lowers the water concentration of the blood. To replace the lost water, the body draws water from surrounding cells. Limit your intake to no more than two ounces per day. Better yet, avoid alcohol altogether.

Earache

7 Sound Ways to Head Off Pain

Most people don't think about their ears much, unless they're self-conscious about their size. But when an earache develops, the affected ear can feel as if it has taken on monster proportions, making it difficult to think of anything else.

For all the unspeakable pain caused by earaches, they are rarely life threatening. Still, they can be serious, especially if they are caused by infection. Signs of an ear infection include ear pain and hearing loss. In a young child, clues that an ear infection may be present include rubbing or tugging at the ear, excessive crying or fussiness, fever, nausea, and vomiting. Since an untreated ear infection can lead to permanent hearing loss, and since ear pain can sometimes reflect a problem in another part of the body (see "Earaches that Aren't"), it is important to have an earache checked out by a doctor. (For information on preventing ear infections, see EAR INFECTION and SWIMMER'S EAR.)

Other than infection, the most common cause of earache is a blocked eustachian tube. The eustachian tube is a thin, membrane-lined tube that connects the inside back portion of the nose with the middle ear. The air in the middle ear is constantly being absorbed by its membranous lining, but the air is never depleted as long as the eustachian tube remains open and able to resupply air during the process of swallowing. In this manner, the air pressure on both sides of the eardrum stays about equal. However, when the eustachian tube is blocked for one reason or another, the pressure in the middle ear can't be equalized. The air that is already there is absorbed and, without an incoming supply, a vacuum occurs in the middle ear, sucking the eardrum inward and stretching it painfully taut.

This type of earache is especially common in people who travel by air, especially when they have a cold or a stuffy nose. As the plane takes off, the air pressure in

EARACHES THAT AREN'T

Sometimes, diseases and disorders in other parts of the head and neck can sound an alarm in the ear. "Referred pain has its origin elsewhere but is felt in the ear," says John W. House, M.D. That's one reason it's important to have ear pain checked out by a doctor.

To otolaryngologists, the most common culprits in referred ear pain are the "five Ts:"

- Tongue
- Teeth
- Throat
- Tonsils
- Temporomandibular joint (TMJ)

the plane's cabin decreases, and as the plane lands, the air pressure in the cabin increases; in each instance, the pressure change occurs very rapidly. While normally the air in the middle ear manages to equalize on its own, if there is congestion in the upper-respiratory tract, air may not be able to flow through the eustachian tube to reach the middle ear. (This type of earache can also occur as a result of pressure changes during an elevator ride in a tall building and during scuba diving.) Fortunately, there are some tricks you can try to ward off ear pain that results from the ups and downs of air travel.

SWALLOW HARD.

"The act of swallowing activates the muscle that opens the eustachian tube," according to James Stankiewicz, M.D., professor and vice-chairperson of the Department of Otolaryngology–Head and Neck Surgery at Loyola University Medical School in Maywood, Illinois. When the pilot makes the announcement that it's time to fasten your seat belts for landing, get your mouth ready to swallow. Swallowing can also bring temporary relief from earache pain until you can get to the doctor.

KEEP YOUR MOUTH MOVING.

You swallow more often when you chew gum or suck on hard candy, so pop some into your mouth just before the plane descends.

DON'T STIFLE A YAWN.

It's not the company, it's the atmospheric conditions. "Yawning is the best way to keep the eustachian tube open," says John W. House, M.D., associate clinical professor in the Department of Otolaryngology, Head and Neck Surgery at the University of Southern California at Los Angeles and an otologist–neurologist at the House Ear Clinic in Los Angeles.

STAY AWAKE.

If you're sleeping, you're not going to be swallowing. "Ask the flight attendant to wake you before descent," suggests Jack J. Wazen, M.D., associate professor of otolaryngology and director of otology and neurotology at Columbia University College of Physicians and Surgeons in New York. "It's much more pleasant than being awakened by a pain in your ear."

WHEN YOUR EARDRUM TAKES A BEATING

If you feel a sudden, sharp pain in your ear following a trauma such as an explosion or a scuba-diving accident, you may have a perforated eardrum, says Jack J. Wazen, M.D.

While the pain may occur only at the time of the accident, the injury itself needs evaluation by a specialist to head off permanent disruption of the middle-ear mechanism. Most injury-related eardrum perforations are small and will heal spontaneously within a few weeks, provided middle-ear infections are prevented or controlled (which is why you still need to see a doctor even for small perforations). Large perforations may require surgery.

HOLD YOUR NOSE.

If your ears still become uncomfortably blocked as the plane descends, the American Academy of Otolaryngology, Head and Neck Surgery suggests that you try this: With your thumb and forefinger, pinch your nostrils tightly closed and block the external opening of the unaffected ear with the forefinger of your other hand. Now, with your mouth closed, try to blow through the pinched nostrils, blowing as forcefully as you would blow your nose. Repeat if necessary. You should experience a cracking sensation or a loud pop and a relief of the pain if the maneuver works. Don't try this trick if you have a sore throat or fever, however, because the infection might be forced into your ears. And don't attempt it if you have a heart or circulatory disorder.

REACH FOR RELIEF.
Frequent flyers should tuck away a decongestant pill or nasal spray to use an hour or so before landing. This shrinks the membranes, making it easier to keep the eustachian tube open. "If you suffer from allergies or sinusitis, you must be sure to take your medication at the beginning of the flight," says Stankiewicz. Over-the-counter medications like this are not for everyone, however. People with heart disease, high blood pressure, irregular heart rhythms, or thyroid disease should avoid them. Pregnant women and individuals who are subject to anxiety should stay away from them, as well.

TAKE THE TRAIN.
If, despite all your best efforts, you still end up with an uncomfortable stuffed feeling and pain following air travel, you might consider taking the scenic route.

Ear infection

9 Tips for Prevention and Treatment

S tep into a pediatrician's waiting room, and you're likely to find that one of every three children there under the age of three has an ear infection. Some one-third of all children have more than three middle-ear infections (or otitis media) during the first three years of life, resulting in 30 million doctor visits a year.

Of course, children aren't the only ones who get ear infections. But they are, by far, the most common victims. Adults are more likely to get an infection of the outer ear, which is aptly referred to as "swimmer's ear" because it usually gets its start when water containing bacteria or fungi seeps into the ear and gets trapped in the ear canal (see SWIMMER'S EAR).

In order to understand how middle-ear infections develop, it helps to know how healthy ears function. The outer ear is connected to an air-containing space called the middle ear. The eardrum, a thin membrane, is stretched across the entrance to the space, and three sound-conducting bones are suspended within it. The pressure within the middle-ear space is equalized with the atmosphere through a narrow tube called the eustachian tube. The eustachian tube opens into a space behind the nose where air or fluid may enter or escape. The air pressure in the middle ear is equalized more than one thousand times a day—every time you swallow— usually without your noticing it. The eustachian tube also carries fluid away from the middle ear.

When a cold or an allergy is present, the eustachian tube swells and air is absorbed by the lining of the middle ear, creating a partial vacuum. The eardrum then gets pulled inward, and fluid weeps from the lining of the middle ear. Bacteria or viruses from the nose and throat can travel up the eustachian tube and infect the stagnant, warm fluid in the middle ear, which provides a perfect environment for them to live and multiply. When this happens, an infection is underway.

Children may be more prone to middle-ear infections than adults. Their eustachian tubes are shorter and straighter, which may make it easier for germs to penetrate. Children also get more colds than adults.

PREVENTING EAR INFECTIONS

There are some things you can do to decrease the chance that your child will develop a middle-ear infection.

STEER YOUR CHILD CLEAR.

"The entire process starts with a cold, allergic reaction, or infection of the tonsils or adenoids," says James Stankiewicz, M.D., professor and vice-chairman of the Department of Otolaryngology–Head and Neck Surgery at Loyola University Medical School in Maywood, Illinois. "If you can keep your child out of contact with children who have colds and other respiratory infections and make sure that allergies are under control, then there is a better chance of avoiding ear infection." If you are in the process of choosing a day-care facility for your child, check the center's policy for dealing with sick children.

TEACH PROPER NOSE-BLOWING TECHNIQUE.

Once your child is old enough, teach him or her to blow his or her nose softly rather than with excessive force, so as not to drive infection into the ears. And teach your child not to stifle a sneeze by pinching the nostrils, since this, too, may force the infection up into the ears.

DON'T SMOKE.

Here's another reason not to smoke: Children who live with smokers seem to be more susceptible to middle-ear infections than are those who live in smokefree homes. Cigarette smoke irritates the linings of the nasal passages and middle-ear cavity, which interferes with the normal functioning of the eustachian tube. If you cannot quit, at least take your habit outside.

BE CAREFUL WITH BOTTLE-FEEDING.

Avoid giving a bottle of milk or formula to a baby who is lying on his or her back, because the milk can flow into the eustachian tube during swallowing and initiate a middle-ear infection.

STAY ALERT TO THE SIGNS.

It is essential to get your child to the doctor as soon as you suspect an ear infection, but to do that, you need to be aware of the symptoms that can signal an ear infection. An older child may complain of ear pain or aching or a stuffiness in the ear. In a younger child who cannot yet describe an earache, you need to be alert to other signs that may signal an imminent ear infection. "One of the first signs is that the child pulls or rubs his or her ears frequently. This is before real pain sets in but indicates that something is amiss," says John W. House, M.D., associate clinical professor in the Department of Otolaryngology, Head and Neck Surgery at the University of Southern California at Los Angeles. "You may also notice that your child does not seem to hear you. Then come the real signs of infection: fever, crying and other signs of pain, nausea, and vomiting."

TREATING AN EAR INFECTION

"It is most important that a child showing signs of ear infection be taken to a doctor immediately," advises

Daniel Kuriloff, M.D., associate director of the Department of Otolaryngology–Head and Neck Surgery at St. Luke's–Roosevelt Hospital Center and associate professor at Columbia University College of Physicians and Surgeons, both in New York. If a middle-ear infection is treated promptly, it is not serious. If not treated right away, your child might suffer hearing loss and, as a result, a delay in learning and speech development. Once your child has seen the doctor, however, there are some things you can do to help make your little one more comfortable.

FOLLOW THROUGH ON THE DOCTOR'S INSTRUCTIONS.

Be sure that your child receives the medication prescribed by the doctor. The one medication that the pediatrician will almost certainly prescribe is an antibiotic. "You must be sure that your child takes the medication for the full time prescribed—usually 10 to 14 days," says Kuriloff. "Read the label on the prescription bottle carefully and follow directions." The doctor may also prescribe an antihistamine and/or a decongestant if your child has a cold or allergy. If you have any questions about the medication, call your doctor or pharmacist.

KEEP YOUR CHILD'S CHIN UP.

If your child is lying down, prop his or her head up on pillows. Elevating the head will help to keep the eustachian tubes draining into the back of the throat.

TRY MILD HEAT.

Applying a heating pad set on warm—not hot—may make your child more comfortable.

GIVE ACETAMINOPHEN.

Try giving your child acetaminophen to help relieve pain and fever. Do not, however, give your child aspirin. Aspirin use in children with a viral illness has been associated with Reye's syndrome, an often fatal condition characterized by severe, sudden deterioration of liver and brain function.

Excessive perspiration

8 Dry Ideas

Following a spicy dinner at your favorite restaurant, you realize that your back and chest are damp. At the end of a very important interview, you reach out to shake hands and notice that your palm is wet. After narrowly missing a collision with a car that has run a red light, you wipe the moisture from your brow.

What's going on here? In a word, it's sweat. Sweat is the by-product of the body's internal thermostat and air-conditioning system, which sometimes responds to spicy foods, anxiety, and danger in the same way that it does to excessive heat. But before you conclude that you would be more comfortable without such sensitive reactions, remember that the system keeps you alive.

There's nothing complicated about the mechanics of sweat (or perspiration, as it is often referred to by those who would rather think they don't do it). The human body contains more than two million sweat glands (women may have more, according to some studies) of two types: eccrine glands and apocrine glands. The eccrines are located almost everywhere on the body's surface—about 400 to the square inch of skin, except in places like the palms of the hands, where as many as 3,000 may be concentrated. The eccrines are the smaller of the two types and originate deep within the skin, with narrow ducts threading to the skin's surface. The task for these glands is primarily temperature control: When things get too hot, the sweat glands go into high gear, drawing fluid from the blood to produce sweat and transporting it through the pores to the skin surface. Once on the surface, sweat evaporates, cooling the skin. This, in turn, cools the blood, which has also been rushed to the surface by temperature-control cells in the brain. The cooled blood then returns to the internal organs and muscles, cooling them.

Apocrine glands are larger, fewer in number, and attached to hair follicles in the genital area and armpits. The apocrines become active after puberty and are exquisitely sensitive to emotional stress and sexual stimulation.

Even the most inactive person sweats as much as a quart a day. Marathon runners, on the other hand, may produce up to two gallons during the course of a race. Such extreme sweat production is still considered quite normal under the circumstances; one would hardly grant it a passing thought except for the fact that it can make its presence known in most embarrassing ways (see BODY ODOR). On the other hand, if you have a body that beads up like a cold seltzer can on a hot day—even

ANTIPERSPIRANT PRIMER

Here are some tips from the FDA Consumer that will help you get more protection and less irritation from your underarm antiperspirant:

• Repeat applications regularly. Antiperspirants work for only a certain length of time. Check the label to see how often yours should be applied.

• Dry the underarms thoroughly before applying an antiperspirant. Dryness enhances penetration of the active ingredient.

• To avoid irritation, don't apply an antiperspirant to freshly shaved skin. (Try shaving at night, so you won't have to apply the antiperspirant until the following morning.)

• Try another product with a different active ingredient if one product doesn't work. What works for one person may not work for someone else.

when you're sitting perfectly still in the shade—you have what is known, in medical terms, as hyperhidrosis. Here's what you can do about it:

STAY OUT OF THE MIDDAY SUN.

When the sun is at its highest and hottest, your body will quickly become overheated, sending your thermoregulatory response into high gear. "One of the most logical ways to avoid excessive sweating is to avoid excessive overheating," says Allan L. Lorincz, M.D., professor of dermatology at the University of Chicago Medical Center. A warm, humid day is even worse. "With high humidity, the percentage of water suspended in the air rises, reducing the amount of sweat that can be taken up by the air from the skin," adds Lorincz.

DRESS RIGHT.

Most synthetic materials appear to increase sweating because they do not absorb moisture. "Try wearing natural fibers such as cotton in summer months and wool during the winter," advises Donald Rudikoff, M.D., assistant clinical professor of dermatology at Mount Sinai School of Medicine in New York.

STAY "DRY."

Since alcohol stimulates blood flow to the skin, alcoholic beverages can cause increased sweating—even before you begin to feel any other effects on your body. "Stick to nonalcoholic beverages on hot, humid days," advises Rudikoff. Cold (but not ice-cold) water is best for quenching thirst and replacing lost fluids.

CUT THE CAFFEINE.

Caffeine speeds up the heart, making it behave as it would in response to overheating. "Reduce your intake of caffeine—coffee, tea, cola drinks—it will benefit your heart as well as your peace of mind," says Rudikoff.

WATCH WHAT YOU EAT.

Eating hot, spicy foods can trigger perspiration, so avoid them at times when staying dry is a priority.

SLIM DOWN.

If you are overweight, even the most moderate activities make your heart strain harder to pump blood around your body. "Reaching and maintaining your desirable body weight may go a long way toward easing a problem of excessive sweating," notes Lorincz.

COOL IT.

Increased anxiety—even if it is temporary—can cause excessive sweating. In anxiety-prone people, even the merest stress—or none at all—can bring on an anxiety attack with accompanying sweating. "If you frequently become anxious, try to divert the symptoms with physical activity, such as jogging, walking, or swimming, or relaxation exercises such as deep breathing," suggests Alan R. Shalita, M.D., chairman of the Department of Dermatology at State University of New York Health Science Center at Brooklyn.

SPRAY, STROKE, DAB.

To add an extra layer of confidence, you can use an antiperspirant under your arms and even on the palms of your hands and soles of your feet (if they are trouble areas). "Antiperspirants inhibit production of eccrine perspiration," says Rudikoff. Most of these products contain an aluminum salt, which is thought to work by causing a slight swelling around the sweat-gland ducts that decreases the outflow of perspiration. Aluminum chlorohydrate is the mildest of the salts; aluminum chloride and aluminum sulfate are even more effective but are also more acidic and, when mixed with perspiration, tend to irritate the skin and stain clothing, particularly linen and cotton.

261

Eye redness

7 Ways to Look Bright-Eyed

What do a long day at the office, a night on the town, and an afternoon of gardening have in common? They can all have you seeing red—when you look in the mirror, that is.

"Eye redness can be caused by a lot of things," says Carol Ziel, M.D., an ophthalmologist with the Eye Clinic of Wausau in Wisconsin. "A red eye may simply be dry or slightly irritated, or it may be a sign of chronic or acute glaucoma, inflammation of the eye, or a conjunctivitis."

"In the case of acute glaucoma, which most often occurs in children but can also occur in adults, there tends to be red eyes in conjunction with dilated pupils, blurring of vision, and pain," says Charles Boylan, M.D., a pediatric ophthalmologist at A Children's Eye Clinic of Seattle.

"You can get red eyes from certain diseases such as chronic glaucoma, blood diseases, gout, thyroid diseases, and even a tumor," warns Jon H. Bosland, M.D., a general ophthalmologist in private practice in Bellevue, Washington. "You can also get red eyes from iritis, an inflammatory disease which is usually inside the eye. It is often associated with discomfort and increased pressure within the eye as well. And it can be very serious if not treated with cortisone," says Boylan.

For these reasons, the experts recommend that you have your eyes checked if the redness persists for more than a couple of days, if there is any pain or change of vision associated with the redness, if your eyes suddenly become sensitive to light, if you notice redness or blood over the pupil (the dark center of the eye), or if you have any discharge from one or both eyes.

For red eyes caused by everyday irritants, you can do some things to help get the red out and relieve irritation.

GIVE YOUR EYES A "LUBE" JOB.

"Lubricating eye drops such as Visine can help to relieve some of the dryness and make the eye feel better," says Bosland. "But don't use them any longer than a few days at most," he adds (see "Eye-Drop Alert"). Eye drops and artificial tears can be especially helpful to older individuals. "Older people don't produce as many tears as they should, which can make the eyes red," says Boylan.

APPLY COOL OR WARM COMPRESSES.

"It doesn't really matter which kind you use. Whatever feels best to you is fine," says Ziel. "A washcloth soaked in cool water feels good, as does simply cupping cool water in your hand and holding it under the eye," adds Bosland.

USE AN OVER-THE-COUNTER ANTIHISTAMINE.

If your red, itchy eyes are the result of an allergy, then treating the allergy itself will tend to help your eyes, too.

GET A GOOD NIGHT'S REST.

"This is often enough to clear up red eyes that are the result of too little sleep," says Bosland. But if 40 winks don't help, then the redness is probably due to some other cause and should be checked by a doctor.

EYE-DROP ALERT

Sometimes, the continual use of over-the-counter eye drops can actually cause red eyes, rather than alleviating them. According to Jon H. Bosland, M.D., there are a couple of reasons for this. "Many of the over-the-counter eye drops have preservatives in them, which can further irritate sensitive eyes," he says. "And certain decongestant eye drops that claim to whiten your eye are pretty mild but can cause a rebound effect similar to the kind you can get with nose drops," he warns. "What happens is that the decongestant in these fluids causes the little arteries to shrink up, making the eye look whiter. This works well at first, but with continued use of these drops, the arteries can become dependent on the chemical in order to stay shrunken. So when the chemical wears off, the arteries dilate again and make the eye appear red," he explains.

While using over-the-counter eye drops for a few days to soothe and whiten eyes is generally OK, using them regularly can be counterproductive. Be sure to read the label for instructions on proper use.

WEAR GOGGLES IN THE POOL.
If you plan to take a splash in the swimming pool, protect your eyes from the irritating effects of chlorine with a pair of well-fitting swimming goggles, available at sporting goods stores.

USE EYE DROPS IN THE AIR.

"The air in the cabin of an airplane is extremely dry and contains less oxygen, both of which can irritate and redden the eyes," says Bosland. Over-the-counter lubricating drops add moisture to the eye, which helps to keep them from getting dried out.

SPORT SHADES.

Wear a pair of good-quality sunglasses whenever you go out during the day. This is especially important if you'll be skiing, boating, or sunbathing on a bright day. "Snow blindness and ultraviolet burns can result when the eyes are unprotected in the sunlight," warns Bosland. "And both conditions can be extremely painful," he adds. "I've also seen skiers get red eyes from going down the hill without protective eye wear and ending up with extremely dry eyes from the wind," says Boylan. "Usually, it's the not-so-good skiers like myself who keep their eyes wide open on the way down so as not to hit anything," he says.

Eyestrain

20 Eye Savers

Y ou simply can't read another word. Your eyes have had it. They're tired, dry, and sore. You're suffering from eyestrain.

There are numerous causes of eyestrain—from stress to astigmatism to jaw disorders. "Most people have a tiny bit of astigmatism and do not even know they have it," says Andrew S. Farber, M.D., F.A.C.S., an ophthalmologist in private practice in Terre Haute, Indiana. "But it may show itself as eyestrain." Astigmatism is a defect in vision caused by an abnormal curvature of the cornea or lens of the eye, both of which help the eye to focus an image; it can usually be corrected with eyeglasses or contact lenses.

Tension in the neck and back muscles—from sitting at a computer all day, for instance—can also cause the eyes to tire.

Numerous diseases may show themselves as eyestrain. Glaucoma, a condition in which pressure within the eye becomes elevated, is one such condition. Even diseases not directly related to the eye may show up as eyestrain. In rare instances, the jaw disorder called temporomandibular joint syndrome, or TMJ, which causes facial pain (see TMJ), can lead to aching eyes.

One of the reasons eyestrain is so common is that the lens in the eye gradually loses some of its ability to change shape—and thus focus an image clearly—as we age. This condition, referred to as presbyopia, becomes most pronounced after age 40. It affects the eye's ability to focus on an image up close, which is why older individuals often need to hold reading material at arm's length.

Because there are so many causes of eyestrain, it's best to consult an eye-care professional for a complete diagnosis if you've been suffering from eyestrain for a month or more or if it seems to have become more frequent or bothersome, advises Henry D. Perry, M.D., clinical associate professor of ophthalmology at Cornell Medical College in New York. An eye examination should be performed once a year, especially for people 35 years of age and older and for anyone with a family history of glaucoma or diabetes.

In the meantime, here are some ways to ease the strain on your eyes.

MAKE THE LIGHT RIGHT.

"Working in dim or harsh light won't harm the eyes, but it may be more demanding," says Farber. Too much light can result in too much glare, while too little light may simply make it too difficult to read or see clearly, says Farber. Try to keep the lighting at a comfortable level—not too dark or too bright.

TRY INDIRECT LIGHTING.

Fixtures that face upward, allowing their light to bounce off a ceiling or wall, create a comfortable, diffusely lighted environment that's not as hard on the eyes as lights that shine down directly on you.

BUY A PAIR OF READING GLASSES.

Especially for those over 40 years of age, reading glasses may do the trick by magnifying the printed page and other close work. Reading glasses can be purchased without a prescription in drugstores and pharmacies; you simply try on several pairs until you find the magnification that provides you with the sharpest vision.

GET GLARE-BUSTING GLASSES.

Prescription lenses made with polarized ultraviolet (UV) filters reduce glare by filtering out certain wavelengths of light. These can be especially good for computer users.

(Continued on page 270)

HOW COMPUTER USERS CAN STOP THE STRAIN

"Computer users often find themselves in a visually demanding job in a visually unfriendly environment," says James E. Sheedy, O.D., Ph.D., associate clinical professor of the School of Optometry at the University of California in Berkeley and chief of the Video Display Terminal Eye Clinic. One result: eyestrain. Here are Sheedy's suggestions for preventing it.

Keep all light at the same level. Ideally, the brightness of the computer screen should be the same as the light in the room.

Get a glare-resistant screen. These filters that fit on your computer screen help decrease eye-straining reflections and glare. "Antireflection screens made of glass are better than the ones made of meshed material for proper imagery," says Sheedy. Check your local computer store or office-supply store for these.

Lighten the background, darken the letters. This contrast on the computer screen is most pleasing to the eye, says Sheedy. Make the background white or near white and the letters a darker color. Although you may not be consciously aware of it, your computer screen flickers, and your eyes see this flickering. Lightening the background of your computer screen makes this flickering less discernible to your eyes.

Place your terminal slightly lower than the top of your head. "Your eyes should be looking at the computer at about a 15-degree angle," says Sheedy. The eyes are most comfortable viewing the screen at this angle rather than straight on.

Use a document holder. These metal stands decrease eyestrain by getting your work off a flat surface and putting it in the same line of sight as your computer screen.

Wear a visor. This may sound a little weird, but a visor can actually help to block overhead light that is too strong and that interferes with your peripheral vision, which can cause eyestrain.

Shut off a light. Many office environments are overlit," according to Sheedy. "The lighting was originally set up for people looking down at work on their desks all day. But nowadays, people are often looking straight ahead at their computers and getting too much light in their eyes." If possible, shut off every other fluorescent ceiling fixture (if there are four fixtures in a row, for example, you can shut off the second and the fourth one) or at least remove one or two of the four tubes from each fixture.

Move your desk. If it isn't possible for you to shut the lights off, perhaps you can rotate the position of your desk in such a way as to get the too-bright lighting out of your line of sight.

Get prescription glasses specially made for computer use. People with bifocals and trifocals often have a problem using a computer because the section of lens they need to use to focus on the computer screen is either too high or too low for working comfortably. If you need to wear bifocals, consult an optometrist, who can fashion lenses specifically for computer use.

TAKE A BREAK.

Whether you're reading, writing, sewing, or tapping away on a computer, it's a good idea to take a break from such close work or switch to a task that isn't so visually demanding for a few minutes each hour, says Farber. Take a walk, make a phone call, talk to someone, focus on objects at a distance, or just close your eyes. Taking a break will give your neck and shoulders, as well as your eyes, a rest; tenseness in these areas can also aggravate eyestrain.

TRY A SALTWATER SOAK.

Perry recommends adding half a teaspoon of salt to a quart of warm water. Then, moisten cotton balls in the water, close your eyes, and place the cotton balls on your eyelids for about ten minutes.

TRY A COOL-WATER SPLASH.

For some people, splashing the face with cool water or laying a cool, damp towel across the eyes helps relieve eyestrain. If nothing else, it provides a break for overworked eyes.

THINK TO BLINK.

Dry eyes can result from tasks such as continuous reading or computer use. "The eyes blink less frequently, so they're not getting as lubricated as they should," explains Arnold Prywes, M.D., an assistant clinical professor of ophthalmology at the Albert Einstein Medical College in New York and chief of ophthalmology at Mid-Island Hospital in Bethpage, New York. When you're doing close work or concentrating on a computer screen for long hours, remember to blink frequently.

SHOULD YOU EXERCISE YOUR EYES?

Eye exercises, primarily developed by a turn-of-the-century ophthalmologist, William Bates, are generally regarded as a worthless practice. The Bates Method promotes such techniques as laying warmed hands over the closed eyes and alternating blinking with squeezing to keep the eyes in shape.

Most eye-care professionals agree that instead of a workout, resting your eyes is one of the best things you can do. Your eyes work all day, every day. Giving them the relief of only having to look at the inside of your eyelids for even a few minutes can make quite a difference. And, if you can take a nap or get a sufficient amount of sleep at night, all the better for your hard-working eyes.

KNOW YOUR DROPS.

Eye drops that decrease redness are not meant to be used for eyestrain, says Farber. Besides, the drops remove the redness by constricting the blood vessels in the eyes, and repeated use will actually have a rebound effect and make the eyes redder in the long run. On the other hand, if you know you're suffering from a case of dry eye, a drop or two of an over-the-counter eye lubricant, commonly referred to as artificial tears, may give you relief.

BUY A PLANT.

Increasing the humidity in your home or office can help a case of dry eyes. Using a humidifier is an obvious way to do this. But setting a pot of water on your home radiator can also increase the humidity level in your home. Potted plants in your home or office can also act as inexpensive—and attractive—humidifiers.

CLEAR THE AIR.

Cigarette smoke can irritate the eyes and make them sore. So give your eyes a break and put out that cigarette for good.

Fever

7 Ways to Manage the Ups and Downs

You're drenched in sweat. Your head is filled with a dull, throbbing ache, and, worse, you feel like someone is pressing their thumbs against your eyelids. One minute you feel afire; the next minute you are overcome with shaking chills. You put a thermometer under your tongue, and the mercury climbs to 101 degrees Fahrenheit. Yep, you have a fever.

To understand what having a fever means, and what you should or shouldn't do about it, it helps to know something about how the body controls temperature. There is quite a range in what is considered normal in body temperature. (By the way, *everyone* has a *temper-*

ature; when it rises above what is considered normal and stays there, it is termed a *fever.*) The body's natural temperature-control system, located in a tiny structure at the base of the brain called the hypothalamus, is normally set somewhere around 98.6 degrees Fahrenheit. A normal temperature measured orally ranges from 96.7 to 99.0 degrees Fahrenheit (taken rectally, it measures one degree Fahrenheit higher). Your own temperature probably varies by more than two degrees during the course of a day, with the lowest reading usually occurring in the early morning and the highest in the evening.

Fever is not a disease in itself but a symptom of some other condition, usually an infection caused by bacteria, fungi, a virus, or parasites, or even an allergic reaction. When this enemy invades, white blood cells are triggered to attack, releasing a protein called endogenous pyrogen. When endogenous pyrogen reaches the brain, it signals the hypothalamus to set itself at a higher point; if that new set point is over 100 degrees Fahrenheit, you have a fever.

When that happens, what should you do? Here's some advice:

LET IT BE.
The fact is, fever may do the body some good. An untreated fever tends to be self limited, relatively benign, and—contrary to popular belief—not likely to escalate to the point that it causes harm. Nor does lowering fever mean that you are lessening the severity of the illness; indeed, fever may be the body's way of mobilizing itself against invading organisms. "Over more than a decade of research, studies show that elevated body temperatures can enhance the immune response," says Matthew

HOW TO READ A FEVER

"Feeling your forehead doesn't even give a good guess about your body temperature," says Harold Neu, M.D. "You must use a fever thermometer to get an accurate reading."

There are two basic types of glass fever thermometers—oral and rectal—with the only difference being in the shape of the bulb: thin and long on the oral and short and stubby on the rectal. Rectal temperatures are the most accurate; oral temperatures can be thrown off by breathing through the mouth, smoking, or having just had a drink of something hot or cold. Rectal readings are, in general, one degree Fahrenheit higher than oral temperatures. (If neither of these methods is convenient, temperature can also be taken by placing an oral thermometer under the armpit for at least two minutes, which will give a reading about one degree Fahrenheit lower than an oral temperature.)

Glass thermometers have several disadvantages: They may break in handling or even in the mouth. If a thermometer breaks in the mouth, don't worry; there is only a tiny amount of mercury in the tube. Just be sure to

J. Kluger, Ph.D., professor of physiology at the University of Michigan Medical School in Ann Arbor. This heightened immune response is brought about by pyrogen, the same protein that causes the hypothalamus to reset itself. And pyrogen also has the ability to withhold iron from the blood, which apparently keeps infectious organisms from feasting and flourishing. "By leaving a fever remove any slivers of glass from the mouth. Glass thermometers also need to be shaken down to 96 degrees Fahrenheit in order to allow the body's true temperature to register. On the other hand, glass thermometers have a big advantage: They are very inexpensive; you can readily purchase one in a local pharmacy or supermarket for about three dollars.

More convenient—and somewhat more expensive (costing about seven to ten dollars)—are newer digital thermometers, which register temperatures accurately within a tenth of a degree. These thermometers are also fast. It takes less than a minute for the temperature to register as compared to three minutes with glass thermometers. Most digital thermometers run on a "button" (or hearing-aid type) battery that boasts a two- to three-year life under normal use.

Pharmacies generally carry a selection of both glass and digital thermometers. If you have any questions regarding which type of thermometer would be best suited to your needs, talk to your pharmacist.

untreated, you may be following Mother Nature's way of dealing with infection," says Kluger. There are, however, some noteworthy exceptions to this "let it be" approach (see "Hello, Doctor?" for more information on when to call the doctor). In addition, if you are feeling truly miserable, there are some steps you can try to make yourself more comfortable when you have a fever.

DRESS COMFORTABLY.

Let your body tell you what to wear. If, as the fever is developing, you get the chills, bundle up until you feel more comfortable. On the other hand, if you feel uncomfortably warm, shed some clothing. With your body exposed as much as possible, your sweat glands will be better able to release moisture, which will make you feel more comfortable. "The fewer the clothes, the faster the fever will go down," says Pascal James Imperato, M.D., professor and chairman of the Department of Preventive Medicine and Community Health at State University of New York Health Science Center at Brooklyn. Avoid overbundling an infant.

DON'T GO UNDER COVER.

Unless you have the chills, bundling yourself in bed under a pile of blankets or quilts will only hold the heat in and make you more uncomfortable. "Forget everything you've heard about 'sweating the fever out' by piling on the covers," advises Harold Neu, M.D., professor of medicine and pharmacology at Columbia University College of Physicians and Surgeons in New York. Once again, let your body be your guide. If a light sheet makes you feel more comfortable, don't feel that you have to bury yourself under blankets.

DIP.

If you feel uncomfortably warm, sponge yourself with tepid water or sit in a tub of shallow, tepid water and splash the water over your body. Don't fill the tub with water, since it's the evaporation of the water from the skin that helps cool you down. "Make sure the water is not ice cold, which can be counterproductive, since it

....

HELLO, DOCTOR?

Letting a fever run its course is not the best idea for everyone. While a fever of 102 to 103 degrees Fahrenheit is not usually dangerous in an otherwise healthy adult, it can be risky for very young children, who can develop seizures, and very elderly individuals, in whom fever can aggravate an underlying illness, such as a heart arrhythmia or respiratory ailment. Infants, young children, and very elderly individuals should be monitored carefully, and a physician should be called if the temperature continues to rise. Even in otherwise healthy adults, if a high fever (above 102 degrees Fahrenheit) lasts for more than a couple of days, a doctor should be consulted. Keep in mind, too, that if you or your child has a fever or other symptom that worries you, it never hurts to contact your doctor for advice.

....

will cause shaking and make the fever rise again. Avoid alcohol altogether because it can be absorbed into the skin and cause intoxication and dehydration," advises Imperato.

SIP.

Fever, especially if it is accompanied by vomiting or diarrhea, can lead to fluid loss and an electrolyte imbalance. "Keep yourself well hydrated," says Neu. Cool water is best, but unsweetened juices are OK if that's what tastes good. Getting a child to drink plenty of water is sometimes difficult; try Popsicles or flavored ices, which are primarily water.

DON'T FORCE FOOD DOWN.

"Don't force yourself to eat if you don't feel like it when you have a fever," says Imperato. Your body will tell you when it's time to eat. Be sure, however, to keep up your fluid intake.

TAKE TWO ASPIRIN.

Drugs known as antipyretics seek out the pyrogen and put it out of commission. Aspirin and acetaminophen are both antipyretics. However, "do not give aspirin to a child who has or is suspected to have chicken pox, influenza, or even a minor respiratory illness," warns Imperato. "This may trigger a potentially fatal condition known as Reye's syndrome," he adds. Stick with acetaminophen for children, and follow package directions.

Fingernail problems

14 Tips for Healthier Nails

Scratch an itch. Strum a guitar. Peel an orange. Your fingernails come in handy all day long, but too much use—or misuse—can cause problems ranging from nasty fungal infections to brittle, broken nails.

Your nails are made of keratin, the same type of protein that goes into your hair. Each nail actually consists of several parts, all of which play an important role in its health and growth:

• **Nail plate:** This is what you see as the fingernail.

• **Nail bed:** This lies below the nail plate; the two are attached. The capillaries in the nail bed nourish the nail and give it its pinkish color.

• **Nail matrix:** You don't see most of this, yet it may be the most important. It's below the cuticle at the base of the nail. Cells in the matrix produce the fingernail. If the matrix gets damaged, your nail will be distorted or may even stop growing completely.

• **Lunula:** This is the part of the matrix that you can see. It's the moon-shaped portion at the bottom of your nail.

• **Cuticle:** This fold of skin, made of dead cells, keeps foreign substances, like infection-causing bacteria, out.

• **Nail fold:** The nail fold is the ridge of skin around the nail.

Although plenty can go wrong with the nails, one of the most common complaints dermatologists hear is that fingernails are brittle—"whether they're soft and brittle or hard and brittle," says Lawrence A. Norton, M.D., clinical professor of dermatology at Boston University School of Medicine.

"Brittle nails can be compared to dry skin of the nails," explains Richard K. Scher, M.D., professor of clinical dermatology and nail specialist at Columbia University School of Medicine in New York. "You treat them like dry skin—use moisturizers and avoid harsh chemicals and detergents that are drying."

"Such nails are often shingling—they split like roof shingles at the end of the nail," says Norton. He blames the condition on nails dried out from indoor heat, exposure to detergents, and too frequent use of nail polish removers.

Nails that are soft and brittle, on the other hand, need to be kept dry. "You've used too much lotion or kept your hands in water too long," says C. Ralph Daniel III, M.D., clinical professor of medicine (dermatology) at the University of Mississippi Medical Center in Jackson.

Trauma, the doctors' term for injury, is another major problem for fingernails. "You hit your fingernail with the hammer," says Daniel. If a bruise forms beneath the nail, a doctor may have to relieve the pressure that builds up.

Injuries also open the door to infections, especially fungal infections. Although these generally plague toenails more often than fingernails (because of athlete's foot), fungal infections can strike the nails on the hands, with some unpleasant consequences.

And finally, certain skin diseases, such as psoriasis, can show up in your nails.

What you don't want to occur: Separation of the nail plate from the nail bed, a condition called onycholysis. It can occur after an injury, infections, allergies to nail cosmetics, exposure to chemicals, or diseases like psoriasis. If the nail appears white, it may have separated. You'll need to see your doctor and you'll want to be careful not to aggravate the problem further. Unfortunately, once the nail separates, it won't reattach until a new nail has grown out.

You also want to take good care of the nail matrix. If this is damaged, it will start producing a deformed nail or, even worse, no nail at all.

Here's what the experts recommend you do to keep your nails as healthy and attractive as possible:

AVOID THE CULPRITS.

The housewife or househusband is exposed to detergents and cleansers, the janitor to strong cleaning fluids, the bartender to citrus fruits, and so on, says Daniel. If you can't stay away from these substances, wear gloves whenever possible. Otherwise, you risk brittle nails and even nail separation, or infection, which could lead to a deformed nail or even the loss of it.

WEAR VINYL GLOVES FOR WET WORK.

That's vinyl, not latex or rubber, stresses Daniel, which will make hands sweat. In fact, Scher recommends wearing cotton gloves under the vinyl gloves.

WEAR COTTON GLOVES FOR DRY WORK.

You'll help protect nails from damage or possible injury.

KEEP YOUR NAILS SHORT.

Try giving that advice to actress/singer Barbra Streisand or Olympic star Florence Griffith Joyner. But face it, the shorter your nails, the less the risk of damaging them.

BE CAREFUL OF NAIL BANGERS.

Don't use your nail in place of a screwdriver, says Daniel. Try not to hit it with a hammer. Such actions can injure your nails, opening the door to infections, stopping nail growth, or causing bruises. "If your nail turns black and blue, go to your doctor or the emergency room," says Daniel. The pressure should be relieved on the blood vessel that's been injured underneath the nail.

STOP NAIL BITING

"There's not a lot that parents can do actively," says Bruce Epstein, M.D., a pediatrician in St. Petersburg, Florida, and a spokesperson for the American Academy of Pediatrics.

"You don't want to engage in a battle you can't win," he points out. His advice to parents: Tell your children that they can chew or bite on their nails all they want as long as they do it in the privacy of their bedrooms and not in front of you. That way, you've expressed your disapproval but you're not forcing your child to stop completely.

Those nasty medicines you can paint on the nails rarely work with kids, Epstein says. "They'll learn to like the taste."

Your child may eventually give up the habit, especially if peer pressure comes into play.

MOISTURIZE YOUR NAILS.
"Soak them in tepid water," says Norton. "Then massage in a moisturizer to hold the water. There's no fat in your nails to hold the moisture in." He suggests trying any product with phospholipids, urea, or lactic acid—all are "humectants," which will hold water; two he recommends are Complex 15 or Aquaderm. Daniel suggests white petrolatum or Moisturel.

PROTECT YOUR TOENAILS, TOO

Toenails are most likely to fall prey to fungal infections. That's because the fungus that causes athlete's foot can invade the toenail after it's been injured. "Use topical antifungals with clotrimazole or miconazole to decrease athlete's foot," recommends C. Ralph Daniel III, M.D. These medications are available without a prescription at your local pharmacy.

AVOID MOISTURE.

Sounds like a contradiction, right? If your nail becomes infected, particularly with a yeast organism, it's important to keep it as dry as possible. The nail plate may look chalky white, yellowish, brownish, or even green when an infection has set in. The nail may separate from the bed, or the nail fold may be red and irritated looking. See your doctor if you're not sure what's happening.

CARE FOR YOUR CUTICLES.

But not the way you may think. "Don't use mechanical instruments and cut them," warns Scher. Soak them first, then push them back with a moist towel. He warns against orange sticks and cuticle scissors. "When you clip cuticles, you're breaking down the normal barrier to bacteria and moisture," says Norton, "and that can lead to an infection."

SECRETS YOUR NAILS REVEAL

The eyes may be the window to the soul, but your fingernails may provide a peek into the status of your health. Remember, the symptoms listed here may possibly signal the health problems listed; they do not provide definite diagnoses. But if you notice any of these, let your doctor know.

- **Pale or bluish nails:** This may indicate anemia.
- **Pink color slow in returning when nail is squeezed:** This may indicate decreased or slowed blood circulation.
- **White spots:** These occur as the result of an injury to the nail; they're not due to zinc deficiency, as some people believe.
- **Beau's lines:** These horizontal depressions occur after a traumatic event, such as a high fever. "You can actually date the event by measuring the nail and figuring in the growth rate," explains C. Ralph Daniel III, M.D.

DON'T PICK OR TEAR AT HANGNAILS.

Otherwise, you're opening the door to infection by making a break in the skin where bacteria can enter. Daniel suggests clipping the dry part of the hangnail with fine scissors and applying an over-the-counter antibiotic ointment. Keeping your hands, nails, and cuticles moisturized will help prevent future hangnails.

REALIZE THE RISK WITH NAIL COSMETICS.

Sculptured nails can hold in too much moisture, says Norton. The glues used in nail wraps can cause reactions

- **White lines parallel to the lunula (and not the cuticle):** These usually indicate some sort of systemic (bodywide) insult.
- **Clubbed nails:** These nails are shaped like the backside of a spoon and may indicate cardiopulmonary disease or asthma.
- **Spoon nails:** These dip inward and could mean certain types of anemia or injury.
- **Pitted nails:** These punched-out looking spots may signify psoriasis.
- **Anything resembling a wart around the nail:** This could be a skin cancer and needs to be examined by a doctor.
- **Dark spot:** This could be melanoma, the most dangerous of the three main types of skin cancer. If the spot "bleeds" into the cuticle or the nail folds or if you're fair-skinned, this is a serious warning sign that requires immediate medical attention.

resulting in permanent damage to the nail bed and root, says Daniel. The most common problem is separation of the nail from the bed. But if you notice any pain or tenderness, you're probably reacting to the glue, and you need medical attention, stresses Daniel.

FORGET FORMALDEHYDE.

Although most fingernail polishes and nail hardeners are not supposed to contain formaldehyde, some still do. And if they cause an allergy or irritation, you can end up with nail separation.

CUT DOWN ON POLISH REMOVER.

"Apply and remove polish no more often than once a week," advises Daniel. "The acetone in polish remover dehydrates the nails."

DON'T EAT GELATIN HOPING TO BUILD STRONG NAILS.

It just doesn't work.

DITTO FOR CALCIUM.

"Calcium has very little, if anything, to do with how hard your nails are," Daniel says. Unless you are crash dieting or suffering from a malabsorption problem, your nails are not influenced that much by what you eat, says Scher.

Flatulence

11 Ways to Combat Gas

For stand-up comedians, the subject of flatulence is sure to generate lots of snickering, giggles, and guffaws. But for those who suffer from this distressing—not to mention embarrassing—problem, it's no laughing matter.

Everyone passes a certain amount of flatus—or "breaks wind," as we delicately describe it. Normally, from 400 to 2,000 milliliters of oxygen, nitrogen, carbon dioxide, hydrogen, and methane are expelled each day from the anus. Most of the time, this happens without inviting notice through sound or smell. But under some circumstances and in some people, undigested food products pass from the small intestine into the large intestine (colon), where the mass is fermented by large amounts of bacteria that are normally present there. The benign bugs of the colon are not choosy. Whatever comes their way goes right on their menu. It is the bacterially produced gas that gives flatus its characteristic odor when expelled.

If you are a stoic or a recluse, you may simply be able to ignore that gaseous excess and its audible effects. If you're neither, there are some things you can do to prevent or relieve flatulence. Here's how:

EAT TO BEAT IT.

"Carbohydrates may be problematic for some people," says Lawrence S. Friedman, M.D., associate professor of medicine at Jefferson Medical College in Philadelphia. But before you cut out nutritious carbohydrates, try eliminating simple carbohydrates—those refined sugars, like fructose and sucrose, and white-flour foods that may taste good but are not very good for you, especially if you have a flatulence problem.

MINIMIZE MILK CONSUMPTION.

"Milk—the so-called perfect food—does cause gas for *some* people," says Sharon Fleming, Ph.D., associate professor of food science in the Department of Nutritional Sciences at the University of California at Berkeley. Some people don't have enough of the enzyme lactase in their gut or intestine to digest the milk sugar lactose. Drinking skim milk and buttermilk instead won't solve the problem either; the lactose is in the nonfat part. Cultured buttermilk may have a little less lactose, but the taste doesn't agree with everyone. If you cut down on or eliminate milk for a few days and you still have a flatulence problem, however, you can feel assured that milk is not the cause.

ADD A LITTLE ENZYME.

If you are lactose intolerant but don't want to give up milk, you can try one of the over-the-counter products, such as Lactaid and Dairy Ease, that contain lactase enzyme, which helps to break down lactose. Be sure to follow the package directions carefully.

BANISH THE OFFENDERS.

"Some foods are known to be flatulogenics—or flatus producers," says Norton Rosensweig, M.D., associate clinical professor of medicine at Columbia University College of Physicians and Surgeons in New York. He recommends giving up the most common ones (see "Gassers" for a list of these) and then when you feel that the flatulence problem has been relieved, start adding the foods back one by one. If your body can tolerate small quantities, you can gradually increase your intake.

SOAK YOUR BEANS.

Beans are a great source of fiber and protein, but for many people, eating them can be an "explosive" enterprise. Rather than give up beans, however, you can try adjusting the way you prepare them. Mindy Hermann, R.D., a registered dietitian and spokesperson for the American Dietetic Association, suggests the following technique for decreasing the flatulogenic effects of beans: Soak the beans overnight, then dump the water out. Pour

GASSERS

"People who suffer with chronic flatulence may be able to control the problem by eliminating foods that increase fermentation activity, thereby producing gas," says Norton Rosensweig, M.D. Here are some possible culprits:

Extremely flatulogenic:

Beans	Beer (dark)
Bran	Broccoli
Brussels sprouts	Cabbage
Carbonated beverages	Cauliflower
Onions	Milk (for those who are lactose intolerant)

Mildly Flatulogenic:

Apples (raw)	Apricots
Bananas	Bread and other products containing wheat
Carrots	Celery
Citrus fruits	Coffee
Cucumbers	Eggplant
Lettuce	Potatoes
Pretzels	Prunes
Radishes	Raisins
Soybeans	Spinach

new water in, and cook the beans for about half an hour. Throw that water out, put in new water, and cook for another 30 minutes. Drain the water out for the last time, put new water in, and finish cooking.

TRY BEANO.

This over-the-counter food modifier contains an enzyme that breaks down some of the sugars that can cause gassiness. You may find that it helps make foods such as beans, cabbage, broccoli, carrots, oats, and other vegetables and legumes more tolerable. Follow the package directions.

STAY CALM.

Emotional stress can play a major role in worsening a flatulence problem. The gastrointestinal tract is exquisitely sensitive to anxiety, anger, and depression. A network of nerves connects this area of the body to the brain, and when you are under stress, muscles in the abdomen tighten. The results are painful spasms. "Eating while under stress also makes you swallow air, which can worsen the problem," says Friedman.

GET PHYSICAL.

Sometimes, flatulence is less a matter of a faulty diet than of a faulty digestive process; the smooth passage of foods down the digestive tract may be hindered. Exercise helps to regulate the process, notes Friedman, who recommends taking a walk when things get uncomfortable. You can also apply pressure to your abdomen or lie face down on the floor with a pillow bunched up under your abdomen to help relieve discomfort. Rocking back and forth on the floor with your knees drawn up to your chest and your arms wrapped around your legs may also help. So might a heating pad placed on your abdomen.

BUST THE BELCH.
Habits that can lead to excessive belching can also cause problems with flatulence (see BELCHING).

GET ACTIVATED.
Activated charcoal tablets, available without a prescription, may help to absorb some excess gas and calm flatulence. If you are taking any prescription medications, however, ask your pharmacist whether the activated charcoal will interfere with them.

REACH FOR RELIEF.
Nonprescription preparations containing simethicone (such as Mylanta and Maalox) may ease gassiness.

Flu

6 Ways to Cope with the Flu-Bug Blahs

Yesterday, you felt fantastic. Today, you feel 100 years old and counting. Your head aches, your skin feels sore to the touch, and you're chilled to the bone even though your forehead is on fire. Welcome to the wonderful world of the flu virus.

HELLO, DOCTOR?

Signs that it's time to see your doctor include a high fever that lasts more than three days, a cough that persists or gets worse (especially if associated with severe chest pain or shortness of breath), or a general inability to recover. These things could signal a secondary bacterial infection that would need to be treated with prescription antibiotics. Marcia Kielhofner, M.D., also urges individuals with underlying lung or heart disease to consult their physician at the first sign of the flu.

"People use the term 'flu' to describe any viral, upper-respiratory-tract infection. But strictly speaking, influenza is a very distinctive viral agent," says Marcia Kielhofner, M.D., a clinical assistant professor of medicine at Baylor College of Medicine in Houston, Texas. "Flu viruses occur yearly and attack almost exclusively between the months of October and April," she continues.

Flu occurs initially in children. "We'll start to see an increasing level of absenteeism within the schools and an increasing number of children hospitalized for some sort of respiratory illness. Following that, we'll see adults being hospitalized with pneumonia or with worsening of an underlying heart or lung problem," she says.

While there are two major strains of the flu virus—influenza A and influenza B—each strain changes slightly from year to year, so being infected one year doesn't guarantee protection against the flu the following year. "Every once in a while, we'll get what's referred to as a 'pandemic.' This is when we see an entirely new type of influenza virus that is associated with a much higher rate of infection and death. The last one reported in the United States was in 1977," says Kielhofner.

Regardless of the strain, the symptoms are generally the same. They include a high fever, sore throat, dry cough, severe muscle aches and pains, fatigue, and loss of appetite. Some people even experience pain and stiffness in the joints. Usually, the aches, pains, and fever last only three to five days. The fatigue and cough, however, can hang on for several weeks.

The change in flu strains from year to year also makes it hard to develop 100 percent effective flu vaccines. "We tend to make vaccines that contain antibodies to the previous year's strain, which presents a real obstacle to fully protecting people from the flu each year," explains W. Paul Glezen, M.D., pediatrician in the Influenza Research Center, professor of microbiology and immunology and of pediatrics, and chief epidemiologist at Baylor College of Medicine in Houston, Texas. Still, flu vaccines manage to be about 80 percent effective when received before the flu season begins (ideally in September or October). So, if you really can't afford to get sick, a flu shot may not be a bad idea. And, if you fall into a high-risk group (see "Should You Get a Flu Shot?"), a flu shot is a priority.

On the other hand, if you don't manage to outrun this relentless bug, you can do a few things to ease some of the discomforts and give your body a chance to fight back.

SHOULD YOU GET A FLU SHOT?

Anyone who wants to reduce their chance of getting the flu should consider being vaccinated against the flu. However, it is especially important for the following groups of individuals to get a flu shot, according to Evan T. Bell, M.D., and Marcia Kielhofner, M.D.:

• **Individuals with chronic heart and lung disease.** The flu virus can aggravate these conditions to the point of causing serious complications and even death.

• **People over the age of 65, especially if living in a nursing home or chronic-care facility.** Viruses spread more rapidly in such environments. What's more, the flu virus attacks the already weakened immune systems of elderly people, which can lead to pneumonia and even death.

• **People with other chronic diseases, such as asthma, diabetes, kidney disease, or cancer.** Any time the body is fighting one disease, getting another illness can cause serious problems.

• **Children who take aspirin regularly for problems such as chronic arthritis.** Again, Reye's syndrome may be triggered by the flu virus in children taking aspirin.

• **Health-care providers.** While catching the flu may not seriously endanger these individuals, it can be deadly to the patients they are treating.

• **Pregnant women in any of the high-risk groups mentioned.** The vaccine must be given after the first trimester of the pregnancy to prevent of harming the fetus.

GET PLENTY OF REST.

"This is especially important due to the high fever that accompanies the flu," says Evan T. Bell, M.D., a specialist in infectious diseases at Lenox Hill Hospital in New York. This shouldn't be hard to do considering fatigue is one of the main symptoms. You won't feel like doing much other than lounging in bed or on the couch. Consider it a good excuse to take a needed break from the daily stresses of life. And if you absolutely must continue to work, at least get to bed earlier than usual and try to go into the office a little later in the morning.

TAKE ASPIRIN, ACETAMINOPHEN, OR IBUPROFEN—IF YOU MUST.

"One of the characteristic symptoms of influenza is a high fever that ranges anywhere from 102 to 106 degrees Fahrenheit," says Kielhofner. "Headaches are also seen almost universally with influenza," she adds. Lowering the fever will help to prevent dehydration and will cut down on the severe, shaking chills associated with fever. On the other hand, since a fever may actually help your body fight the influenza bug (see "Influenza Myths"), you may want to try to let the fever run its course if you can. "The aspirin- and ibuprofen-containing drugs tend to work better against the aches and pains, while the acetaminophen works best on the fever," says Bell. But both doctors warn that people who have a history of gastrointestinal problems and/or ulcer disease should avoid taking aspirin and ibuprofen, because these medications have been shown to further complicate these conditions. And Glezen adds that individuals aged 21 and under should avoid taking aspirin during the flu season because the combination of aspirin and the flu in this age group

INFLUENZA MYTHS

Despite evidence to the contrary, there are still a few myths about the flu. One has to do with what people often refer to as the "24-hour flu." This is an illness characterized by the sudden onset of vomiting and diarrhea, and a general feeling of malaise. It can be quite intense in the first few hours but tends to subside completely after 24 hours. While this illness is caused by a viral agent, it is not the influenza virus, and is not a form of the flu, notes Evan T. Bell, M.D. This is "gastroenteritis," an infection of the gastrointestinal tract.

Another common myth about influenza is that being cold or chilled makes us more susceptible to it (as well as to the common cold). According to W. Paul Glezen, M.D., several scientific studies on humans have shown that those exposed to severe temperatures for several hours fare no worse as far as becoming ill than those who are kept warm and dry. The myth is perpetuated because severe chills are one of the first symptoms of the flu, leading people to believe that they somehow "caught a chill" that led to the illness.

An additional myth is the belief that using medicine to keep the fever down helps us to get over the illness. "Experimental studies on the flu in animals show that more of the virus is excreted over a longer period of time when the body temperature is lowered with medication," says Glezen. "So while such treatments may make you feel better, they don't necessarily help you get over the virus."

has been associated with Reye's syndrome, an often fatal illness characterized by sudden, severe deterioration of brain and liver function.

DRINK, DRINK, DRINK.
Drinking plenty of nonalcoholic, decaffeinated liquid (caffeine actually increases fluid loss) to keep you hydrated and will also keep any mucous secretions you have more liquid. "Clear broth that is salty and warm tends to agree with people when they have the flu and are experiencing a general loss of appetite," says Glezen. Juices are also good for keeping some nutrients coming in when you're not eating much else.

HUMIDIFY YOUR HOME IN WINTER.
"Influenza viruses survive better when the humidity is low, which explains why they tend to show up more during the winter, when we use artificial heat to warm our homes," says Glezen. Humidifying your home in the winter not only helps to prevent the spread of flu, it also makes you feel better once you have it. "When you are really sick, a little extra humidity in the form of a warm- or cool-mist humidifier works wonders," he adds.

SUPPRESS A DRY COUGH.
For a dry, hacking cough that's keeping you from getting the rest you need, you can reach for over-the-counter relief. "Cough remedies containing dextromethorphan are best for a dry cough," says Kielhofner.

ENCOURAGE A "PRODUCTIVE" COUGH.
A cough that brings up mucus, on the other hand, is considered productive and should not be suppressed with

cough medicines. Drinking fluids will help bring the mucus of a productive cough up and will ease the cough a little as well, according to Glezen.

Food poisoning

8 Coping Tips

As anyone who's had a bad case of food poisoning can testify, it is an experience so thoroughly awful that you wouldn't wish it upon your worst enemy. Not only does everything you've eaten for the last 24 hours seem to want to escape out of both ends of your body simultaneously, but the cramps and pain you experience can make you want to crawl into a hole and die.

The good news is that food poisoning is rarely life-threatening. In most cases, it will pass within 24 hours, leaving you as good as new. The bad news is that once it's started, there's no real way to put the brakes on it until it has run its course.

The following tips, however, may help minimize your discomfort and shorten the duration of your symptoms.

REPLACE YOUR BODY'S FLUIDS.

If your stomach will tolerate it, be sure to keep taking liquids, especially if you have diarrhea, says Zachary T. Bloomgarden, M.D., an internist and assistant clinical professor of medicine at Mount Sinai School of Medicine in New York. "Sometimes people feel that if they drink more, they'll throw up more or have more diarrhea," he

PREVENTION IS THE BEST MEDICINE

The best way to treat food poisoning is to avoid getting it in the first place. Although you can't control the conditions in the restaurants you patronize, you can take several precautions in your own home, say John C. Johnson, M.D., and David Posner, M.D.

"Mixed foods, such as potato salads, creamy coleslaws, and other foods containing dairy products, are likely to breed bacteria, especially if they are not kept well refrigerated or if they get warm and are later refrigerated," Johnson says. Summer picnics are notorious for such conditions, he adds.

Another problem arises at holiday times when people tend to thaw and stuff turkeys or roasts hours before guests arrive, leaving them out of the refrigerator for long periods of time, according to Johnson.

"Make sure that perishables are kept cold," Posner says. "Cook chicken, pork, and beef very thoroughly, and wash hands and utensils in very hot water and soap after using them to cut meat."

says. "However, these illnesses require acute hydration. Even if you do have a little more diarrhea, you'll still be ahead of the game if you've been drinking more. Also, you feel worse if you are dehydrated." He recommends gelatin, decaffeinated soda, or water.

AVOID RICH OR SPICY FOODS.

When your stomach is feeling irritated, eating fatty or highly seasoned foods may send you right back to the toilet bowl, says John C. Johnson, M.D., past president of the American College of Emergency Physicians and director of the Emergency Department of Porter Memorial Hospital in Valparaiso, Indiana. If you feel hungry, it's probably best to restrict yourself to clear liquids, plain toast, mashed potatoes, bananas, gelatin, or other bland foods.

GO WITH THE FLOW—LITERALLY.

If you've been poisoned by contaminated food and your body is reacting with diarrhea or vomiting, you can trust your body's impulses, according to Johnson. "Don't run out and buy antidiarrheal medications," he says. "If there's something in your system, you may feel better sooner if you let it out. The same goes for vomiting— wait a while before you take anything orally. Your stomach doesn't want anything more down there. If you give it a chance to rest, it will usually take care of itself."

BE CAREFUL WITH PAIN MEDICATIONS.

Some people make the mistake of taking prescription or over-the-counter pain medications to reduce the discomfort of intestinal cramps, says Johnson. "The side effect of many of these drugs is to irritate the stomach or gastrointestinal tract," he says. The one exception is acetaminophen, says David Posner, M.D., a gastroenterologist and assistant professor of medicine at the University of Maryland School of Medicine in Baltimore. Drugs containing aspirin or ibuprofen are definitely out when your stomach is irritated.

HELLO, DOCTOR?

In rare instances, food poisoning may be downright dangerous. It's time to head for the doctor's office or the emergency room if you are experiencing severe cramps, if you are weak or dizzy, or if you can't keep anything at all down, says John C. Johnson, M.D. Ditto if you have a fever of over 102, if you faint, if the symptoms persist longer than 48 hours, or if you see any blood in your stool or vomitus, says David Posner, M.D. Other symptoms that signal an emergency are paralysis, double vision, breathlessness, or weakness in a limb, Posner says.

TRY A HOT-WATER BOTTLE.
One thing that may help cramps is a hot-water bottle placed on the stomach, according to Posner. "Make sure it's not too hot to the touch," he cautions.

TREAT IT LIKE THE STOMACH FLU.
Just like with the stomach flu, there's really not a whole lot you can do, except to be good to yourself and wait it out, says Bloomgarden. Cancel your appointments, rest, take it easy, and take solace in the fact that it's guaranteed to pass, most likely within 24 hours.

REPLACE YOUR POTASSIUM.
Vomiting and diarrhea may lead to a depletion in your body's supply of potassium, which may leave you feel-

ing even worse, according to Johnson. Twenty-four hours after your symptoms started, a sports drink or a banana "may perk you up," he says.

REPORT IT TO THE HEALTH DEPARTMENT.
If you were the only person affected by food that may have been contaminated, reporting your condition may not be necessary, according to Posner. However, if you were one of a group of people who ate at a restaurant or other food establishment and more than one of you became ill, tell the restaurant, your physician, or your local health department, he says. "If it turns out to be an infection, such as dysentery, the health department may want to track it down," he adds.

Foot aches

22 Ways to Ease the Agony

Our poor, overworked feet. In a single day, they absorb about 1,000 pounds of force as they carry us from place to place. And we mistreat them terribly—we stand on them for hours; we walk on hard, unyielding surfaces; and we cram them into shoes that may be fashionable, but often uncomfortable. It's no wonder that four out of five adults eventually suffer from foot problems.

Foot pain is so common, podiatrist Andrew Schink, D.P.M., past president of the Oregon Podiatric Medical

Association and podiatrist in private practice in Eugene, quips, "At parties, I've stopped telling people what I do for a living."

While certainly not as glamorous as the heart or the brain, the feet are amazing pieces of engineering, perfectly designed to give years of service—if you treat them right. Each foot has 26 bones—together the feet have almost one-quarter of the bones in the entire body. Thirty-three joints make the feet flexible and 19 muscles control movement of foot parts. Tendons stretch tautly between muscles and bones, moving parts of the feet as the muscles contract. Two arches in the midfoot and forefoot, constructed like small bridges, support each foot and provide a springy, elastic structure to absorb shock. Numerous nerve endings in the feet make them sensitive (and ticklish). And the whole structure is held together by more than 100 ligaments.

As incredible as our feet may be, few of us ever think about them until they hurt. And when they do hurt, it's difficult to think of anything else. Fortunately, if your dogs are barking, there are several things you can do to soothe and pamper your tired, aching, overworked feet. There are also some simple steps you can take to prevent serious foot problems from developing in the first place. Here are some suggestions:

TAKE A LOAD OFF.

Much of the foot pain we experience comes from tired muscles. "The leg has four basic muscle groups that move the foot up, down, and from side to side," explains Schink. "After a period of time, the foot flattens out because the muscles get overly fatigued from trying to hold up the foot."

If you have to stand a great deal, take breaks to take the weight off your feet. The same advice applies if you do a lot of walking. Whenever you can, elevate your feet at a 45-degree angle to your body, and relax for 10 to 15 minutes. Elevating your feet will move blood away from the feet and help reduce swelling.

GIVE THEM A SOAK.

Put two tablespoons of Epsom salts (available without a prescription at your local drugstore) into a basin of comfortably warm water and give your aching feet a relaxing bath for 15 minutes, says Schink. Then, pat your feet dry with a soft towel, and don't forget the moisturizer.

ALTERNATE HOT AND COLD.

Sit on the edge of the bathtub and alternately run cold water, then (comfortably) hot water (for one minute each) on the feet; end with cold water. If you are diabetic, do not try this without your doctor's OK.

GIVE THEM THE SQUEEZE.

There's nothing quite as relaxing as a foot massage. Have a partner massage your feet with massage oil, baby oil, or moisturizing lotion. Or treat yourself by massaging your own feet. First, apply oil, and condition the foot with medium-light strokes, using your thumbs and fingers. Next, starting with the ball of the foot, work across and down the entire foot using the thumbs to make small, circular motions. Use the thumbs to make long, deep strokes along the arch of the foot, moving in the direction of the toes. Gently squeeze, rotate, and pull each toe. End by cupping the foot between both hands and gently squeezing up and down the length of each foot.

ICE 'EM.

A cool way to refresh your feet after a long, hard day is to ice them down with a washcloth filled with ice cubes. It will make them feel wonderful and it will also decrease swelling.

EXERCISE YOUR FEET.

Like any part of the body, the feet stay healthiest if they're kept strong and flexible with regular exercise. Walking in shoes that provide good support and cushioning is excellent exercise for the feet.

Feet also benefit from specific foot exercises. Michael Martindale, L.P.T., a physical therapist at the Sports Medicine Center at Portland Adventist Medical Center in Oregon who specializes in athletic injuries, suggests the following:

• **Golf-Ball Roll:** With your shoe off, place your foot on top of a golf ball, and roll (don't stand) on the ball using only the weight of the foot.

• **Spill the Beans:** Scatter beans or marbles on the floor, and pick them up with your toes.

• **Circle and Stretch:** Sit in a chair with your feet out in front of you, and make four or five small circles in both directions with your feet. Next, stretch your toes out as far as you can; then stretch them up toward you. Repeat six times.

TRIM YOUR TOENAILS.

Ingrown toenails may be inherited, but improper nail trimming can make the problem worse. Trim the nails straight across and only to the end of the toe, then file the corners to remove sharp edges that might cut the skin (see INGROWN TOENAILS).

HIGH-HEEL HELL

Remember your grandmother's feet? Chances are good they were misshapen with corns, bunions, calluses, and curled toes. Chances are equally good your grandfather had long, well-formed feet. A genetic difference? No, it's probably high-heel hell, the purgatory women's feet are put through by high-heeled shoes.

"The body can tolerate a heel up to about an inch," says Kathleen Galligan, D.C., who frequently sees the results of high-heeled shoes in her chiropractic practice. "But over an inch rocks all your weight onto the ball of your foot. It causes the Achilles tendon to shorten and the pelvis to shift forward."

The result of this precarious sliding forward can cause all kinds of structural problems, including back pain and foot pain. Podiatrists often see women for "forefoot shock"—

MAINTAIN IDEAL WEIGHT.

Being overweight puts excess strain on your feet, as well as on all of the other weight-bearing joints of the body.

BUY SHOES THAT FIT.

Too often, people buy shoes that don't fit their feet. They opt for fashion rather than fit or comfort. "I could make almost any foot problem feel better with the right pair of shoes," says Schink.

He says to look for shoes that:

• Have plenty of room in the toe area (toe box).

pain, fatigue, and a wobbly gait caused by the body's weight being centered on the ball of the foot.

Sometimes, we just can't get around the convention of wearing high-heeled shoes at work or social gatherings. But here are a few ideas to help you minimize the strain on your feet.

• Wear the lowest heel you can find.

• If you must wear high-heeled shoes, wear lower-heeled or flat shoes to and from work and during lunch and breaks.

• Look for shoes that are more rounded in the toe area; avoid pointy shoes that pinch the toes.

• Buy shoes that are large enough to accommodate added padding or an arch support. A half insole can help keep your foot in place when you wear heeled shoes. Experiment and see what works for you.

• Buy the thickest heel possible for the greatest stability.

• Don't slip. The foot should not slide around in the shoe.
• Are wide enough. Your foot shouldn't bulge over the edges of the shoe.
• Fit in the store. Don't buy shoes that are too small for your feet believing that you'll "stretch them out" with wearing.

KNOW YOUR FEET.

Different types of feet require different kinds of shoes, according to Martyn Shorten, Ph.D., former director of NIKE's Sports Research Laboratory. "High-arched feet tend to be rigid and need shoes that provide good cushioning and absorb shock," he says. "Flat feet have lots of flexibility so they need shoes that can control excess motion."

To find out what kind of foot you have, wet your bare feet and stand on a concrete floor or piece of paper. If you have high arches, the outline of your foot will appear very narrow and curved like a half-moon. If the outline looks like a slab, you're probably flat-footed.

WEAR THE RIGHT SHOE FOR THE ACTIVITY.

"The wrong shoe can cause injuries such as tendinitis in the knees, chronic foot pain, heel spurs, and stress fractures," says Kathleen Galligan, D.C., a chiropractor in Lake Oswego, Oregon, who specializes in sports injuries.

She says each activity has its own set of repetitive movements that require special support and cushioning. You wouldn't play basketball in a pair of heels. Likewise, don't rely on that old pair of sneakers if you're going climbing or hiking. Spend the extra money to buy shoes that are specific for the activity you're doing. The investment could save you and your feet a good deal of discomfort.

REPLACE WORN SHOES.

It's tough to give up those old favorite shoes, but often we wear shoes long after they've lost their ability to support and cushion the foot. "Shoes are often worn out before you can see the wear," says Galligan.

She advises paying attention to the worn-out-shoe messages from your body. "If your feet hurt, your legs feel tired, your knees are sore, or your hips hurt, it's definitely time to buy a new pair of shoes."

Foot odor

13 Steps to Sweeter-Smelling Feet

I f removing your footwear at the end of the day calls to mind the scent of a postgame locker room, you may be suffering from what is scientifically known as bromhidrosis—sweaty, smelly feet.

While neither painful nor contagious, foot odor causes unmitigated social suffering to those who have it. Normally, each of your feet produces half a pint of sweat a day by means of some 20,000 sweat glands. In most people, this perspiration evaporates. In people with bromhidrosis, however, more sweat is produced, and it doesn't evaporate as easily. The result: odoriferous feet.

If you suffer from this problem, don't worry. You don't have to stand for it anymore. Simply follow these suggestions for keeping your feet drier and sweeter smelling.

WASH WELL.

Those sweat glands on the soles of your feet produce perspiration composed of water, sodium chloride, fat, minerals, and various acids that are end products of your body's metabolism. In the presence of certain bacteria, these sweaty secretions break down, generating a foul smell. Obviously, washing away the bacteria will short-circuit this process. "Washing your feet often with a deodorant soap and drying very carefully can *temporarily* make your feet smell sweet," says Joseph C. D'Amico, D.P.M., a podiatrist in private practice in New York.

WASH WISELY.

How often should you wash your feet? Enough to remove the offending bacteria but not so often that you remove all the protective oils from your skin. For strong foot odor, you may need to bathe your feet several times a day. However, if you notice that your feet are becoming scaly and cracked, cut back on the number of washings.

SOAK THE SWEAT OUT OF THEM.

Suzanne M. Levine, D.P.M., a podiatrist in private practice in New York, suggests the following treatment for sweaty feet. First, alternate footbaths of hot and cold water to help decrease blood flow to your feet and reduce perspiration. Next, dip your feet into another footbath containing ice cubes and lemon juice. Finally, rub your feet with alcohol. In hot weather, when your feet tend to perspire more, this form of treatment should be repeated daily. If you have diabetes or any other condition that causes decreased circulation, do not try this treatment at all.

SALT YOUR TOOTSIES.

For extra-sweaty feet, try adding half a cup of kosher salt (it has larger crystals than ordinary table salt) to a quart of water and soaking your feet in the solution. After soaking, don't rinse your feet; just dry them thoroughly.

TREAT THEM LIKE UNDERARMS.

"The key to controlling foot odor is to use either an antiperspirant or a deodorant right on your feet," advises Levine. Foot deodorants, like underarm deodorants, contain antibacterial agents that can kill bacteria. They won't stop the sweat, but they will eliminate the odor that ensues when sweat meets bacteria. Antiperspirants, however, stop the sweat and the smell simultaneously.

TAKE A POWDER.
Spray or put on foot-deodorant powder. Be sure it contains aluminum chloride hexahydrate, advises Levine.

SOCK 'EM AWAY.
"Clean feet need clean coverings," remarks Mary Papadopoulos, D.P.M., a podiatrist in private practice in Alexandria, Virginia. Wear socks that let your feet breathe. (Some experts advise cotton or wool, others suggest acrylic; try different fabrics until you find the one that seems to keep your feet driest.) If possible, change your socks at least once during the day, and don't wear the same pair two days in a row. Contrary to popular belief, white socks are not sterile and do contain dye, so they are not preferable to colored socks.

SHOE IT AWAY.
"Stay away from solid-rubber or synthetically lined shoes, because they don't allow your feet to breathe easily, allowing odor-producing bacteria to flourish," says Levine.

WASH YOUR SNEAKERS.
Some shoes—such as sneakers—should go right in the washing machine, says D'Amico. Let them air dry rather than throwing them in the dryer.

LET YOUR SHOES BREATHE.
Try airing out your shoes between wearings, too. If you can, alternate shoes on a daily basis so that you don't wear the same pair two days in a row. Loosen the laces

and pull up the tongue on the pair you're not wearing, and let them dry out in the sunshine.

SPRINKLE YOUR SHOES.
Sprinkle the inside of your shoes with cornstarch to help absorb moisture and keep your feet drier.

EAT WISELY.
"Eating certain strong foods, such as onions, garlic, scallions, peppers, and even curry, can cause strong foot odor," says D'Amico. The odoriferous products pass through the bloodstream and eventually concentrate in the perspiration. While this effect is not restricted to foot perspiration, it certainly won't help a case of smelly feet.

KEEP CALM.
Stress and anxiety increase production of sweat, giving those nasty little bacteria even more to feed on. "A level of stress so high that it produces foot odor should be dealt with right away, because other parts of the body are probably feeling the toll, as well," says Levine.

Grinding teeth
11 Ways to Conquer the Daily Grind

Everybody handles excess stress differently. Some people develop an ulcer, some develop high blood pressure, and some people grind or clench their teeth.

Stress, it's now believed, is the major cause of grinding and clenching, say dental researchers. In the past, a malocclusion (the way your teeth fit together) got the blame, and dentists would grind the teeth down, trying to readjust the bite.

In a small percentage of cases, sleep patterns are responsible, says Daniel M. Laskin, D.D.S., M.S., professor and chairman of the Department of Oral and Maxillofacial Surgery and director of the TMJ and Facial Pain Research Center at the Medical College of Virginia in Richmond. The reasons children grind remain unclear.

The problem with bruxism, as the habit of grinding and clenching is called, is the wear and tear on your teeth. "It can wear away tooth enamel, causing decay and sensitive teeth," says Laskin. Expensive dental work can get destroyed in the process, too. "And, you can get aching jaw muscles, which may be confused with pain in the joint and the symptoms of temporomandibular [jaw] joint [TMJ] disorder," Laskin adds. (See TEMPOROMANDIBULAR JOINT SYNDROME.)

Prolonged grinding may damage the jaw joint enough to cause osteoarthritis, says John D. Rugh, Ph.D., professor in the Department of Orthodontics and director of research for the Dental School at the University of Texas Health Science Center at San Antonio. And it can increase bone loss in periodontal (gum) disease, although it does not actually cause gum disease.

You may inherit the tendency to grind your teeth, says Rugh. Three times as many women as men grind their teeth, says Thomas F. Truhe, D.D.S., codirector of the Princeton Dental Resource Center in New Jersey. Bruxism is most common in those between 20 and 40 years of age.

Ironically, the regular grinder may do less harm than the intermittent grinder—sort of like the weekend athlete who's not in shape for intense activity. The regular grinder can wear down teeth, but his or her muscles get stronger from the habit, says Laskin.

Clenching may do more harm than grinding, adds Laskin. "Your jaws are constructed for bruxing, or chewing, but clenching loads the joint isometrically and can end up causing degenerative changes in the joint."

People who grind are usually aware of their habit, too, says Laskin. They wake up with a stiff or tired jaw, or their spouse hears the noise during the night. Clenchers, on the other hand, may be ignorant of their problem. "If you notice the pain gets worse as the day goes on, then you're doing something in the daytime," says Laskin.

Here's what you can do to try to stop bruxing and to cope with discomfort until you do:

WEAR A NIGHT GUARD.

Your dentist can make a plastic or acrylic appliance for you to wear at night. It will redistribute the forces from grinding and protect your teeth from damage. "It's a little like banging your head against the wall and putting a pillow between your head and the wall so it doesn't hurt anymore," says Rugh. Opinions are divided as to whether it will actually keep you from grinding. Your dentist will want to see you regularly to check for any tooth movement or cavities that might result from wearing it.

KEEP YOUR LIPS SEALED, TEETH APART.

Your teeth should be touching only when you're chewing or swallowing. Drop your jaw and feel the muscles relax—then try to maintain that feeling.

TAKE A WARM BATH BEFORE BEDTIME.

You may temporarily relax your jaw muscles, although they may not stay that way, says Laskin.

EXERCISE.

Your body, not your jaw, that is. A walk or other mild exercise may help relieve some of the tension and stress that's causing bruxism, says Rugh.

REMIND YOURSELF.

If you're a daytime clencher, you can put a red dot on your phone, stickers on your wristwatch, or even a string on your finger to remind you to keep your jaw relaxed, says Rugh.

RELIEVE STRESS.

"Change jobs, get a divorce, get married, move the kids out, but if you can relieve stress, you can relieve the bruxism," says Rugh.

"Don't forget that good things as well as bad things can cause stress," says Laskin. "I've had patients say they don't have any stress, then they go on to say they've got a wonderful husband, two kids, a great job, they're active in the PTA, they do this and that, and it's all good, but it's overload."

LEARN COPING SKILLS.

See a psychologist or psychiatrist. Take an assertiveness training course. Practice techniques such as progressive relaxation or guided imagery or self-hypnosis. Listen to relaxation tapes. In other words, find something that helps you to better handle the stress in your life and stick with it.

TAKE A MILD ANALGESIC.

Ibuprofen, for example, can dull the pain and help relax stiff muscles.

APPLY HEAT.

Warm, moist heat is best. The simplest method: Soak a washcloth in hot water, wring it out, and hold it up to your jaw. You can use a heating pad, although moist heat will penetrate better. A hot shower's nice, too. "Think of these muscles like the baseball pitcher treats the sore muscles in his pitching arm," suggests Truhe.

MASSAGE.

It works for the rest of your body, so try a gentle massage to your jaw muscles.

GIVE YOUR JAW MUSCLES A BREAK.

Avoid the steak, the hard-crusted bread, and the popcorn for a while. "Your muscles aren't able to tolerate that much activity," says Laskin. Chewing gum's a no-no, too, if your jaw muscles ache.

Headaches

16 Ways to Keep the Pain at Bay

Headaches. We've all had them. From the morning-after-celebrating-too-much headache to the tough-day-at-the-office headache to the you-might-as-well-kill-me-now-because-I'm-going-to-die-anyway headache. Sometimes, an aspirin or other analgesic may ease the pain; at other times, nothing short of waiting it out seems to help.

If you suffer from frequent, severe headaches that put you out of commission several times a month, you need to seek medical attention. Likewise, if your headaches are associated with physical exertion, changes in vision, or weakness, numbness, or paralysis of the limbs, skip the urge to self-treat and see a doctor. If you're already seeing a physician and aren't getting relief, think about getting a referral to a headache specialist or headache clinic.

However, if you are prone to occasional headache pain, read on. The tips that follow can help you feel a lot better—fast.

DON'T OVERDO THE PAIN PILLS.

Although an occasional dose of an over-the-counter analgesic may help alleviate your headache for a few hours, taking these drugs too often may actually worsen the pain, according to Sabiha Ali, M.D., a neurologist at the Houston Headache Clinic in Texas. "These drugs are OK in limited quantities," she says, "but if you need to take more than two doses a day, you should see a doctor."

LIE DOWN.

Lying down and closing your eyes for half an hour or more may be one of the best treatments for a bad headache. For some types of headaches, such as migraines, sleep is the only thing that seems to interrupt the pain cycle. "The most important thing is to recognize that the faster the patient with a severe headache stops what they're doing and goes to bed and rests, the faster the headache will go away," says James R. Couch, Jr., M.D., Ph.D., professor and chairman of the Department of Neurology at the University of Oklahoma Health Sciences Center in Oklahoma City. "You need to recognize when the big headache is coming. That's the time to give up and go to bed."

DON'T LET THE SUN SHINE IN.

Especially if your symptoms resemble those of a migraine (such as severe pain on one side of the head, nausea, blurred vision, and extreme sensitivity to light), resting in a darkened room may alleviate the pain. Bright light may also cause headaches, according to Seymour Diamond, M.D., founder of Diamond Headache Clinic in Chicago. "Sometimes, looking at a computer screen may bring on a headache," he says. "Tinted glasses may help."

USE A COLD COMPRESS.

A washcloth dipped in ice-cold water and placed over the eyes or an ice pack placed on the site of the pain are other good ways of relieving a headache, says Fred D. Sheftell, M.D., director and founder of The New England Center for Headache in Stamford, Connecticut. "Other good solutions are the 'headache hat,' which is an ice pack that surrounds the head, and the ice pillow, which is a frozen gel pack that is inserted into a special pillow," he says. (These special ice packs can be found in some pharmacies; if you don't see them at yours, ask your pharmacist about ordering them.) Using ice as soon as possible after the onset of the headache will relieve the pain within 20 minutes for most people, according to Sheftell.

TRY HEAT.

If ice feels uncomfortable to you, or if it doesn't seem to help your headache, you can try placing a warm washcloth over your eyes or on the site of the pain, Ali says. She recommends leaving the compress on for half an hour, rewarming it once or twice if the washcloth gets cool.

THINK PLEASANT THOUGHTS.

Many headaches are brought on or worsened by stress and tension, according to Couch. Learning to handle life's difficulties in a calm way may keep the volume down on a bad headache, he says. "Turn off all thoughts of unpleasant, crisis-provoking things," he says. "Think about pleasant things. Just for the moment, try to forget about the confrontation with the boss or the coworker. Try to relax while you work out a strategy to cope with the problem."

CHECK FOR TENSION.

Along with the preceding tip, Sheftell recommends that patients periodically check their body for tension throughout the day. "If you notice that you get these headaches frequently, check the body for signs of tension," he says. "Are your jaws set very tightly? Are you scrunching your forehead? You want to check to see if your fists are clenched. Also, when you stop at a red light, are your hands gripping the wheel very tightly?" If the answer to any of the questions is yes—stop, relax, and take a deep breath or two (don't go beyond a couple of deep breaths, though; otherwise, you may begin to hyperventilate).

(Continued on page 322)

....

RECIPES FOR RELAXATION

In addition to being given an antityramine diet (see Diamond Antiheadache Diet"), patients at Diamond Headache Clinic in Chicago are instructed in relaxation techniques. The following is a typical relaxation exercise. The exercise can be memorized, or the written instructions can be recorded on a cassette tape. The entire exercise, which relaxes the facial area, neck, shoulders, and upper back, takes about five minutes. Before you begin, make sure you won't be disturbed—close the door and take the phone off the hook.

1. Settle back quietly and comfortably into a favorite chair or sofa. Let your muscles become loose and heavy.

2. Wrinkle up your forehead, hold it, then smooth it out, picturing the entire forehead becoming smoother as the relaxation increases.

3. Frown, creasing your eyebrows tightly, feeling the tension. Let go of the tension, smoothing out your forehead once more.

4. Close your eyes more and more tightly. Feel the tension as you hold them shut. Relax your eyes until they are closed gently and comfortably.

5. Clench your jaws and teeth together. Feel the tension build, then let go and relax, letting the lips part slightly. Allow yourself to feel relief in the relaxation.

6. Press your tongue hard against the roof of your mouth. Again, feel the tension, then relax.

7. Purse your lips together more and more tightly, then relax. Notice the contrast between tension and relaxation.

Feel the relaxation all over your face, forehead and scalp, eyes, jaws, lips, and tongue.

8. Press your head back against your chair, concentrating on the tension in the neck. Roll your head to the right and feel the tension shift. Repeat to the left. Then straighten your head and bring it forward, pressing your chin to your chest. Finally, allow your head to return to a comfortable upright position.

9. Shrug your shoulders up to your ears, holding the tension, then drop. Repeat the shrug, then move the shoulders forward and backward, feeling the tension in your shoulders and upper back. Drop the shoulders and relax.

10. Allow the relaxation to spread deep into the shoulders, into your back. Relax your neck and throat. Relax your jaws and face. Allow the relaxation to take over and grow deeper and deeper. When you are ready, slowly open your eyes.

Fred D. Sheftell, M.D., recommends the following relaxation exercise to his headache patients:

Lie down and relax your muscles. Place your hand on your stomach and take a deep breath. As you inhale to the count of five, feel your stomach rise. Allow yourself to slowly exhale to the count of five, letting your stomach fall. Imagine that you are breathing in relaxation and breathing out tension. As you breathe, visualize the muscles in your head and neck as if they were scrunched up, tense. Then, picture them becoming relaxed and smooth, parallel to one another. Continue the deep breathing for five minutes, then slowly open your eyes.

QUIT SMOKING.

Smoking may bring on or worsen a headache, Couch says, especially if you suffer from cluster headaches—extremely painful headaches that last from 5 to 20 minutes and come in groups.

DON'T DRINK.

Alcohol, aside from its notorious morning-after effect, may also bring on migraines and cluster headaches, according to Diamond. Alcoholic beverages contain tyramine, an amino acid that may stimulate headaches (see "Diamond Antiheadache Diet" for other foods and beverages that contain tyramine).

START A PROGRAM OF REGULAR EXERCISE.

Regular exercise helps to release the physical and emotional tension that may lead to headaches, according to Ali. She recommends walking or jogging. These and other aerobic activities, she says, help to boost the body's production of endorphins (natural pain-relieving substances).

CUT DOWN ON CAFFEINE.

"Caffeine can increase muscle tension and your anxiety level," Sheftell says. "It also creates difficulties in sleeping, which can cause headaches." Another problem is that many people drink several cups of coffee a day during their work week but cut their consumption on weekends. This can lead to weekend caffeine-withdrawal headaches, according to Sheftell. "My advice to those people is for them to slowly decaffeinate themselves," he says. "Decrease your caffeine intake by one-half cup per week. I suggest that people who are prone to headaches cut down to the equivalent of one cup of caffeinated coffee per day," says Sheftell. One five-ounce cup of drip coffee contains about 150 milligrams of caffeine. A five-ounce cup of tea brewed for three to five minutes may contain 20 to 50 milligrams of caffeine. And cola drinks contain about 35 to 45 milligrams of caffeine per 12-ounce serving. (Try substituting decaffeinated varieties of coffee, tea, or soft drinks.) Sheftell also recommends checking the caffeine content of any over-the-counter drugs in your medicine cabinet.

FIGHT THE NAUSEA FIRST.

Some headaches may be accompanied by nausea, which can make you feel even worse. What's more, the gastric juices produced by stomach upset may hinder the absorption of certain over-the-counter and prescription analgesics, which may make these drugs less effective at relieving the pain of your headache. So, by first taking care of the nausea, the pain of the headache may be easier to treat, says Sheftell. He says that many of his patients have found that drinking peach juice, apricot nectar, or flat cola has helped alleviate nausea. Over-the-counter antinauseants such as Emetrol and Dramamine may also be useful.

RISE AND RETIRE AT THE SAME TIME EVERY DAY.

Going to bed and getting up at the same time every day also helps prevent headaches, according to Diamond. "Changes in body chemistry that occur when you oversleep can precipitate migraines or other headaches," he says.

(Continued on page 326)

DIAMOND ANTIHEADACHE DIET

At Diamond Headache Clinic in Chicago, patients are advised to eat foods low in tyramine, an amino acid that is known to promote headaches, nausea, and high blood pressure. People who take certain antidepressant drugs called monoamine oxidase inhibitors are especially prone to accumulating high amounts of tyramine. The following diet keeps tyramine levels to a minimum.

BEVERAGES

Foods allowed: Decaffeinated coffee, fruit juices, club soda, noncola sodas.

Foods to avoid: Caffeine: coffee, tea, colas in excess of two cups per day. Cocoa, alcoholic beverages.

DAIRY

Foods allowed: Milk: homogenized, low-fat, or skim. Cheese: American, cottage, farmer, ricotta, cream cheese. Yogurt: limit to one-half cup per day.

Foods to avoid: Cultured dairy, such as buttermilk, sour cream, chocolate milk. Cheese: not listed above.

MEAT, FISH, POULTRY

Foods allowed: Fresh or frozen turkey, chicken, fish, beef, lamb, veal, pork, eggs (three per week), tuna fish.

Foods to avoid: Aged, canned, cured, or processed meats; pickled herring; salted, dried fish; chicken liver; aged game; hot dogs; fermented sausages (no nitrates or nitrites allowed), including bologna, salami, pepperoni, summer sausage; any meat prepared with meat tenderizer, soy sauce, or yeast extracts.

BREADS AND CEREALS

Foods allowed: Commercial breads: white, whole wheat, rye, French, Italian, English muffins, melba toast, crackers, bagels. All hot and dry cereals.

Foods to avoid: Hot, fresh, homemade yeast breads; breads and crackers containing cheese; fresh yeast coffee cake, doughnuts, sourdough breads; any breads or cereals containing chocolate or nuts.

STARCHES

Foods allowed: Potatoes, sweet potatoes, rice, macaroni, spaghetti, noodles.

VEGETABLES, LEGUMES, AND SEEDS

Foods allowed: All except those listed below.

Foods to avoid: Pole, broad, lima, or Italian beans; lentils; snow peas; fava, navy, or pinto beans; pea pods; sauerkraut; garbanzo beans; onions (except as a condiment); olives; pickles; peanuts; sunflower, sesame, or pumpkin seeds.

FRUIT

Foods allowed: Prunes, apples, cherries, apricots, peaches, pears. Citrus fruits and juices: Limit to one-half cup per day of orange, grapefruit, tangerine, pineapple, lemon, or lime.

Foods to avoid: Avocados, bananas (one-half allowed per day), figs, raisins, papaya, passion fruit, red plums.

DESSERTS

Foods allowed: Fruits listed above, ice cream, cakes and cookies without chocolate or yeast, gelatin.

Foods to avoid: Chocolate-flavored ice cream, pudding, cookies, or cakes; mincemeat pies.

HEADACHE RESOURCES

The following associations provide support and information for headache sufferers:

The American Council for Headache Education (ACHE). ACHE provides patient information and referrals to headache specialists. The organization also sends out free informational pamphlets about headache treatment. In the future, ACHE plans to set up patient-support groups around the country. You can contact ACHE at 1-800-255-ACHE.

The National Headache Foundation. This organization sends out free headache information to patients and publishes a headache newsletter. You can contact the Foundation at 1-800-843-2256.

KEEP A HEADACHE DIARY.

If you get frequent headaches, try to tease out the factors that seem to be responsible, says Sheftell. "Pick up patterns. Figure out a way to record headaches and rate them on a zero-to-three scale of intensity: no headache, mild headache, moderate to severe headache, incapacitating headache. Start to look at what foods you are eating. Women should begin tracking their periods, as well as their use of hormone-replacement medications or oral contraceptives. You can show this calendar to your doctor."

Heartburn

21 Ways to Beat the Burn

Heartburn. The word evokes a frightening picture: Your heart on fire, sizzling and smoking, without a fire fighter in sight. Fortunately, the word is a misnomer. It's not your heart that's on fire, it's your esophagus. But heartburn is easier to say than "esophagusburn."

The "burn" part, however, they got right. Your esophagus, the food tube that carries what you swallow down to your stomach, can literally be burned by the acids released by your stomach. Those acids are industrial-strength stuff and are meant to stay where the tough stomach lining can handle them.

Unfortunately, we can experience something called reflux. That's when some of the stomach contents, including the acid, slip back up through the esophageal sphincter, the valve that's supposed to prevent the stomach's contents from reversing course.

David M. Taylor, M.D., a gastroenterologist and assistant professor of medicine at Emory University in Atlanta and at the Medical College of Georgia in Augusta, puts it plainly: "If it goes south, that's good; if it goes north, you're in trouble."

Reflux causes an uncomfortable burning sensation between the stomach and the neck. Most people feel the discomfort right below the breastbone.

The easy way to avoid a simple case of heartburn? Moderation. Heartburn is generally the result of eating too much too fast. But if it's too late for moderation, here are some ways to put out that fire and keep it from flaring up again.

TAKE AN ANTACID.

Over-the-counter antacids in tablet or liquid form can help cool the burn. Take a dose about every six hours as needed, says Nalin M. Patel, M.D., a gastroenterologist in private practice and clinical instructor at the University of Illinois at Urbana-Champaign. Don't overdo it, though, because too much antacid can cause constipation or diarrhea.

DON'T FORGET YOUR BEDTIME DOSE.

Even if you forget to take an antacid during the day, try to remember to take one at bedtime to protect yourself from the pooling of stomach acids. "Nighttime damage is probably the worst that will occur, because you're bathing your esophagus in acid, and you're much more prone to burn it," says Douglas C. Walta, M.D., a gastroenterologist in private practice in Portland, Oregon. Try keeping a bottle of antacid on your nightstand so that you remember to take your nightly dose.

HAVE A GLASS OF MILK.

Milk can sometimes cut the acid and decrease heartburn, says Taylor.

KEEP YOUR HEAD UP.

Another way to protect your esophagus while you sleep is to elevate the head of your bed. That way, you'll be sleeping on a slope, and gravity will work for you in keeping your stomach contents where they belong. Put

HEIMLICH MANEUVER WON'T HELP THIS

Heartburn can become very serious, says Douglas C. Walta, M.D. The acid reflux of heartburn can sometimes burn the lining of the esophagus so badly that scar tissue will build up. The resulting strictures can cause food to get stuck in the esophagus.

A person with a piece of food stuck in his or her esophagus can still breathe and talk, says Walta. "It doesn't interfere with breathing, but if it totally occludes, all of a sudden you can't swallow your saliva."

The Heimlich maneuver, used for dislodging an object that is obstructing the airway, is not the appropriate treatment in this case. Usually, a doctor must use a special instrument that is inserted into the esophagus to dislodge the food. So if it feels as if you have food stuck in your esophagus or if you are having trouble swallowing your saliva, see a doctor.

---

wooden blocks or bricks under the legs at the head of your bed in order to bring it up about six inches, advises Patel.

GET RID OF YOUR WATER BED.
"People with water beds who have reflux have to get rid of their water beds," says Walta. "They don't like to hear

that." The problem with a water bed is that your body basically lies flat on the water-filled mattress. You can't effectively elevate your chest and so can't keep your stomach contents from heading north.

SAY NO TO THE COUCH.

Tempting as it may look, the couch is not your friend after eating a meal. People who lie down with a full stomach are asking for trouble. "Stay upright for one hour after meals," says Patel.

DON'T EAT BEFORE BED.

Heading from the dinner table to bed is a no-no for heartburn sufferers. In fact, doctors recommend warding off sleepy time for two to three hours after a meal. And by that, they mean staying upright for that amount of time. "You should stay upright until the gastric contents are emptied," says Walta.

PASS ON SECONDS.

"If you overeat, it's kind of like a balloon," says Walta. "If you blow it up real tense, it's more likely to empty quickly if you release the valve." A stomach, ballooned by too much food and drink, may partly empty in the wrong direction.

LOOSEN YOUR BELT.

"Avoid tight clothing around the waist," says Patel. "This tends to increase acid backing up into the esophagus."

LOSE THE FAT.

If you're fat on the outside, you can be sure you're fat on the inside, too, says Walta. "The fat competes for space with your stomach." Fat pressing against the stomach can cause the contents to reflux.

DON'T BLAME THE BABY.

For the same reason that fat can impede normal digestion—competition for space—pregnancy can cause heartburn. That's all the more reason expectant mothers should watch what they eat and give up that nonsense about eating for two. Remember, pregnant or not, you only have one stomach. Be sure to discuss with your doctor any questions you may have about proper diet and weight gain during pregnancy.

GET IN SHAPE.

"Couch potatoes have heartburn," according to Taylor. "You almost never have heartburn when you exercise." Even mild exercise done on a regular basis, such as a daily walk around the neighborhood, may help ease digestive woes. However, avoid working out strenuously immediately after a meal. You'd be better off to wait a couple of hours.

WATCH YOUR DIET.

"A high-carbohydrate, low-fat, high-bulk diet is the best thing," says Taylor. Fried foods and fatty foods should be avoided, he says, because they take longer to digest. Highly spiced foods sometimes contribute to heartburn as well.

DON'T SMOKE.

Nicotine from cigarette smoke irritates the valve between the stomach and the esophagus, as well as the stomach lining, so smokers tend to get more heartburn.

··

IS IT REALLY HEARTBURN?

If symptoms don't subside, you may have something other than a simple case of heartburn.

"Persistent heartburn can be a sign of significant disease," warns David M. Taylor, M.D. "They [persistent-heartburn sufferers] can have hiatal hernia or esophagitis [inflammation of the esophagus], they can have an ulcer in their stomach, they can have an ulcer in the duodenum [part of the small intestine], and in an older person, they can even have cancer. And sometimes heartburn can mimic coronary disease, and they can have heart trouble."

The best advice: If symptoms persist, see your doctor.

··

BE CAREFUL OF COFFEE.
It may not be the caffeine that's the problem. The oils contained in both regular *and* decaffeinated coffee may play a role in heartburn. Try cutting your coffee intake to see if your heartburn troubles subside.

BE WARY OF PEPPERMINT.
For some people, peppermint seems to cause heartburn. Try skipping the after-dinner mints and see if it helps.

HOLD THE PEPPER.
For people with heartburn problems, using pepper is not such a hot idea, says Kimra Warren, R.D., a registered dietitian at St. Vincent Hospital and Medical Center in

Portland, Oregon. Whether red or black, pepper may contribute to heartburn, so go easy.

TAKE IT EASY.
"A big contributor to heartburn is stress," says Taylor. Stress can create increased acid secretion and can cause the esophageal sphincter to malfunction.

DON'T CRACK OPEN A COLD ONE.
Alcohol can relax the sphincter, notes Taylor. It can irritate the stomach, too, which can lead to reflux.

SLOW DOWN ON SODA.
Carbonated drinks can lead to heartburn. "Carbonation causes stomach distention due to gas, and that causes acid rolling back up into the esophagus," Patel says.

CHECK YOUR PAINKILLER.
If you're about to pop a couple of aspirin in your mouth, think again. Aspirin, ibuprofen, and products that contain them can burn the esophagus as well as the stomach, warns Walta. Opt for acetaminophen instead.

Hemorrhoids

14 Ways to End the Torment

When was the last time you heard a party conversation turn to the subject of hemorrhoids? The condition is rarely discussed, even between close friends and relatives, although Americans spend $150 million a year on remedies that promise relief.

Hemorrhoids are swollen and stretched-out veins that line the anal canal and lower rectum. Internal hemorrhoids may either bulge into the anal canal or protrude out through the anus, in which case they are called "prolapsed." External hemorrhoids occur under the surface of the skin at the anal opening. Regardless of type, hemorrhoids cause cruel distress: They hurt, burn, itch, irritate the anal area, and, very often, bleed.

About one-half to three-fourths of all Americans will develop hemorrhoids at some time in their lives. The following factors contribute to them, and some can be avoided.

• **Gravity.** Humans stand upright, which causes a downward pressure on all veins in the body, including those in the anal canal and rectum.

• **Genes.** If one parent has hemorrhoids, it is more likely that his or her child will develop them in adult life; if both parents have hemorrhoids, it is an almost certain outcome.

• **Age.** While hemorrhoids usually begin to develop when an individual is twenty years old or even earlier, symptoms usually do not appear until the thirties and beyond.

• **Constipation.** Difficulty in passing fecal matter creates pressure and possible injury to veins in the anal canal and rectum.

• **Low-fiber diet.** Highly refined foods (white flour products, sugar, foods high in fat and protein and low in complex carbohydrate) result in a fiber-deficient diet, with resulting constipation and hemorrhoids.

- **Obesity.** Added pounds put more pressure on veins. What's more, overweight individuals may be more likely to favor refined foods and a sedentary lifestyle.

- **Laxatives.** Improper use of these products is a major cause of constipation and, as such, it may also be considered a prime factor in the development of hemorrhoids.

- **Pregnancy.** As the fetus grows, it puts additional pressure on the rectal area. Pregnancy-related hemorrhoids usually retract after the baby is born, unless they were present beforehand.

- **Sexual practices.** Anal intercourse also puts pressure on veins in the anal canal.

- **Prolonged sitting.** Without some form of exercise, the heart muscle works more slowly in returning blood in the body's veins to the heart.

- **Prolonged standing.** The pull of gravity continues unabated on the body's veins in individuals who are on their feet all day.

Fortunately, most cases of hemorrhoids respond to basic self-care methods, so you may never have to tell a soul about them. (If you notice blood, see "Could It Be Something Else?") Here are the most effective steps you can take to soothe your achy bottom.

ROUGH UP YOUR DIET.

"People who consume large amounts of food containing fiber—or what grandmothers used to call 'roughage'—rarely have problems with hemorrhoids," says Thomas J. Stahl, M.D., assistant professor of general surgery at Georgetown University Medical Center in Washington, D.C. Fiber passes through the human digestive tract untouched by digestive enzymes. As it travels, it has the

COULD IT BE SOMETHING ELSE?

"Often people attribute symptoms to hemorrhoids when other conditions are to blame," notes Norton Rosensweig, M.D. Itching may be the result of poor anal hygiene, perianal warts, intestinal worms, medication allergies, psoriasis, other forms of dermatitis or local infection, or too much coffee. Pain can result from fissures—small cracks in the skin around the anus.

Erroneously attributing bleeding to hemorrhoids can be a serious mistake. Bleeding can be a symptom of colorectal cancer, which kills 60,000 people every year. "Rectal bleeding must be followed up promptly," cautions Rosensweig. While bright-red bleeding usually heralds hemorrhoids, don't try to make a diagnosis yourself. If you notice blood, see your doctor.

capacity to absorb many times its weight in water; by the time it reaches the colon in combination with digestive waste, it produces a stool that is bulky, heavy, and soft—all factors that make it easier to eliminate. "Straining to have a bowel movement day after day because of constipation is probably the main cause of hemorrhoids," says Norton Rosensweig, M.D., associate clinical professor of medicine at Columbia University College of Physicians and Surgeons in New York. Adding fiber to the diet is all that's necessary for about half the hemorrhoid cases (see "An Apple a Day").

AN APPLE A DAY

One of the most important moves toward healing hemorrhoids is a change in diet. "By all means, increase your intake of fiber-rich foods—but do it gradually," advises Norton Rosensweig, M.D. Too rapid an increase can cause gas, abdominal cramps, or diarrhea. As it is, you can expect some increase in intestinal gas at first, but this will subside in a week or two as your system and the bacteria that inhabit your colon adjust to your new diet.

Here are some foods that can increase the fiber content of your diet when eaten regularly:

Vegetables
 Carrots
 Brussels sprouts
 Eggplant
 Cabbage
 Corn
 Green beans
 Lettuce
Fruits
 Apples
 Figs
 Prunes
 Apricots
 Raisins
 Oranges

Grains
 Wheat, whole
 Rye, whole
 Rice, brown
 Corn, milled
 Oatmeal, unprocessed
 Oats, rolled Bran, unprocessed
  miller's
Legumes
 Lima beans
 Soy beans
 Kidney beans
 Lentils
 Chickpeas

THOSE OVER-THE-COUNTER "SHRINKS"

Drugstore remedies for hemorrhoidal discomfort usually achieve part of what they promise: temporary relief of pain and itching. Claims that they can shrink hemorrhoids or reduce inflamed tissue, however, don't hold up when put to the test, say the experts.

Over-the-counter aids are available in three forms: cleansers, suppositories, and creams and ointments. The cleansers, although effective, are more costly than ordinary warm water, which works very well. Suppositories may be of little use, according to some experts, because they may slip up into the upper rectum, bypassing the area they are meant to soothe. Ointments are greasy and tend to retain moisture, which can lead to increased irritation. Creams, especially hydrocortisone creams, are effective; however, their prolonged use may lead to dependency and can also cause thinning of the skin.

Furthermore, while some drugstore remedies may feel good, they may cause more harm than good in the long run. Some of these products should not be used by individuals with certain medical conditions, such as heart disease or diabetes, so you'll need to check the label of any product you are considering. In addition, many preparations contain a number of ingredients, including anesthetics, astringents,

DRINK UP.
Be sure to drink lots of water to keep the digestive process moving right along. A minimum of eight large

counterirritants, and skin protectants, which may cause an allergic reaction in some persons that is far worse than the discomfort of the hemorrhoids themselves.

The Food and Drug Administration has also made some specific rulings about products that are marketed for hemorrhoidal use.

• Boric acid is no longer allowed. While it's safe enough for ordinary skin, it is toxic if absorbed by the mucous membranes.

• Painkilling ingredients are out, too, because rectal nerves don't sense pain and, therefore, such ingredients are unnecessary.

• Lanolin alcohols, cod liver oil, and Peruvian balsam are banned as ineffective rather than unsafe.

• Product labels must say "If your condition worsens or does not improve in seven days, consult your doctor."

• Product labels claiming to shrink tissue must also caution: "Do not use this product if you have heart disease, high blood pressure, thyroid disease, diabetes, or difficulty in urinating due to an enlarged prostate gland unless directed by a doctor."

Keep in mind that, according to the experts, using petroleum jelly or zinc oxide ointment or powder may be as beneficial as any of the special "hemorrhoid preparations" you can buy.

glasses of water or other fluid a day is recommended, says Gayle Randall, M.D., assistant professor of medicine in the Department of Medicine at the University of

California Los Angeles School of Medicine. And remember, fruits and vegetables, which are important sources of dietary fiber, come packaged in their own water.

AVOID SWEAT AND STRAIN.

Don't try to move your bowels unless you feel the urge to do so. And don't spend any more time on the toilet than it takes to defecate without straining. "You should not try to catch up on yesterday's reading while sitting on the toilet," advises Rosensweig. Once your bowels have moved, don't strain to produce more.

HEED THE CALL OF NATURE.

On the other hand, don't wait too long before responding to the urge to eliminate. The longer the stool stays in the lower portion of the digestive tract, the more chance there is for moisture to be lost, making the stool hard and dry. "The frenzied pace many people follow today can lead to elimination always getting low priority," says Stahl.

TRY A DIFFERENT POSITION.

It has been suggested that squatting is a more natural position than sitting for moving one's bowels; unfortunately, Western toilets are not designed to make this possible for most people. "Try putting your feet on a small footstool to raise your knees closer to your chest," advises Randall.

SOFTEN IT.

Sometimes, eating more fiber-packed food and increasing water intake aren't enough to solve a severe constipation problem. In this case, you might want to ask your doctor to recommend a laxative known as a stool softener (such as Colace or Correctol) or one that contains a natural bulking agent (such as Metamucil and Effer-Syllium). Experts agree, however, that the safest and best way to add fiber to the diet is through foods. Don't—repeat don't—use laxatives that act on the muscles of the colon and rectum; prolonged use of these products can cause permanent malfunction of the bowel in addition to severe irritation of the anal area. Avoid mineral oil, as well, since it can interfere with the absorption of some essential nutrients such as vitamin A. "Ordinary laxatives are short-term solutions that lead to long-term problems," says Rosensweig.

TAKE A WALK.

Regular exercise helps your digestive system work more efficiently. No need for strenuous aerobics, however; a lengthy walk at a brisk pace will do the job quite adequately.

KEEP IT CLEAN.

Keep your rectal area clean at all times. Residual fecal matter can irritate the skin, but so can vigorous rubbing with dry toilet paper. Randall's suggested solution: "Gently rinse the area with plain water while sitting on the toilet. Then pat the area dry and dust with powder, preferably nontalc and unperfumed." More convenient, but also more expensive, are premoistened wipes designed for anal care. These wipes, however, may cause irritation in some people, says Randall. If you want to try them, they are available without a prescription at pharmacies and drugstores.

RINSE WELL.

Soap residue can also irritate the anal area. "Be sure to rinse the anal area completely after a bath or shower," says Randall.

SKIP THE SOAP.

If you find that, even with thorough rinsing, soap still irritates the anal area, look for a special perianal cleansing lotion in your drugstore. Follow the package directions.

SOFTEN YOUR SEAT.

If your job demands that you sit all day, try sitting on a donut-shaped cushion—an inexpensive device that takes the pressure off the sensitive area. "But it's still important to get up and walk around whenever possible," says Stahl.

SITZ AROUND.

Sit in six inches of warm water on your donut cushion or a towel twisted into a circle big enough to support your bottom. "Taken three or four times daily, a half-hour sitz bath will soothe inflamed tissues and relax muscle spasms," says Randall.

TAKE THE HEAT.

Even if you can't manage a full-scale sitz bath, applying a washcloth moistened with warm water can soothe the painful area.

SLIM DOWN.

If you are overweight, you'll be doing your bottom a favor by getting your weight closer to the desirable range. Of course, you'll be doing the rest of your body good, too.

Hiccups

13 Techniques Worth a Try

"It's a reflex similar to your leg jerking when a doctor hits a hammer to your knee." So says George Triadafilopoulos, M.D., a gastroenterologist and associate professor of medicine at the University of California at Davis, in describing hiccups. Hiccups result when the vagus nerve or one of its branches, which run from the brain to the abdomen, is irritated. And the vagus lets you know by tweaking the phrenic nerve, which leads to the diaphragm, the muscle below the lungs that helps you breathe. The diaphragm then spasms, causing the "hic."

Experts say hiccups are most often a reaction to common digestive disturbances. And luckily, they're usually more a nuisance than anything else. But what about the times when we seem to hiccup for no apparent reason? No one knows for sure why these seemingly innocuous bouts occur. What experts do know is that even infants hiccup, and the reflex continues, about three to five times a year, throughout life.

The home remedies used to stop a hiccuping bout are believed to work on two principles. Some basically rely on overstimulating the vagus nerve. "Nerves deal with a number of different sensations, from temperature to taste," Triadafilopoulos explains. "When one sensation is more overwhelming than another, the vagus nerve tells the brain that there's something more important to deal with. The brain then shuts off the hiccup response."

Other methods, which interfere with breathing, increase the amount of carbon dioxide in the blood, probably causing the body to become more concerned with getting rid of the carbon dioxide than making hiccups. Here are some tried-and-true remedies from both "camps."

SWEETEN THE HICCUPS.

Mary Poppins sang that a spoonful of sugar helps the medicine go down. But does it help hiccups? Many experts think so. "The nerve endings in the mouth become overloaded with the sweet sensation," Triadafilopoulos explains. Have a teaspoonful of sugar, and if you can, place the sugar on the back of the tongue, where "sour" is tasted. This way, the sugar will pack the most punch.

PLAY "HEAR NO EVIL."

Some doctors recommend that you put your fingers in your ears. It seems that branches of the vagus nerve also reach into the auditory system, and by stimulating the nerve endings there, the vagus nerve goes into action. "The pressure you create in the ears," says Triadafilopoulos, "is similar to the gag reflex caused when you put a finger in the back of your mouth." Of course, other doctors insist that you should never put anything smaller than your elbow in your ear in order to avoid irritating or damaging the ear canal. So if you do decide to try this hiccup reliever, be gentle, and don't stick your fingers too far into your ears.

GET SCARED SILLY.

Having someone surprise you may be the one method that overwhelms the vagus nerve more than anything else. "It's similar to the method an adult uses to quiet a

WHEN YOU CAN'T STOP THE HICCUPS

Though thankfully rare, "chronic or consistent hiccups can be a sign of a more serious problem," says George Triadafilopoulos, M.D. He estimates that the number of causes of hiccups may be as many as 100. Among the medical reasons for this affliction are infection; renal (kidney) failure; liver disease; cancer, including lung cancer; nervous system or abdominal problems, such as ulcers; and even heart attacks. Virtually anything that affects the head, chest, or abdomen can be implicated as causing hiccups, reports the National Heart, Lung, and Blood Institute in Bethesda, Maryland.

"Normally, people get hiccups about three to five times a year," according to Howard Goldin, M.D. A common bout usually lasts no more than an hour, and the hiccups occur at a rhythmic interval of about every 30 seconds. It's time to worry if the hiccups continue with frequency for more than an hour or as many as 12 hours plus, with no relief from home remedies. And "hiccups that keep you awake at night should be diagnosed," says Allan Burke, M.D.

In some cases, a physician will prescribe antacids or a sedative to help calm the digestive system. And in instances of severe, nonstop hiccuping, surgery may be performed to cut the link between the phrenic nerve and the diaphragm, as a means of stopping the spasms.

child who's crying endlessly. Out of frustration, a parent may yell at the child to stop, and sure enough, the child will stop, almost as if on cue," Triadafilopoulos says. Scaring the vagus may shut it up.

DRINK WATER.
Swallowing water interrupts the hiccuping cycle, which can quiet the nerves. Gargling with water may also help.

PULL ON YOUR TONGUE.
Sticking out your tongue and yanking on it may stop hiccups, says Howard Goldin, M.D., clinical professor of medicine at The New York Hospital–Cornell Medical Center in New York.

TICKLE IT AWAY.
Tickling the soft palate of the roof of your mouth with a cotton swab may do the trick. Or, if you enjoy getting tickled, have someone find your ticklish spots.

HOLD YOUR BREATH.
Hold your nose and close your mouth—like when you jump in a pool.

BAG THOSE HICCUPS.
Breathing into a paper bag is believed to work on the same principle as breath-holding. They increase the amount of carbon dioxide in the bloodstream, and the body becomes preoccupied with getting rid of it.

TAKE AN ANTACID.
"One or two tablets should help, especially if you take the kind that contains magnesium," says Allan Burke,

M.D., assistant professor of clinical neurology at Northwestern University School of Medicine in Chicago. Magnesium tends to decrease the irritation and quiet the nerves, he says.

EAT MORE SLOWLY.

"People who eat too fast tend not to chew well, which can cause hiccups," says Triadafilopoulos. And besides that, you swallow more than the meal. "Air gets entrapped between pieces of food," he explains. Chew deliberately and take smaller sips of drinks.

DON'T PIG OUT.

Overloading the stomach with food is another cause of hiccups. Triadafilopoulos has a theory as to why some digestive disturbances trigger a bout: "If you're eating too much or too fast, hiccups may be the body's way of stopping you from continuing to binge, which gives the digestive system a chance to catch up and recover."

AVOID SPICY FOODS.

Some spices can irritate the lining of the esophagus (the food pipe) and stomach. At the same time, they can also cause acid from the stomach to leak into the esophagus. The extra acid can bring on a bout.

DRINK ONLY IN MODERATION.

Like spices, alcoholic beverages can cause a simultaneous irritation of the esophagus and the stomach. And with time, excessive drinking can damage the lining of the food pipe. But long-time alcoholism isn't the only cause. Parties, like the kind some college students attend, where people are sometimes dared to consume a lot of alcohol as quickly as possible, can lead to what is called acute ingestion. The digestive system not only becomes irritated by the alcohol, but big gulps of it cause the esophagus to expand rapidly, resulting in hiccups.

High blood cholesterol

21 Heart-Healthy Ways to Lower It

Heart attacks are the leading cause of death in the United States. In 1989 alone, says the American Heart Association (AHA), heart attacks claimed the lives of 497,850 American men and women.

What causes a heart attack? In most cases, an attack occurs when the blood supply to part of the heart muscle is severely reduced or stopped, according to the AHA. This stoppage is caused when one of the arteries that supply blood to the heart is obstructed, usually by the fatty plaques that characterize atherosclerosis, a result of coronary-artery disease.

Although it's not clear where the plaques come from in each individual case, the most common causes are a blood cholesterol level that's too high, a hereditary tendency to develop atherosclerosis, and increasing age (55 percent of all heart attack victims are 65 or older, 45 percent are under 65 years of age, and 5 percent are under 40). Other factors that contribute to the likelihood that heart disease will develop are cigarette smoking, high blood pressure, and male sex (although after menopause, a woman's risk rises to almost equal that of a man), according to the AHA.

You can't change your age, your gender, or your genes, but you can make positive lifestyle changes that can sharply reduce your risk of developing heart disease. Getting your blood cholesterol down to a level that's considered low risk (see "Low, Borderline, High—What Do the Numbers Mean?") is an important first step. The following tips are designed to help you take that step.

ADOPT A NEW LIFESTYLE.

Making a commitment to lowering blood cholesterol and improving your heart health requires a change of mindset, not a temporary fad diet, according to Henry Blackburn, M.D., Mayo Professor of Public Health and a professor of medicine at the University of Minnesota in Minneapolis. "You need to adopt a healthy lifestyle, a familywide lifestyle," he says. "Even if one member of your family has a low risk of developing heart disease, that doesn't mean his or her risk will stay low. Our risk rises as we get older, and it takes a lifetime to establish good habits." Lifetime good habits also mean avoiding "yo-yo" dieting—losing weight and gaining it back repeatedly. Yo-yo dieting has been shown to cause cholesterol levels to rise.

KNOW IT'S NEVER TOO EARLY TO ACT.

Although much of the emphasis on heart disease risk is placed on people with a total blood cholesterol level over 240, the numbers can be a bit misleading, says William P. Castelli, M.D., director of the Framingham

LOW, BORDERLINE, HIGH—WHAT DO THE NUMBERS MEAN?

According to the American Heart Association (AHA), total levels of blood cholesterol under 200 milligrams per deciliter represent a low risk for coronary heart disease. Levels between 200 and 240 are considered borderline, and over 240 is considered dangerously high.

While total blood cholesterol is important, other factors count, too. For example, if someone has a borderline-high total cholesterol but has very low levels of HDL, or "good" cholesterol, he or she may still have a high risk of heart disease. In general, doctors worry about the ratio of LDL ("bad" cholesterol) to HDL.

A desirable HDL level is over 50, according to W. Virgil Brown, M.D. For LDL, a level below 130 is desirable, 130 to 160 is borderline high, and over 160 represents a high risk of heart disease, he says. Although these numbers aren't absolute (for example, levels of triglycerides, another fatty acid, also enter into the big picture), they do represent a fairly good predictor of heart disease risk, according to Brown. "We know that, on average, for every one percent increase in total blood cholesterol, there is a two to three percent increase in heart disease rates," he says. That means a person with a total cholesterol of 220 has a 20 percent higher risk than a person with a total cholesterol of 200. And a person with a level of 250 has a 50 percent higher risk than a person with a level of 200.

Heart Study in Massachusetts, the oldest and largest heart disease study in the United States. "Most heart attacks occur in people with a total cholesterol level between 150 and 250," he says. "Many doctors don't understand that. That group up at the top, the highest-risk group (with cholesterol levels above 240), only produces about 20 percent of the heart attacks." Even if you're in a low or borderline group, you still need to pay attention to your lifestyle habits, he advises.

IGNORE THE MAGIC BULLETS.

This week it's rice bran, last week it was oat bran and fish oil. All were touted as the solution to your cholesterol problem. While it's the American way to search for shortcuts, such an approach just doesn't cut it when you're dealing with your health, according to Basil M. Rifkind, M.D., F.C.R.P., chief of the Lipid Metabolism and Atherogenesis Branch at the National Heart, Lung, and Blood Institute in Bethesda, Maryland. "We are very cautionary about these magic-bullet remedies," he says. "If someone's cholesterol is high, we know that it comes about by eating a bunch of foods that are higher than the optimum in fat and cholesterol. We need to address the source of the problem, instead of paying attention to garlic, fiber, or fish oil."

STAY AWAY FROM SATURATED FATS.

Many people make the mistake of believing that if their blood cholesterol level is high that it's because they ate too many foods containing cholesterol. Not exactly true, says W. Virgil Brown, M.D., past president of the AHA and professor of medicine and director of the Division of Arteriosclerosis and Lipid Metabolism at Emory

University School of Medicine in Atlanta. The number-one cause of high serum cholesterol is eating too much saturated fat, the kind of fat that is found in full-fat dairy products and animal fat, he says. Another culprit is partially hydrogenated vegetable oil, which contains *trans* fatty acids, substances that increase the cholesterol-raising properties of a fat. The best rule of thumb is to stick with fats that are as liquid as possible at room temperature, according to Brown. "For example," he says, "if you are going to use margarine, use the most liquid kinds, such as the tubs or squeeze bottles."

READ YOUR MEAT.

The small orange labels stuck to packages of meat at the grocery store aren't advertisements or promotions; they're actually grades of meat, says Castelli. "Prime," "Choice," and "Select" are official U.S. Department of Agriculture shorthand for "fatty," "less fatty," and "lean," he explains. "Prime is about 40 percent to 45 percent fat by weight, Choice is from 30 percent to 40 percent fat, and Select, or diet lean, is from 15 percent to 20 percent fat," he says. You could have a hamburger made from Select ground beef for breakfast, lunch, and dinner and still not exceed your daily saturated fat limit, he adds.

LEARN TO COUNT GRAMS OF FAT.

The AHA's dietary guidelines outline the percentages of daily calories that should come from fat (see "The American Heart Association Diet"). However, since most package labels show grams of fat, not percentages, it can be difficult to figure out exactly what you're eating, Castelli says. Instead, he recommends counting grams of fat. How many grams of fat, and how many grams of saturated fat, can you have each day? Multiply your total number of calories per day by .30, then divide by 9 to find the number of grams of total fat allowed. (You divide by 9 because each gram of fat provides 9 calories.) Multiply your total number of calories per day by .10 and divide by 9 to find the number of grams of saturated fat allowed each day.

"If you're on a 2,000-calorie-per-day diet, you should eat no more than 22 grams of saturated fat a day," Castelli says. "The average American eats twice as much."

What can you eat for 22 grams of fat? One serving of Choice beef contains from 12 to 15 grams of fat, whereas a serving of Select contains 4 to 10. One tablespoon of butter is just under seven grams, while many brands of low-fat margarine contain only one gram per tablespoon. Whole milk has a whopping five grams per cup; skim milk just one. You add it up. After all, if you choose the lower-fat versions of each item, maybe you'll have enough saturated fat calories left in your daily budget to indulge in some low-fat frozen yogurt, a cup of which may contain as little as two grams of saturated fat.

GO TO THE EXTREME.

Although the AHA recommends deriving less than 30 percent of your daily calories from fat, some heart specialists believe it's not only safer, but better, to go even lower than that. (The average American derives about 37 percent to 40 percent of his or her calories from fat.) "It's quite appropriate for a person with a high degree of risk for heart disease to go to these sort of extremes," says Blackburn. "That means reducing fats way down. You can go down even to five percent of your calories

THE AMERICAN HEART ASSOCIATION DIET

The following dietary guidelines of the American Heart Association are designed to prevent heart attacks, stroke, and other cardiovascular diseases from occurring in healthy adults.

1. Total fat intake should be less than 30 percent of daily calories.

2. Saturated fat intake should be less than ten percent of daily calories.

3. Polyunsaturated fat intake should not exceed ten percent of daily calories.

4. Cholesterol intake should not exceed 300 milligrams per day.

5. Carbohydrates, especially complex carbohydrates, should comprise 50 percent or more of daily calories.

6. Protein should provide the remainding calories.

7. Sodium intake should not exceed three grams (3,000 milligrams) per day.

8. Alcohol consumption should not exceed one to two ounces of ethanol per day. Two ounces of 100-proof whisky, 8 ounces of wine, and 24 ounces of beer each contain 1 ounce of ethanol.

9. Total calories should be sufficient to maintain the individual's recommended body weight, as defined by the Metropolitan Tables of Height and Weight (Metropolitan Life Insurance Company, New York, 1959).

10. A wide variety of foods should be consumed.

from fat without hurting yourself. We've examined populations in Japan who consume 9 percent to 12 percent of their calories from fat and they are perfectly healthy and have very low cholesterol. It's worth the effort."

EAT AS MUCH LIKE A VEGETARIAN AS POSSIBLE.

Dietary cholesterol is found only in animal products; animal products also tend to be higher in fat (skim-milk products are exceptions), especially saturated fat. Foods derived from plant sources, on the other hand, contain no cholesterol and tend to be lower in fat. The fats they do contain tend to be polyunsaturated and monounsaturated, which are more healthful than the saturated kind, says Peter F. Cohn, M.D., chief of cardiology at the State University of New York at Stony Brook. (The exceptions are coconut oil, palm oil, palm kernel oil, and partially hydrogenated oils, which contain higher amounts of saturated fatty acids.) You'll be doing your arteries a favor if you increase your intake of vegetable proteins, such as beans, whole grains, and tofu, and keep servings of high-fat animal products to a minimum.

INCREASE YOUR CARBOHYDRATE INTAKE.

Adding extra servings of complex carbohydrates into your diet will fill you up and make you feel more satisfied, leaving less room for fatty meats and desserts, says Cohn. Complex carbohydrates include fruits, vegetables, pasta, whole grains, and rice.

GRILL IT.

Grilling, broiling, and steaming are heart-smart ways to cook. Unlike frying, they require no added fat.

SKIN A (DEAD) CHICKEN.

The skin of chicken (and turkey, too, for that matter), is an absolute "no-no" for people who are watching their fat intake, according to Cohn. The skin contains high amounts of saturated fat, he says.

SKIP THE PASTRY.

One hidden source of saturated fat is pastry—donuts, Danishes, pie crust, éclairs, and so on, says Brown. These confections are often made with shortening or butter— two things that should be limited by people who are working to reduce their saturated fat intake. Stick with whole-grain bread and rolls, and read labels to be sure you know what's in the package, he suggests.

EAT FISH.

Fish oil, as a cholesterol reducer, has gotten a lot of play in the media in the past few years. And it is true that the slimy stuff contains high levels of omega-3 fatty acids, substances that have been associated with lower cholesterol levels, according to Blackburn. However, the greatest benefit has been achieved in people who frequently substitute their intake of higher-fat meats with fish. Also, fish oil itself tends to be high in fat, Blackburn says. His advice is to add more servings of fish into the diet (as substitutes for some of the meat dishes) and reap the oil's benefits naturally.

GO EASY ON YOLKS.

You can have all the eggs you like, as long as you leave the yolks behind. Egg yolks are more than 50 percent fat and also contain high amounts of cholesterol. Egg yolks may also be hidden inside processed foods, so be sure to read labels carefully. The AHA recommends limiting egg yolks to no more than three per week, including those found in processed foods or used in cooking.

EAT SMALLER MEAT PORTIONS.

One way to cut down on saturated fat without giving up steaks is to keep your portions small, says Brown. "Reduce the size of the meat portions, even chicken, to about three ounces per serving," he advises. "Try to have a vegetarian lunch. Then you can have six ounces at dinner." A three-ounce serving is about the size of a deck of cards, Brown says.

GIVE UP ORGAN MEATS.

Like eggs, organ meats are something best left behind as a memory of foods gone by, says Brown. Although rich in iron and protein, these meats are also tremendously high in fat and cholesterol. And remember—pâté is made from liver, so it, too, should be restricted.

INCREASE YOUR FIBER INTAKE.

Soluble fiber, the kind found in fruits and brans, has been shown to be effective in lowering cholesterol levels, says Brown. However, to exert this effect, it must be consumed in high amounts; a bowl of oatmeal a day probably won't make much difference. "You have to eat about a quarter pound of oatmeal per day to get ten grams of soluble fiber a day, the amount that can lower cholesterol," he says. He recommends a daily one-teaspoon dose of a psyllium-husk powder, such as Metamucil, which provides a lot more bang for your buck. "For the person whose cholesterol is still borderline high after changing their diet, psyllium may give them another eight

HEART-SMART GLOSSARY

The following are definitions of terms commonly used in discussions of cholesterol and cardiovascular health:

LDL: Low-density lipoprotein, the "bad" cholesterol often implicated in the development of atherosclerosis.

HDL: High-density lipoprotein, the "good" cholesterol thought to protect against atherosclerosis.

Triglycerides: Another type of fatty acid found in the blood that doctors measure when they evaluate heart-disease risk.

percent to ten percent reduction in their LDL," he says. And no need to go overboard, either. More than ten grams a day won't make much more of a difference, he says. It's also prudent to increase your fiber intake gradually in order to give your system time to adjust.

EAT LIKE THE REST OF THE WORLD.
"Four billion of the 5.3 billion people on this earth eat 15 grams of saturated fat or less each day," says Castelli. "Where do they live? Asia, Africa, and Latin America. They are the four billion people that never get atherosclerosis. We want our 250 million people to eat like those 4 billion. If we accomplished this, we could get rid of heart attacks, stroke, and other manifestations of cardiovascular disease. We could live five years longer,

which isn't much. However, we wouldn't have heart attacks in our 40s, 50s, 60s, 70s, or 80s. That is the vision for America."

QUIT SMOKING.

Most of us are aware that smoking can cause lung cancer and raise the risk of heart attack, but few people know that smoking can actually affect your cholesterol levels, says Brown. "When you stop smoking, your HDL levels rise significantly," he explains. "A two-pack-a-day smoker who quits may have an eight-point rise in their HDL cholesterol."

ADD EXERCISE TO YOUR DAILY ROUTINE.

Studies have shown that regular aerobic exercise can boost levels of HDL, says Brown. "Exercise can be very useful in reducing body weight, which can help cholesterol levels," he says. "When you engage in even modest amounts of exercise, your triglycerides come down, your LDL comes down, and your HDL goes up after several months." He recommends 30 to 45 minutes of moderate exercise, such as walking, five days per week. It is important to accelerate your heart rate and keep it up for at least 20 minutes, he says. However, he adds, it is not necessary to do your exercise all at once. Try parking your car a quarter mile from work and walk it twice a day. Take the stairs instead of the elevator. All these things add up.

KNOW IT'S NEVER TOO LATE.

Even if you've had a heart attack or have other evidence of heart disease, changing your lifestyle can still dramatically reduce your risk of a recurrence, says Rifkind.

In the past, heart specialists thought that lifestyle changes couldn't make much of a difference for people who already had heart disease. They now believe differently. "We want the cholesterol to be much lower in these people than in their healthy counterparts," he says. "For these people, the target levels of total serum [blood] cholesterol are between 160 and 170."

High blood pressure

13 Ways to Reduce It

At last count, 62,770,000 Americans had or were being treated for high blood pressure, according to the American Heart Association (AHA). That's almost one-quarter of our country's population. Every year, 31,630 of these individuals die as a direct result of the condition, the AHA says. An additional 147,470 deaths every year occur from stroke (a blood clot that travels to the brain), making it the number-one fatality related to high blood pressure. Another 2,980,000 Americans have had a stroke and lived. Many of these people are now severely disabled and unable to care for themselves.

High blood pressure, or hypertension, is defined as having blood pressure (the force that is created by the heart as it pumps blood into the arteries and through the circulatory system) equal to or higher than 160 systolic (the top number) over 95 diastolic (the bottom number), according to William P. Castelli, M.D., director of the Framingham Heart Study in Framingham, Massachusetts, the oldest and largest heart-disease study in the United States. Between 140 and 159 systolic over 90 to 94 diastolic is considered "borderline" high. Below these numbers is considered normal.

In addition to strokes, high blood pressure can cause blindness, kidney failure, and a swelling of the heart that may lead to heart failure.

Who's at risk for high blood pressure? People with a family history of the condition, blacks (they have an almost one-third greater chance of having high blood pressure than whites), overweight individuals, and aging individuals. Also at risk are women who are pregnant or who are taking oral contraceptives.

The good news is that, together with your doctor, you can control hypertension. It won't be easy—you'll have to change the way you think and act. You may have to take medication for the rest of your life. You'll definitely have to cut out some bad habits and begin some new, more healthful ones. However, your efforts are likely to pay off in a longer, healthier life. Here's to your health!

JOIN THE CLUB.

It may sound trivial, but the first step toward controlling your blood pressure is actually accepting that you've got a problem to begin with, says David B. Carmichael, M.D., medical director of the Cardiovascular Institute at Scripps Memorial Hospital in La Jolla, California. "People must accept the fact that they've got hypertension," he says. "The worst person in the world is an aggressive 40-year-old male who comes in feeling fine and is told he has hypertension and will have to monitor his blood pressure. They often just won't believe it. In fact, if I ask myself what type of patient has left my practice over the years, I would say it has been the hypertensives." Carmichael likens this type of acceptance to joining a fraternal lodge. "You've got to do certain things: go to the doctor, take your medications faithfully, modify your diet, report bizarre symptoms. You have got to join the club."

LOSE WEIGHT.

"At all levels of blood pressure, increased weight contributes to the degree of blood pressure elevation," according to Robert A. Phillips, M.D., Ph.D., director of the Hypertension Section and associate director of the Cardiovascular Training Program in the Division of Cardiology at Mount Sinai Medical Center in New York. He adds, "Weight loss lowers blood pressure—not in everybody, but in many people. It's worth a try." Phillips explains why losing weight impacts so heavily on blood pressure levels by noting the fact that for each pound of excess body weight that is lost, blood pressure may drop by two points. "It's always a good thing to do, even if you are severely hypertensive," he continues. "If you are mildly hypertensive, that weight loss may enable you to stay off of medication." Even a modest amount of weight loss is better than none at all, according to Castelli. "The most common problem in hypertension is borderline hypertension—between 140 and 159 systolic and 90 to 94 diastolic," explains Castelli. "That level of blood pressure increases the risk of stroke three times. And yet, virtually all of those people would be cured with a ten-pound weight loss."

INVEST IN A HOME BLOOD PRESSURE MONITOR.

If you have been diagnosed as hypertensive, or if your doctor wanted more blood pressure readings before making a definitive diagnosis, he or she may have prescribed you a home blood pressure monitor. At-home monitoring has several benefits—first and foremost, warning you if your pressure becomes dangerously high, so you can get medical attention early. Second, a monitor can save you money, because it will save you trips to the doctor. "This is now very common," says Carmichael. "It is also easy to do. If the patient is afraid to use the monitor [some people become panicky if they find their pressure is high], another person, such as a spouse, can do it for them. The blood pressure should be checked at close to the same time of day, under the same conditions." Carmichael says that most insurance companies will cover the purchase of such devices if prescribed by a physician.

START AN EXERCISE PROGRAM.

Along with helping with weight loss, exercise confers additional benefits for those with high blood pressure, says Phillips. "For people who are severely hypertensive, they shouldn't exercise until their blood pressure is controlled," he says, "but people with mild hypertension can exercise aerobically for 20 to 30 minutes, three times per week, and will benefit with a reduction in blood pressure by about eight points that will last at least half a day." It's best to check with your doctor before beginning any exercise program, especially if you have been sedentary. The types of exercise that are most likely to benefit your blood pressure are walking, jogging, stair-climbing, aerobic dance, swimming, bicycling, tennis, skating, skiing, or anything else that elevates your pulse and sustains the elevation for at least 20 minutes. Nonaerobic exercise, such as weight lifting, push-ups, and chin-ups, may actually be dangerous for hypertensives. These types of exercise should not be done without the explicit consent of your doctor.

TAKE YOUR BLOOD PRESSURE MEDICINE.

The biggest danger with hypertension, Carmichael says, is that it is usually asymptomatic until its final stages, where it becomes fatal. That's why the condition is often labeled "the silent killer." Unlike people who have other chronic illnesses, such as diabetes, you'll probably feel just fine if you don't take your medicine. However, inside your body, the disease will continue to progress, damaging the arteries in your eyes, destroying your kidneys, causing your heart to swell, and so on. Another problem that can occur when you stop taking your blood pressure medicine is a rebound phenomenon, where the blood pressure rises to a higher level than it was before you started taking the medication. The moral of the story? "If you're starting and stopping taking your medication, you haven't joined the club," says Carmichael.

CULTIVATE A TASTE FOR LESS SALTY FOODS.

"There is no question that salt in the diet has a relationship with blood pressure," says Jeffrey A. Cutler, M.D., a hypertension specialist and chief of the Prevention and Demonstration Research Branch of the National Heart, Lung, and Blood Institute in Bethesda, Maryland. "We Americans take in far more salt than we need. We've become accustomed to the taste. However, the fact is that our taste sense is adaptable. People who lower the salt in their diets, after a period of time, have been shown to taste something as salty at a much lower level of salt than before." The average American takes in about eight to ten grams of salt a day, Cutler says. However, studies have shown that by cutting that amount down by a third, blood pressure can be significantly reduced, he says. Ideally, he says, people should cut down to six grams per day as a short-term goal, and to about four-and-a-half grams per day as a long-term goal.

READ LABELS.

So how do you know how much salt you're eating? As far as table salt goes, one teaspoon contains over two grams—almost half of the recommended daily amount. Also, says Cutler, the average American adult takes in somewhere between one-and-a-half to two extra teaspoons of salt a day without knowing it. These insidious salt sources are frozen entrées, canned vegetables, even antacid medications. To avoid this extra salt, read labels. Many labels will express the amount of sodium in milligrams (1,000 milligrams is equivalent to 1 gram). According to Cutler, to calculate the amount of sodium chloride, or salt, multiply the amount of sodium by two-and-a-half.

SAY NO TO A SECOND ROUND.

Restriction of alcohol consumption to one drink (1.5 ounces of hard liquor, 4 ounces of wine, or 12 ounces of beer) per day does not appear to increase the risk of high blood pressure, but consuming two or three drinks per day is associated with an elevated risk of hypertension, according to Phillips.

PREGNANCY AND HYPERTENSION

If you have been diagnosed as having high blood pressure and you become pregnant, you should see your doctor as soon as possible to discuss ways to control your condition during pregnancy.

During pregnancy, your blood volume triples, placing a great deal of additional strain upon the heart. Perhaps because of this increase in blood volume, many women who never had a problem with blood pressure become hypertensive.

The problems of hypertension in pregnancy are twofold: First, the condition is extremely dangerous, posing a risk of stroke, preeclampsia, stillbirth, premature delivery, and low birth weight. Second, blood pressure may be difficult to control without medication, and many medications may endanger the developing fetus.

However, studies have shown that extra calcium lowers blood pressure in pregnant women, says Johns Hopkins researcher John T. Repke, Ph.D. Repke's findings show that pregnant women may need to take between one-and-one-half and two times the recommended daily allowance of calcium to keep their blood pressure at safe levels. However, he cautions that pregnant women should consult their doctors before taking supplements or exceeding the recommended amount of any nutrient.

The recommended daily allowance for calcium during pregnancy is 1,200 milligrams per day, the amount in eight servings of low-fat milk, yogurt, or broccoli.

EAT A BANANA.

One substance (other than prescription medication) that has been proven to reduce blood pressure is potassium, says Cutler. However, it may be difficult to increase your intake of potassium enough to lower blood pressure, he adds. While supplements may help, they are not recommended without the permission of a doctor, since they may be hazardous in individuals with certain medical conditions. "The average person needs three to four servings of potassium-rich fruits and vegetables per day," he says. "It would probably benefit your blood pressure in a detectable way if you could double that number of servings. A little more may be a little better, and a lot more may be a lot better." Potassium-rich foods include bananas, raisins, currants, milk, yogurt, and orange juice.

DRINK YOUR MILK.

Some studies have shown that extra calcium added to the diet may have a modest effect on blood pressure, says Phillips. Although the effect may not be significant, there's certainly no harm in adding a few extra glasses of skim milk, low-fat yogurt, or leafy green vegetables to the daily diet, he says.

ADD POLYUNSATURATED OILS TO YOUR DIET.

Most people know that by substituting polyunsaturated oils for saturated fats in their diets they can reduce their level of blood cholesterol. However, what most people don't know is that polyunsaturates can also reduce blood pressure, according to James A. Hearn, M.D., an assistant professor of medicine at the University of Alabama at Birmingham. "Switching to canola and safflower oils in cooking can cut your blood pressure by ten points."

SYMPTOMS OF A STROKE

If you are experiencing any of the following stroke symptoms, call your doctor or an ambulance at once. Waiting too long or not recognizing the signs could mean the difference between life and death. If you experience any of these symptoms and then feel better within 24 hours, you may have had a transient ischemic attack, or TIA. A TIA is a warning sign that a full-blown stroke is on its way. Again—call your doctor at once.

• Sudden weakness or numbness of the face, arm, or leg on one side of the body

• Sudden dimness or loss of vision, particularly in only one eye

• Loss of speech, or trouble talking or understanding speech

• Sudden, severe headaches with no apparent cause

• Unexplained dizziness, unsteadiness, or sudden falls, especially along with any of the previous symptoms

(Source: "1992 Heart and Stroke Facts," by the American Heart Association.)

QUIT SMOKING—NOW.

Cigarette smoking is the number-one taboo for hypertensives, says Phillips. Not only does the nicotine in the smoke cause blood pressure to rise, but it dramatically raises your risk of stroke, he says. According to the AHA, cigarette smoking can thicken the blood and increase its propensity to clot. Blood clots in the arteries leading to the heart can cause a heart attack, while blood clots in the artery leading to the brain may cause a stroke, according to the AHA. The good news is, you get an immediate benefit by giving up the habit right now. "Two years after you quit smoking, your risk of developing coronary artery disease has dropped to the same level as someone who never smoked," Phillips says. In contrast, it can take much longer for a person's risk of lung cancer to drop to that level. Your doctor can be a great source of help to you in quitting smoking. He or she may prescribe nicotine gum or skin patches to reduce withdrawal discomfort. Your local Heart Association may also be able to provide you with resources.

LEARN TO RELAX.

Many people misunderstand the term hypertension, believing it to mean a condition where the patient is overly tense. This isn't true. The term is defined solely by blood pressure levels. However, many hypertensives are the consummate "Type A" personality—aggressive, workaholic, hostile, frustrated, or angry, says Carmichael. For these people, some form of relaxation, be it prayer, yoga, biofeedback, or just resting, may be an important component of treatment, he says. "People need to recognize their personality traits and do their best to change," he says. Some chronically stressed-out individuals release a lot of adrenaline into their systems. That rush of hormone can constrict the arterioles (tiny blood vessels), causing them to go into spasm. It is difficult for the heart to push blood through constricted arterioles. The effect? Higher blood pressure, says Carmichael.

Hives

14 Methods for Relieving Them

Just about anything can make you break out in hives: Foods such as peanuts or strawberries, drugs such as penicillin or aspirin, vitamin supplements, heat, cold, sunlight, exercise, fever, stress, and even scratching or rubbing the skin are among some of the possibilities.

Some substances cause an allergic reaction that results in hives; others have nothing to do with allergies. Strawberries, for example, contain a chemical that can cause cells in your body to release histamine, a chemical also produced in allergies, which allows blood plasma to leak into the skin and form hives, says Philip C. Anderson, M.D., chairman of dermatology at the University of Missouri–Columbia School of Medicine.

And sometimes only a tiny amount of the culprit is needed to set off a reaction. "You can be sensitive to fish and order something completely different in a restaurant. But it's cooked in a pan that was previously used to fry fish, and you break out in hives," explains Larry Borish, M.D., staff physician at National Jewish Center for Immunology and Respiratory Medicine in Denver.

Don't confuse hives with other skin eruptions. Hives (or urticaria) occur when blood plasma leaks into the skin, causing "wheals," or swollen areas. They can be as small as a pencil eraser or as large as a dinner plate, and they usually last only a few hours. But new hives may form continuously. And as they form, they often itch.

An attack of hives generally lasts a short time, often just a few days. (Some people, however, may be plagued with recurrent outbreaks or with hives that persist for years.) If you are burdened with hives, here are some tips for relief.

TAKE AN ORAL ANTIHISTAMINE.

The most recommended remedy is over-the-counter Benadryl, but it may cause drowsiness. "That may not be so bad, since hives are generally worse at night, and the itch is more annoying then," says Borish.

DON'T SCRATCH.

"It's said that with hives, a million scratches are never enough and one is too many," says Borish. Scratching can increase local inflammation and even cause more hives.

WEAR GLOVES TO BED.

If you think you'll scratch in your sleep, gloves will help prevent damage.

WRAP UP THE AFFECTED AREA.

Wrap an elastic bandage around the area with hives or cover it with clothing so you can't reach it with your fingernails.

USE A MILK COMPRESS.

Wet a cloth with cold milk and lay it on the affected area for 10 to 15 minutes at a time. "Don't freeze the skin," warns Judy Jordan, M.D., a dermatologist in San Antonio and a spokesperson for the American Academy of Dermatology. "Just cool it."

TOP TRIGGERS OF HIVES

According to the American Academy of Dermatology, the most common **foods** that cause hives are*:

- Peanuts
- Eggs
- Nuts
- Beans
- Chocolate
- Strawberries
- Tomatoes
- Seasonings such as mustard, ketchup, mayonnaise, and spices
- Fresh fruits, especially citrus
- Corn
- Fish
- Pork

The **drugs** most likely to cause hives are*:

- Aspirin (check the labels on over-the-counter drugs, which may contain aspirin)
- Penicillin
- Sulfa drugs
- Tetracyclines
- Codeine

*This is not an all-inclusive list.

CHILL THE ITCH.

Hold an ice pack or ice cubes in a thin towel on the skin for five minutes at a time, three to four times a day.

TAKE A BATH.
Put half a box of baking soda or one cup of oatmeal in the water first, says Jordan.

TRY CORTISONE.
A one percent cortisone preparation, available without a prescription, may help.

TRY TO FERRET OUT THE CAUSE.
"In the overwhelming number of patients, there's no explanation found," says Borish. "We only find the cause 20 to 30 percent of the time." Do remember that hives generally show up within half an hour of eating. "You don't get hives the next day from something you ate the night before," he says.

AVOID THE TRIGGER.
This one's pretty obvious, but if you know that cold sets off hives, don't put your hands in the freezer. In fact, jumping into cold water could be life-threatening, points out Borish. And there's no question, he says, that if you're prone to hives, stress will trigger them.

TREAT THE UNDERLYING INFECTION.
If hives turn into a chronic problem, they may be caused by an infection. "You can have a tooth or yeast infection and not be aware of it," points out Jordan. Consider these possibilities and have them checked out by your physician.

RELIEVE THE PRESSURE.
Hives often form where clothing is tight, such as under bra straps or waistbands.

HELLO, DOCTOR?

Many episodes of hives are short-lived inconveniences that go away on their own in a day or two. But sometimes hives become a long-term problem or indicate a more serious condition. See your doctor or visit the emergency room if you:

- Have a lot of swelling around your face and throat
- Feel nauseated or dizzy
- Have trouble breathing
- Have a fever
- Are losing weight or suffering from malaise
- Have hives that persist for four to six weeks

In some cases, diseases like thyroid disorders, hepatitis, lupus, or even some cancers can have hives as a symptom. Don't ignore hives that won't go away. "If you're sick otherwise and you're suffering from hives, you need to see the doctor," says Philip C. Anderson, M.D. "Hives could signal a serious internal disease in that case."

USE A MOISTURIZER.
If dry skin contributes to the itch, apply a moisturizer to relieve it.

DON'T MAKE THE PROBLEM WORSE.
Nonprescription anti-itch lotions or creams can cause allergic reactions. If you react to topical Benadryl and

topical products ending in "-caine," you'll be in worse shape after using them. Calamine lotion, that old standby for so many itches, doesn't do much for hives either.

Incontinence
20 Steps to Greater Security

Have you stopped taking an aerobics class because you're afraid you might have an "accident"? Do you worry when it's time to take a long car trip on highways with few roadside rest areas? Do you dread sneezing, coughing, laughing, because you may not stay dry?

Rest assured, you're not alone. Help for Incontinent People (HIP), a not-for-profit organization in Union, South Carolina, estimates that at least 12 million, and perhaps as many as 20 million, people in the United States and Canada suffer with urinary incontinence, oftentimes in silence. Indeed, it's a problem that's only been recognized relatively recently in America as a treatable condition and not merely an unavoidable symptom of old age. As a matter of fact, other cultures in times past seemed to have been much more aware of the problem. The ancient Egyptians developed products for incontinence, and in Great Britain around the turn of the century, it was perfectly acceptable for a woman to hold what was called a "slipper" under her dress to relieve herself during a long church service.

The loss of bladder control is not a disease but a symptom with any of a host of causes. It can affect anyone at any age—from children to the elderly, both women and men. Women, however, are three times more likely than men to be incontinent, due in part to the physical stresses of childbearing and a decrease in estrogen after menopause. The cause of incontinence may be as minor as an infection triggered by a cold or the use of certain prescription or over-the-counter medications. Incontinence may also be the result of sagging pelvic-floor muscles. This set of muscles located at the bottom of the pelvis supports the lower internal organs and helps them maintain their shape and proper function. Childbirth and certain types of surgery, such as a hysterectomy (removal of the uterus) in a woman or a prostatectomy (removal of the prostate gland) in a man, can cause these pelvic-floor muscles to become deficient. (See "Exercises for Incontinence" for help in toning up and strengthening the pelvic-floor muscles.)

Incontinence reveals itself in a number of ways, and one person can suffer from more than one form of it. Stress incontinence occurs from rigorous or spontaneous activity, like playing tennis or sneezing. Urge incontinence is marked by a sudden need to go but possibly not making it to the bathroom in time. Overflow incontinence is a full bladder that begins to dribble. And reflex incontinence is marked by an unawareness of the need to urinate (caused by an enlarged prostate gland, for example), which results in leakage. Here are ways to cope:

KEEP A DIARY.

"This is very helpful in establishing symptom patterns," says Katherine Jeter, Ed.D, E.T., executive director of HIP. By maintaining a voiding diary, or uro-log, you'll have a record of when you urinated and the circumstances causing it. The diary should include: the time of day of urination or leakage; the type and amount of fluid intake that preceded it; the amount voided in ounces (pharmacies carry measuring devices that fit right inside the toilet bowl); the amount of leakage (small, medium, or large); the activity engaged in when leakage occurred; and whether or not an urge to urinate was present. Keeping such a diary for at least four days, if not a full week, before you see a doctor can help him or her to determine what type of incontinence you have and the course of treatment. When you see a doctor, take along a list or the actual bottles of any prescription or over-the-counter medicines you have been taking, because some medications can cause incontinence.

WATCH WHAT YOU DRINK.

Experts are not entirely sure why some beverages seem to irritate the bladder lining and, as a result, cause bladder leakage. But you may want to eliminate certain substances from your diet or at least decrease your intake of them to see if your urine control improves. The caffeine in coffee, for instance, may irritate the bladder, and the ingredients that give coffee its distinct aroma (also found in decaffeinated varieties) can be irritating, too. Tea, another favorite breakfast drink, is not only a diuretic, which means it pulls more water from the kidneys as it passes through, but also a bladder irritant. (HIP recommends substituting hot grain beverages, found in your grocer's coffee and tea aisle.) Citrus fruits and juices, such as grapefruit and tomato, can be a problem. Carbonated sodas may be irritating, too, according to HIP (you might be able to tolerate seltzer water, which is not as highly carbonated as sodas). And, finally, alco-

EXERCISES FOR INCONTINENCE

The pelvic floor is a set of muscles at the bottom of the pelvis that supports the lower internal organs, such as the bladder and uterus, and controls the sphincter muscles, which are the muscles that control the urethra and rectum. When you stop and start your urine stream, you're working these muscles. When this set of muscles becomes weak, incontinence may occur. Since these muscles can be controlled voluntarily, exercises may help strengthen them and in turn help control leakage, especially in cases of stress incontinence. This is true only if the exercises are done properly, however.

The following are a few simple exercises recommended by Help for Incontinent People (HIP). These exercises should be done on a daily basis for the best results. If you need additional instruction, HIP can provide you with manuals and tapes, or you can consult your doctor. In addition, your doctor may be able to recommend exercises of increasing difficulty, depending on your specific case.

holic beverages should be avoided. Your safest bet: water.

TRY THESE JUICES.

Grape juice, cranberry juice, cherry juice, and apple juice are not irritating to the bladder and may, in fact, control the odor of your urine. And surprisingly, orange juice is

1. Lie on your back with your knees bent and feet slightly apart. Contract all the openings in the pelvic floor—the rectum, urethra, and, in women, the vagina, too. To help you isolate the muscles, first squeeze as if trying to keep from passing gas. Then (for women) contract the vagina as if trying not to lose a tampon. Then, proceed forward as if trying to stop urinating. Hold the tension while slowly counting to three. Then slowly release the tension. Repeat five to ten times. You should feel a "lift" inside you. Be sure to breathe smoothly and comfortably and do not tense your stomach, thigh, or buttocks muscles; otherwise, you may be exercising the wrong muscles. Check your abdomen with your hand to make sure the stomach area is relaxed.

2. Repeat the first exercise while using a low stool to support the lower part of your legs. Raising your legs will help further relax the pelvic-floor muscles for the exercise.

3. Third, repeat the first exercise while kneeling on the floor with your elbows resting on a cushion. In this position, the stomach muscles are completely relaxed. If you are unable to kneel, roll up a blanket and place it under your groin while you lie on your stomach.

not an irritant, because it is metabolized by the body into a more alkaline, or less acidic, fluid before it reaches the bladder, says Jeter.

KEEP DRINKING.
"Too often, people who suffer with incontinence limit their fluid intake, believing that the less they take in, the

less they'll urinate. But dehydration can occur," warns Thelma Wells, Ph.D., R.N., F.A.A.N., F.R.C.N., a professor of nursing at the University of Rochester School of Nursing in Rochester, New York. Dehydration can lead to constipation, which in turn can irritate nearby nerves that will trigger the bladder to void. The result: incontinence. Instead of cutting back on how much you drink, schedule the time that you drink. Having liquids at set intervals during the day will keep your bladder from becoming too empty or too full. "The bladder becomes irritated if its fluid level is too low or too high," explains Wells. A normal bladder holds about two cups of fluid; problem bladders may hold as little as half a cup or as much as a quart and a half. If you find yourself constantly waking up in the middle of the night to go to the bathroom, you might try to taper off your fluid intake between dinner and bedtime, says Wells. Experts suggest an average total fluid intake of six to ten 8-ounce cups a day.

WATCH WHAT YOU EAT.

Again, experts are not sure why certain foods aggravate the bladder, but you may want to try cutting back on the following foods to see if it helps: hot spices and the foods they're used in, such as curry powder and chili; tomato-based foods; sugars, such as honey and corn syrup; and chocolate.

TRY A RECIPE FOR SUCCESS.

If you are constipated, adding fiber to your diet may relieve your constipation, and in turn, your incontinence. Here's an easy-to-make-snack recipe from HIP that may help. Combine one cup of applesauce, one cup of oat bran, and a quarter cup of prune juice. Store the mixture in your refrigerator, or freeze premeasured servings in sectioned ice-cube trays. Begin with two tablespoons every evening, followed by a six- to eight-ounce glass of water or juice (one of the acceptable varieties mentioned previously). After seven to ten days, increase this to three tablespoons. Then, at the end of the second or third week, increase your intake to four tablespoons. You should begin to see an improvement in your bowel habits in about two weeks. The extra fiber may cause increased gas or bloating, but this should decrease after a few weeks. Be sure to keep up your daily fluid intake in addition to using this fiber recipe.

LOSE WEIGHT.
Obesity can cause muscles to sag, including the pelvic-floor muscles, which aid in proper voiding.

DO NOT SMOKE.
Here's another reason to give up the habit. Nicotine can irritate the bladder, and for heavy smokers, coughing can contribute to stress incontinence.

BUY YOURSELF SOME INSURANCE.
There are numerous products on the market today that will absorb any accidents, whether urine or a bowel movement, and at the same time, protect your clothing or bedding from wetness. Specially made disposable and reusable briefs, diapers, liners, inserts, and linen protectors can add a measure of confidence. For some people, sanitary napkins or panty liners may be an acceptable alternative that provides enough protection. And a new product may be on the market soon. "Within the

next year or two, urethral plugs, which can block the flow of urine during everyday activities, will be available in the United States," says Peter K. Sand, M.D., associate professor of obstetrics and gynecology at Northwestern University School of Medicine and director of the Evanston Continence Center at Evanston Hospital in Evanston, Illinois. These plugs, now in use in Europe, can be inserted by the user and later removed by means of an attached string.

BE CONFIDENT ON THE ROAD.

External collecting devices that are specially designed for use by females or males can make traveling a little more comfortable. These on-the-go urinals, which are also convenient for bedside use, are available at medical supply stores and pharmacies and through medical-specialty mail order.

GO BEFORE YOU GO.

Empty your bladder before you take a trip of an hour or more, whether you have the urge to go or not.

THEN GO AGAIN.

After voiding, stand up and sit down again. Then lean forward, which will compress the abdomen and put pressure on the bladder, to help empty the bladder completely, suggests Wells.

WEAR CLOTHES THAT ARE EASY TO REMOVE.

Women's clothing, in particular, can pose a problem. Jumpsuits or unitards can slow you down when you're in a hurry to go because these one-piece outfits must be removed from the top down. Skip such suits or look for ones with a snapped opening at the crotch for quick-and-easy removal. Carry extra clothing with you so that you can change if an accident occurs. If your clothes happen to become stained with urine, soak them for three hours in a mixture of one gallon of water and one cup of dishwashing detergent.

WEIGHT FOR RESULTS.

Resistive exercise—when force is exerted against a weight—can be applied to the sphincter muscles of the urethra and rectum, which are important to regaining continence, says Wells. Cones that are about the size of a tampon and that come in varying weights are designed for use in the vagina (women) or rectum (men). When a cone is inserted, the sphincter muscles must contract in order to hold the weight and not let it drop. "Over a few months and with progressive use of the varying weights, the pelvic-floor muscles should get stronger," says Jeter. These weight sets are available from physicians, who can guide your use of the cones, or from medical supply stores. Be sure to carefully read and follow the accompanying instructions on proper use for best results. Start by holding in the lightest weight for 15 minutes, two times a day. Once successful at that weight, try the next heaviest weight for the same amount of time. Some versions of these cones come with an electronic biofeedback system, called a perineometer, which reports on the amount of pressure you're applying to the inserted cone.

TAKE CONTROL OF YOUR MUSCLES EVERY DAY.

To prevent leakage, contract the pelvic-floor muscles when coughing or sneezing. You should also contract them when carrying or lifting something. Do so by standing close to the object to be lifted with your feet slightly apart, one foot just in front of the other. Then, bend your knees but keep your back straight. Lean forward slightly as you contract, or tighten, your pelvic muscles. Then lift the object.

BE WARY OF EXERCISE GIMMICKS.

Carefully investigate any exercise contraption that claims to help decrease incontinence. A company may promote the fact that its gadget will tone the pelvic-floor muscles, but the device may actually exercise an unrelated muscle group, if it does anything at all. An exerciser for use between the thighs, for instance, will not strengthen the pelvic-floor muscles. If you're not sure if a certain exerciser will benefit your incontinence problem, don't waste your time or money. Check first with your health-care provider.

MAKE A PHONE CALL.

Call 1-800-BLADDER, a toll-free number sponsored by HIP, for details on how to receive free information on services and products for incontinent people.

Ingrown hair

10 Ways to Get It Straight

Curly-haired men, particularly blacks, get curls on their cheeks and necks as well as on their heads.

The hair sometimes just curls right back on itself. When the tip of the hair re-enters the skin, it's called an ingrown hair.

Women are not immune to this shaving malady. Women can get something known as bikini bottom, says Jerome Z. Litt, M.D., assistant clinical professor of dermatology at Case Western Reserve University School of Medicine in Cleveland. It happens sometimes after shaving the places a skimpy bikini won't cover.

The solution for both men and women: Stop shaving altogether. Short of that, here are a few other tips to consider:

GO WITH THE GRAIN.
Shave your face in the direction your hair grows. Gordon Scarbrough, a barber for 40 years and owner of Moler Barber College in Portland, Oregon, says hair grows down on the cheeks, straight out on the chin, down below the jawbone, and up along the lower neck, usually below the Adam's apple.

HANG UP YOUR RAZOR.
At least for a day or two. Particularly if your razor bumps have become infected, you will do more damage if you shave over them. Giving the hairs a rest, and meanwhile washing the affected areas with an antibacterial soap, will usually end the inflammation, says Litt.

SHAVE MORE OFTEN.
The choice is up to you. If you don't completely quit shaving to cure your razor bumps, then shave more often. It makes perfect sense to Andrew Lazar, M.D., assistant professor of clinical dermatology at Northwestern

University School of Medicine in Chicago. "It may be better to shave more often and not press quite as hard," he says. This applies especially to young men whose beards are just coming in, says Lazar.

LIFT THEM OUT.
Before shaving, take a straight pin or a beard pick and carefully lift out any ingrown hairs, says Litt. Don't pick or dig at them.

GET READY TO SHAVE.
To lessen the trauma from shaving, prepare your beard and skin. Make sure your skin is softened with warm water or towels and is wet, says Scarbrough. Never apply foam or soap to a dry surface, he says.

AVOID ELECTRIC.
Electric shavers sometimes cause the hair to go in all sorts of directions—up and down, back and forth. That's no help at all when you're trying to shave with the grain, says Lazar.

TRAIN YOUR WHISKERS.
Then they can join a flea circus and support you in your old age. Seriously, whiskers can be trained. "It takes many moons of shaving one way and not shaving too close," says Litt. After a few weeks, lo and behold, your whiskers will be growing out straight. Well, at least they won't be so curly.

CHANGE YOUR BLADE.
If you're using a double-track razor, you're probably shaving too close for the good of your skin. Switch to a single-

track, disposable razor or, better yet, an old-fashioned safety razor, so you can adjust the closeness of your shave, suggests Joseph P. Bark, M.D., chairman of dermatology at St. Joseph Hospital in Lexington, Kentucky.

SHARPEN UP.
A dull razor blade will make the problem worse. Use a new razor blade every time you shave, advises Litt.

CHANGE YOUR COLLAR.
Avoid wearing shirts with stiff, high collars that rub against the skin of your neck, suggests Lazar. The neck is the site of most ingrown hairs and razor bumps, so try not to wear clothing that will aggravate the problem.

Ingrown toenails
13 Ways to Curb Them

H ere's the good news: "Ingrown toenails can be simply solved with a minimum of pain and discomfort," says Donald Skwor, D.P.M., a podiatrist in Memphis and past president of the American Podiatric Medical Association.

Now for the bad news: A simple nail infection, if not treated properly, can swiftly lead to further complications. When a sharp edge of a toenail grows into the skin folds at its edge, it will result in pain and discomfort, especially if the wound gets infected.

Diabetics and people with vascular disease in particular should get immediate medical treatment for ingrown toenails (see "Hello, Doctor?"). People without circulatory problems, however, can usually take care of an ingrown toenail themselves, if they follow these tips from the experts.

GO SOAK YOUR TOE.

To relieve the soreness, soak your foot in warm, not hot, water. Put a tablespoon or two of Epsom salts in a basin of warm water, suggests Raymond Merkin, D.P.M., a podiatrist in Rockville, Maryland. Soak your toe for five to ten minutes, once or twice a day.

TRY A DIFFERENT SOLUTION.

Rock G. Positano, D.P.M., M.Sc., codirector of the Foot and Ankle Orthopedic Institute at the Hospital for Special Surgery in New York, is a fan of something called Domeboro solution, an antibacterial, anti-inflammatory soak that's available without a prescription. Positano recommends nightly soaks of 20 to 30 minutes. Soaking in this solution should help bring down inflammation so that the nail can grow out naturally.

APPLY OINTMENT.

Spread a topical antibiotic dressing, such as Neosporin, on the wound to prevent infection, says Merkin.

DON'T PLAY SURGEON.

You're not helping matters by performing bathroom surgery on your toe. First of all, the implements in your medicine cabinet are probably chock full of bacteria. Secondly, you could hurt yourself. "The first thing to do

HELLO, DOCTOR?

If you are diabetic or have vascular disease or any other condition that affects circulation, don't even think of trying to treat a nail infection yourself. Furthermore, you shouldn't even be doing your own foot care.

"If someone is a diabetic, they shouldn't be cutting their own nails, period," says Rock G. Positano, D.P.M., M.Sc. "They should be going to a health-care professional who's trained in nail care."

Because diabetics have poor circulation in their extremities, any foot wound or infection takes longer to heal. Without proper treatment, an injury could worsen quickly and bring other complications.

"A simple nail infection can be absolutely catastrophic," Positano warns. "It has led to half a foot being amputated."

The reduced circulation also affects the foot's sensitivity to pain, which can delay detection of a minor injury. For this reason, diabetics and others with poor circulation need to examine their feet daily and should not hesitate to call their doctor at the first sign of foot injury.

is not do bathroom surgery," says Positano, "especially with a dirty instrument. You're many times introducing bacteria or foreign bodies." If the nail has grown in so deeply that it is causing serious infection, see a podiatrist.

TOO MUCH NAIL, TOO LITTLE TOE

Raymond Merkin, D.P.M., likens this situation to when a child's teeth grow in and the need for braces is suddenly very obvious. There seem to be too many teeth for the kid's mouth.

Sometimes, a similar thing can happen with toenails. The growth pattern may change for some reason. The nail seems to be growing wider than before. The result may be a persistent problem with ingrown toenails.

Merkin says a podiatrist can solve the problem with minor surgery using a local anesthetic. "Treatment is to try to permanently narrow the nail by removing part of the side nail border and some of the root of the nail—the matrix, a group of cells that line the base of the toenail. By removing some of the matrix cells, that corner that digs down into the skin is eliminated." If you have persistent ingrown toenails, see a podiatrist.

GO STRAIGHT.
Get in the habit of cutting toenails straight across. "You can file the corners if they're sharp," says Merkin.

DON'T CUT TOO SHORT.
When we stand up, pressure pushes the skin up in front of the toenail. "As the nail grows forward, it imbeds into the skin. So it's best to cut the nail to the end of the skin, rather than below the end of the toe," says Merkin.

STEP INTO A DIFFERENT SHOE.

An ingrown toenail may be nature's way of telling you to go shopping. It's time for some new shoes, ones that don't pinch your toes. If you're a woman, avoid high heels. Try a lower heel (about one inch high) to relieve the pressure on your toes, suggests Skwor.

GET SOME SANDALS, TOO.

If the weather allows, wear open-toed sandals to allow your ailing toe to breathe. Positano describes the space inside socks and shoes as "a very hostile environment" for feet, one that's dark, damp, and hot. Healing will be speedier in the open air.

WATCH WHERE YOU WALK.

Now that you're padding around in sandals, be careful where you walk in them. "Don't walk in the city streets," Positano says. Bacteria could enter your hurt toe. Wear your sandals around your home, but choose shoes with closed toes for urban excursions.

GUARD YOUR TOES.

Even while wearing shoes, you can hurt your toes pretty badly by dropping something on your foot. "If you drop something on your toe that causes you to lose your toe-nail, the nail may grow in when it grows back," says Skwor. If dropping things is a problem for you, wear steel-toed shoes, he advises.

DON'T STUB.

Stubbing your toe can result in an injury that affects the nail. Skwor notes, "That can cause your nail to grow in a thickened manner or cause it to grow in."

IGNORE OLD WIVES.

There's an old wives' tale that by cutting a "V" in the top center of the nail, pressure will be relieved. That doesn't make sense, says Skwor, because the nail grows from the base of the toe. Another tale he has heard concerns rubbing coal oil into the affected area. "They say it helps," says Skwor, but he can't imagine why.

PASS ON SOME PEDICURES.

If you intend to have a pedicure, be sure the person who is performing it does not use metallic instruments to remove dead skin, says Positano. Pumice stones are OK.

Insomnia

21 Ways to Sleep Tight

You know the story: It's 5:00 A.M., and the first traces of dawn have begun to appear in the nighttime sky. You've been awake since 2:00 A.M. and are beginning to feel hopeless about ever getting back to sleep. How will you function at work tomorrow (today)? How will you cope with your presentation at the board meeting? How will you keep yourself from yawning through that dinner with your boss? How will you make it through another day after yet another night without sleep?

Insomnia is the most common sleep disorder in North America and in Europe. A whopping one-third of the U.S. population cannot sleep well enough to function well during the day. One-half of those people have only one or two bad nights a week. The other half spend countless sleepless nights tossing and turning, staring at the alarm clock, and feeling miserable. They also spend countless days exhausted.

Insomnia is also one of the least-understood sleep disorders. German Nino-Murcia, M.D., founder and medical director of the Sleep Medicine and Neuroscience Institute in Palo Alto, California, talks about the frustration he feels at not being able to help more patients who suffer from sleepless nights. "Ten years ago, when I was the director of Stanford University's Sleep Disorders Center, I couldn't do a thing for a quarter of the insomniacs I saw," he says. "Twenty-five percent, after treatment, said they weren't sleeping any more than before they first sought help."

Luckily, after many years of study, sleep experts have come up with many tried-and-true strategies for putting an end to insomnia. The results of their work appear in the tips that follow. Try them out, and see what works for you. If nothing has helped after six months—if you're still struggling to get a decent night's sleep—consult your doctor for a referral to a sleep clinic near you, or call the National Sleep Foundation at 213-288-0466 for a referral to a sleep specialist.

MAKE IT AS NONPUNISHING AS POSSIBLE.

The worst thing that an insomniac can do is to lie in bed tossing and turning, says Peter Hauri, Ph.D., a professor of psychology and director of the Mayo Clinic Insomnia Program in Rochester, Minnesota. Hauri, one of the country's leading authorities on insomnia, is coauthor of the book *No More Sleepless Nights*. "Pass your time reading in bed or watching television, rather than lying in bed frustrated," he says. "This goes for everyone. If you are lying in bed, even if you are not sleeping, your body will still get the same amount of recovery as if you had slept. Although your brain doesn't get any recovery, you'll still be better off than if you spend the time watching the clock, tossing and turning. Hide the clock; put it out of view. You'll only watch it getting later and later and get more and more tense."

DON'T NAP.

"Napping tends to make matters worse for the chronic insomniac," says Karl Doghramji, M.D., director of the Sleep Disorders Center at Jefferson Medical College of Thomas Jefferson University in Philadelphia. The concept is similar to the reason you shouldn't stay in bed late the morning after you had trouble sleeping: you'll have more trouble getting to sleep the next night, thereby compounding your insomnia. Let yourself get sleepy so that it will be easier to get to sleep the next night.

CHANGE YOUR INTERPRETATION OF THE PROBLEM.

Several misconceptions about sleep can make people overly concerned about their insomnia and can actually keep them awake, says Nino-Murcia. One example is when people wake up out of what seems like a deep sleep and feel wide awake. They think that because they feel so alert that they will never be able to get back to sleep. However, says Nino-Murcia, this is not the case. "What happens is that if insomnia wakes you from your REM stage [REM stands for Rapid Eye Movements, the stage of sleep in which you dream], you will be very alert.

HOW MUCH SLEEP DO YOU NEED?

The conventional wisdom is that adults need eight hours of sleep per night. But does that wisdom apply to everyone?

The consensus among sleep researchers is a resounding "no."

Peter Hauri, Ph.D., in the book **No More Sleepless Nights,** says that while different individuals have very different sleep needs, the amount remains amazingly constant for each person. He tells the story of a 70-year-old nurse who slept only one hour each night, took no naps during the day, and said that she never felt tired. In fact, she said she didn't understand why other people wasted so much time in bed. She also said that she had averaged the same amount of sleep each night since she was a child.

Other people may need 9, 10 or even 11 hours of sleep per night. There is no "norm."

"Studies demonstrate that people perform just as well cognitively if they are sleep deprived," says German Nino-Murcia, M.D. "What happens is that people start to demonstrate intellectual problems when they are worried about how little they sleep. If you think you will be impaired, you will be. If you sleep for 90 minutes and when you wake up I tell you that you have slept for eight hours, you will feel great. But if you sleep for eight hours and I wake you up and tell you that you have only slept for 45 minutes, you will feel exhausted."

However, all you have to do is wait for 30 minutes and you will easily fall back to sleep." The key is to understand that your awakening is natural and that you just have to wait it out, he says. Another instance of mistaken perception is that when people wake, they often have the feeling they were never asleep at all. But most people sleep longer than they think, says Nino-Murcia.

TRY EARPLUGS.

Sometimes, insomnia is caused by being awakened repeatedly by loud noises. Often, the sleeper is not aware of what awakened him or her, according to Doghramji. "The classic case is a person who lives near an airport," he says. He suggests minimizing ambient noise as much as possible and, failing that, investing in a good pair of earplugs.

TRY A SLEEPING PILL.

You're not admitting defeat by asking your doctor for a prescription sleeping pill or trying an over-the-counter remedy, says J. Christian Gillin, M.D., a professor of psychiatry at the University of California at San Diego and an adjunct professor in the Department of Psychology at San Diego State University. However, prescription pills should not be used for more than a month at a time, says Gillin. They should also not be used for insomnia at high altitudes, since that type of insomnia may be caused by trouble breathing and a lack of oxygen. Taking sleeping pills at high altitudes may slow your breathing rate even further and may be dangerous. (If you often suffer insomnia at high altitudes, ask your doctor for a prescription drug called Diamox, says Gillin. It may make sleep easier.)

Some doctors don't endorse over-the-counter sleeping pills, however, since they can cause side effects such as drying out your mucous membranes (they often have antihistamines as ingredients) and can make you drowsy the next day. Of course, if you are pregnant, are nursing a baby, or have a serious medical problem, you should consult your doctor before taking any drugs. Sleep medications may also worsen snoring and sleep apnea, a dangerous condition in which breathing is labored during sleep.

NEVER TAKE SLEEPING PILLS THROUGHOUT THE NIGHT.

If you do choose to take medication to help you fall asleep, make sure you only take your dose before you go to bed, says Nino-Murcia. If you take the medication when you wake in the middle of the night, it won't have a chance to wear off before morning, and you're likely to end up being sleepy during the day, he says.

GET A COMFORTABLE BED.

Sleep may also be disturbed because the individual is uncomfortable in his or her bed, says Doghramji. In this case, the sleeper will probably be unaware of why he or she was awakened. "Soft beds are usually better for sleeping than firm ones are," he says.

DON'T DRINK ALCOHOL.

Although alcohol can make you feel drowsy and may actually put you to sleep, it has the unpleasant side effect of waking you up later on in the night, says Gillin. "After drinking alcohol, people often wake up in the middle of the night because of headaches, a full bladder, or gastric upset," he says. In addition, once alcohol's sedative effect wears off, there's a rebound effect that actually makes the individual more likely to have trouble falling back to sleep. So skip the nightcap for a better night's sleep.

CUT DOWN ON CAFFEINE.

We all know that too much coffee, tea, or soda with caffeine can impede the ability to go to sleep at night. But how much is too much? Hauri recommends no more than two cups of coffee or other caffeine-containing beverage in the morning and none after noon.

DON'T SWITCH BEDS OR MOVE TO THE COUCH.

It is important to associate your bed, and only your bed, with sleep, according to Doghramji. "We are all creatures of habit," he says. "Regularity has to be enforced to facilitate sleep. Even animals tend to sleep in the same place every night."

TRY TO MAINTAIN A NORMAL SCHEDULE.

Perhaps the most important rule for people with insomnia is to keep a strict sleep-wake schedule, even on weekends, sleep specialists agree. "Many insomniacs become so desperate that they'll go to sleep any time that they can," says Gillin. If you can't sleep one night, simply get up at your usual time the next morning and don't take any naps. Chances are, you'll be ready for a sound sleep by the next night, he says.

CONFINE WORK TO THE OFFICE.

For the same reason that you shouldn't switch beds or move to the couch every night, you shouldn't do work in bed, says Doghramji. It's important to associate your bed with sleep, not with unpleasant things, like work. Relaxing activities, like reading a novel or watching television, are OK bedtime activities.

TAKE A HOT BATH.

A hot bath taken two hours before bedtime is a wonderful way to relax your body and make it ready for sleep, says Hauri. For most people, however, taking a bath closer to bedtime may be stimulating and may delay sleep (of course, there are always exceptions, he says, so be your own guide). Hauri recommends making the water very hot, like a hot tub, and staying in it for at least 20 minutes. Do not bathe in very hot water, however, if you are pregnant or have significant health problems.

ESTABLISH A BEDTIME RELAXATION RITUAL.

When parents bathe their children or read to them every night before bedtime, they are reinforcing a signal that it's time to get ready for sleep. Establishing such a ritual may also be helpful for adults, says Doghramji. "Learn how to relax," he says. "You can try systematic muscle-tension-and-relaxation exercises: Tense all of your muscles, one at a time, then let go. Buy a tape of ocean or bird sounds. There are plenty of things available. Most insomniacs have a problem with not being able to relax prior to bedtime. They worry about the insomnia." Doghramji recommends doing a relaxation exercise of some sort every night before you retire.

DRINK HOT MILK.

Try drinking warm milk or a malted-milk drink before bed. Even if it doesn't help make you drowsy, it can be comforting and certainly can't do any harm (unless you are allergic to milk or are lactose intolerant).

CUT DOWN ON THE TIME YOU SPEND IN BED.

"Drastically curtail your time in bed," says Hauri. "About 90 percent of people I talk to stay in bed too long. If you stay in bed ten hours and you only need seven hours of sleep, you'll sleep ten hours, but it won't be very high-quality sleep. Stay in bed two hours less than you do now. Try it for a week and see if it makes you sleep sounder and increases the restorative value of your sleep."

EVALUATE YOUR MEDICATIONS.

Certain prescription medications, such as those for asthma and thyroid problems, may cause insomnia, says Gillin. Check with your doctor if you suspect that one of your medications is causing your insomnia.

BE YOUR OWN SLEEP SCIENTIST.

There is no one formula for perfect sleep, says Hauri. The important thing is to give everything a fair and persistent trial (at least a week or two). "Think back to 10 or 15 years ago when you were not an insomniac," Hauri says. "How much did you sleep then? What helped you sleep?" He recommends keeping a sleep log, a notebook of what works and doesn't work for you.

NEVER TRY TO GO TO SLEEP.

Sounds counterintuitive, right? Well, it's not. Falling asleep is something that requires the opposite of effort. Effort is work, and work keeps you awake. "The harder you try to go to sleep, the harder it will be to go to sleep,"

Gillin says. Instead, try to just lie still, relax, and let sleep come.

STAY COOL.

For high-quality sleep to occur, the internal body temperature should be a few degrees cooler than it is during the day, says Hauri. However, many insomniacs lack the proper internal controls to regulate their body temperature. That's why a hot bath helps—after raising the body's temperature, it drops it back down within a couple of hours. Exercise, done at least six hours before bedtime, has the same effect, Hauri says. Keeping the bedroom cool may also be helpful.

EAT A SANDWICH.

Although you may have been told that eating before you go to bed may give you nightmares, the reverse is actually true, according to Hauri. Going to bed on a full stomach may actually help you sleep. That may be part of the reason why folks are always nodding off after a big holiday dinner.

Lactose intolerance

10 Ways to Manage It

Many folks relish the thought of downing a frosty-cold glass of milk, polishing off a bowl of creamy ice cream, or biting into a piping-hot slice of cheesy pizza. For close to 50 million Americans, though, the aftereffects of indulging in these dairy delights may force them to forgo such foods or suffer some decidedly unpleasant consequences.

The common condition these people share is lactose intolerance. That means they don't properly digest lactose, which is milk sugar found in all milk products. This problem is usually due to a shortage of the enzyme lactase, which normally breaks down milk sugar in the small intestine into simple parts that can be absorbed into the bloodstream. The end result of this lactase deficiency may be gas, stomach pains, bloating, and diarrhea. The severity of the symptoms varies from person to person.

Who is lactose intolerant? It's not an equal opportunity problem. It affects some ethnic groups much more than others. The National Institute of Diabetes & Digestive & Kidney Diseases estimates that 75 percent of African-American, Jewish, Native-American, and Mexican-American adults and 90 percent of Asian-American adults have this condition. Only about 10 to 15 percent of adult Caucasians are lactase deficient, says David Alpers, M.D., a professor of medicine and chief of the Gastroenterology Division at Washington University School of Medicine in St. Louis. Though you may not fall into any of these categories, keep in mind that as we get older, we all lose some of the ability to digest lactose in milk.

Some people figure out that they are lactose intolerant on their own; for others, it takes a trip to a doctor to pinpoint the problem. "Among the black or Asian community, it's kind of folk wisdom that these people don't do well with milk, so they tend not to drink as much,"

HELLO, DOCTOR?

If you're feeling digestive distress that you think may be lactose intolerance but you're not certain, try this simple test. Lay off all milk products for a few weeks and see if your gut gets better. If things don't improve, it may be time to check in with your doctor. Other glitches in the digestive system may be causing your problems. For instance, you may have irritable bowel syndrome, another common digestive disorder that can produce symptoms similar to lactose intolerance . "Another thing that lactose intolerance can be confused with is an intolerance to caffeine," says David Alpers, M.D. So play it safe and get an expert's opinion, especially if you notice a major change in bowel patterns.

says Alpers. On the other hand, he says, "There's also a significant number of people who are having symptoms from milk sugar and really have no idea of what the problem is."

If you suspect that your problem may be lactose intolerance but you're not entirely sure, it may be worthwhile to visit your physician. He or she will be able to rule out other possible problems (see "Hello, Doctor?"). Once you know that you are indeed lactose intolerant, you may want to follow these helpful tips to ease your symptoms:

DETERMINE YOUR LEVEL OF LACTOSE INTOLERANCE.

The degree of intolerance differs with each person. The easiest way to do this is first to get all lactose out of your system. "That means having no dairy food and no lactose for about three to four weeks," says Jane Zukin, author of *The Dairy-Free Cookbook* and editor of *The Newsletter for People with Lactose Intolerance and Milk Allergies*. Then start with very small quantities of milk or cheese. Monitor your symptoms to see how much or how little dairy food you can handle. Once you know your limits, management becomes a little easier.

STICK WITH SMALL SERVINGS.

While you may not be able to tolerate an eight-ounce glass of milk all at once, you may feel fine drinking a third of a cup in the morning, a third of a cup in the afternoon, and a third of a cup at night. "If you have 'x' amount of lactase enzyme in your body that can only digest 'x' amount of lactose, it will be easier if you take in less lactose over a longer period of time than if you overload," says Zukin.

DON'T EAT DAIRY FOODS ALONE.

If you eat some cheese or drink a little milk, plan to do so with a meal or a snack. "Having more in your stomach to digest slows the digestive process and may ease your symptoms," says Zukin.

COLOR YOUR MILK CHOCOLATE.

A study by researcher Chong Lee at the University of Rhode Island in Kingston found that 35 lactose-intolerant people digested more lactose when they drank milk with cocoa and sugar added than they did when they drank plain milk. They also experienced less bloating and fewer cramps. No one knows why this is so, but Alpers says it may be because "chocolate delays the emptying of your stomach." Slower emptying may mean fewer symptoms.

SUPPLEMENT YOUR DIET.

Lactase-enzyme supplements can supply your body with some of what it lacks. They're sold in tablet or liquid form, without a prescription. The tablets are chewed with or right after you consume a dairy product; you add the drops directly to milk. "These work quite well for some people," says Zukin. You can also try lactose-reduced milk.

TRY YOGURT.

"By and large, lactose intolerant people tolerate yogurt pretty well," says Alpers. This holds true, however, only for yogurt with active cultures, which you may have to buy in a health-food store. If you can tolerate yogurt, it's to your advantage to include it in your diet, because this creamy food is a great source of calcium.

CHOOSE HARD CHEESES.

If you find yourself drawn to the cheese aisle at your grocery store, pick hard, aged cheeses such as Swiss, cheddar, or Colby, advises Elyse Sosin, R.D., Supervisor of Clinical Nutrition at Mount Sinai Medical Center in New York. They contain less lactose than soft cheeses.

AVOID PROCESSED FOODS.

Lactose is used in a lot of processed foods where you might not expect to find it (see "Hidden Sources of

HIDDEN SOURCES OF LACTOSE

Lactose lurks in many prepared foods. Bread, cereals, pancakes, chocolate, soups, puddings, salad dressings, sherbet, instant cocoa mix, candies, frozen dinners, cookie mixes, and hot dogs may all contain lactose. While the amounts of lactose may be small, people with low tolerance levels can be bothered. "People need to read every single label and be careful of what they eat," says author Jane Zukin. When perusing ingredient labels, it's not just milk that you have to watch for. Whey, curds, milk by-products, dry milk solids, nonfat dry milk powder, casein, galactose, skim milk powder, milk sugar, and whey protein concentrate are all buzzwords that indicate the presence of lactose.

Lactose"). "It's best for people to stick to as much fresh food as possible, and skip the cans, frozen foods, and stuff that comes out of a box," says Zukin. One added benefit to this strategy: You'll be eating a healthier diet.

GET CALCIUM FROM OTHER FOODS.

Lactose intolerant people, especially women and children, should make sure their calcium intake doesn't plunge. Green, leafy vegetables, such as collard greens, kale, turnip greens, and chinese cabbage (bok choy), as well as oysters, sardines, canned salmon with the bones, and tofu, provide lots of calcium. If your diet is calcium poor, you may want to take calcium supplements; talk to your doctor for a recommendation on proper dosage.

WATCH OUT FOR MEDICATIONS.

Lactose is used as a filler in more than 20 percent of prescription drugs (including many types of birth control pills) and in about 6 percent of over-the-counter medicines. This may not matter to someone who takes medication only occasionally, but Zukin says, "for the person who takes medication on a regular basis, this can be a problem." Complicating matters is the fact that lactose may not be listed under the inactive ingredients on the label. To find out if what you're taking contains lactose, Zukin advises first seeking help from your doctor. You might also check with your pharmacist or write directly to the drug manufacturer.

Laryngitis

18 Ways to Tame a Hoarse Throat

Your voice sounds more like a frog croaking than a human talking. Chances are, you can figure out why—all the yelling you did at last night's hockey game or that cold you've had for the past couple of days.

Don't confuse laryngitis with a sore throat, though. "Some people say they've got laryngitis when what they really mean is their throat is sore," says Michael S. Benninger, M.D., vice-chairperson of the Department of Otolaryngology at Henry Ford Hospital in Detroit.

LARYNGITIS

True laryngitis is the loss of the voice or hoarseness, and it's the result of inflammation (swelling) of the larynx, or voice box, and the voice folds, explains Gary Y. Shaw, M.D., associate professor of otolaryngology, head and neck surgery at the University of Kansas Medical Center in Kansas City.

The most common cause of temporary laryngitis is an upper-respiratory infection, usually viral, like the common cold. If the infection is bacterial, you may need to see a doctor to get antibiotic treatment.

The second most common cause of laryngitis is voice abuse or overuse. "If you screamed at the top of your lungs at the football game, you'll be hoarse afterward," says Shaw.

The symptoms of acute, or short-term laryngitis, can include pain in the throat or around the larynx, hoarseness, raspiness, the loss of range (noticed especially by singers), easy fatiguability, and a scratchy feeling in the throat. Constantly clearing your throat can be another symptom.

If you suffer from chronic laryngitis, smoking may be the culprit. The smoke increases the mass of the larynx, explains Benninger, lowering the pitch of the voice.

One surprising cause of laryngitis is gastroesophageal reflux. That's a long name for what a lot of us think of as heartburn, except that only about half of its sufferers actually feel any "heartburn," so they're unaware that the acid-rich contents of their stomach are coming back up in their throats, especially during the night. "It's the principal player in laryngitis in the elderly," says Benninger. "People complain there's something sticking in their throat, and they think it's mucus from postnasal drip." Symptoms are worse in the morning. You may

HELLO, DOCTOR?

Laryngitis is usually a temporary inconvenience without serious consequences. But sometimes, persistent hoarseness or voice loss is your body's way of telling you something is wrong. When should you see a doctor?

• If pain is present

• If the hoarseness continues for more than 72 hours

• If you've got an upper-respiratory infection with a fever that lasts more than a couple of days

• If you have trouble breathing

• If you notice a permanent change in the pitch of your voice, especially if you are a smoker

• If you cough up blood

The problem may be as minor as a bacterial infection that needs antibiotics. You could have polyps or nodules on your vocal folds that cause them to vibrate more slowly, changing the sound of your voice. Or you could have cancer of the larynx, which can be treated with radiation if caught early.

wake up with a bad taste in your mouth, do a lot of throat clearing, and have hoarseness that gets better as the day goes on, says Shaw. "And you often feel like there's something in your throat all the time." If you suspect this is causing your laryngitis, see your doctor (also see HEARTBURN).

LARYNGITIS

If you're experiencing laryngitis, here's what you can do to soothe your voice:

DRINK.
Water, that is. Take frequent sips of water to stay hydrated and keep your throat moist. Or choose other fluids, like juices, says Sally Wenzel, M.D., assistant professor of medicine at the National Jewish Center for Immunology and Respiratory Medicine in Denver. She adds that warm drinks may feel more soothing than cold.

SUCK ON LEMON DROPS.
Lemon helps stimulate the flow of saliva.

SIP NONCAFFEINATED TEA WITH LEMON.
Avoid caffeine because it is dehydrating, says Benninger. Make sure the tea isn't too hot or too cold.

USE ARTIFICIAL SALIVA.
It may sound unpleasant, but you can buy over-the-counter products that help keep your mouth moist.

SPEAK SOFTLY.
"Speak in a confidential tone, as if you're telling someone a secret," says Benninger.

DON'T WHISPER.
Whispering is more stressful than speaking softly .

LIMIT CONVERSATION.
"It's sort of like limiting the motion of your knee when it's skinned," says Shaw. "I tell patients to use their voices only if they're getting paid for it," adds Benninger.

DON'T CLEAR YOUR THROAT.

You're actually irritating the situation, setting up "a vicious cycle," says Benninger.

STOP SMOKING.

One more reason to kick the habit. Or at least go without while your throat is healing.

AVOID SMOKERS.

Even passive smoke irritates the larynx. If you live with a smoker, ask him or her to take their habit outside.

FORGET RECREATIONAL DRUGS.

Marijuana and cocaine are extremely rough on the larynx, Benninger says.

ABSTAIN FROM ALCOHOL.

Alcohol dehydrates you, which is the opposite of what your voice needs.

CUT OUT THE CAFFEINE.

Like alcohol, the caffeine in coffee, tea, and colas dehydrates you.

HUMIDIFY THE AIR.

Indoor heating takes moisture out of winter air. Use a humidifier or portable steamer. If nothing else, breathe in the steam from a teapot or pan of boiling water, suggests Shaw.

AVOID DUSTY ENVIRONMENTS.

The dust is irritating, and such places are often also dry, which compounds the problem.

BEWARE OF CERTAIN DRYING DRUGS.

Medications such as antihistamines and diuretics can dry your mouth and throat. You shouldn't stop diuretics (they're often prescribed for high blood pressure), but think twice about taking over-the-counter antihistamines. Talk to your doctor or pharmacist if you have any questions about any medications you may be taking.

GARGLE WITH SALT WATER.

Add one-half teaspoon salt to a cup of warm (about body temperature) water, advises Wenzel. You don't want it too salty, warns Benninger. "It's not like ocean water. And too much salt could cause more irritation."

PROTECT YOUR VOICE.

To help your voice heal and to prevent future attacks of laryngitis, learn how to take care of your voice. Staying well hydrated is the first step. Avoiding voice abuse is the next. And if you depend on your voice in your career, you may want to invest in voice training, suggests Benninger.

Menopause

11 Tips for Coping with "the Change"

For most women, menopause, the cessation of the menstrual cycle, is fraught with rumor and misinformation. Stories of menopausal hot flashes, vaginal dryness, wrinkles, weight gain, depression, anxiety, thinning hair, and loss of sex drive may have you dreading "the change." Relax. Most of the stories you've heard probably aren't true.

Too often, women confuse natural aging changes with menopause. The few symptoms actually associated with the hormonal changes during menopause can usually be handled with a few minor lifestyle changes. Contrary to what most women have heard about menopause, it's a natural period of transition that gives rise to an exciting and challenging period in life.

Menopause is a period of four or five years, usually two years before the last menstrual period and two to three years after it. For most women, menopause occurs between the ages of 45 and 53, although some women experience it earlier and others go through it at a later age. A woman generally experiences menopause at about the same age as her mother did.

Menopause begins with changes in the menstrual cycle—shorter or longer periods, heavier or lighter bleeding, decreased or increased premenstrual symptoms—until the menstrual periods cease altogether. Women should keep track of their irregular bleeding so their physician can help them determine whether these changes are normal or whether they indicate some abnormal changes in the uterine lining.

Although there is much talk about menopausal "symptoms," the only symptoms that have been clearly demonstrated to be associated with the hormonal changes of menopause are hot flashes and vaginal dryness. Mood swings or depression aren't related to hormonal changes as much as they are to fatigue caused from sleep disturbances due to hot flashes, according to Amanda Clark,

M.D., assistant professor of obstetrics and gynecology at Oregon Health Sciences University in Portland. "The hormonal fluctuations of menopause aren't believed to cause any major psychological depression," she says.

But menopause signals more than hormonal changes. It is the doorway to a new life. Postmenopausal women are free of the discomforts of menstruation, free of the need for contraceptives, and, in many cases, free of child-rearing responsibilities. For the first time, many women find they can concentrate on their own agendas and do the things *they* want to do.

Here are some tips about how to make the most of this exciting transition called menopause:

DRESS FOR HOT FLASHES.

Eight in ten women experience periods of sudden, intense heat and accompanying sweating often called "flushes" or "hot flashes," according to Sadja Greenwood, M.D., an assistant clinical professor in the Department of Obstetrics, Gynecology, and Reproductive Sciences at the University of California at San Francisco. "Hot flashes are the body's response to lower-than-usual estrogen levels," says Greenwood. She recommends wearing loose clothing that is easily removed.

DOUSE IT.

If it's convenient, you can "spritz" your face with cool water from a squeeze bottle or blot with a cool wash-cloth or moist towelette.

AVOID CAFFEINE AND ALCOHOL.

If hot flashes seem to be triggered by caffeine and alcohol consumption, Greenwood advises women to avoid them completely. Try substituting noncaffeinated teas or decaffeinated coffee for caffeinated beverages. (Keep in mind that caffeine withdrawal may cause headaches and fatigue for several days.) Greenwood says excess caffeine also causes the kidneys to excrete more calcium, a factor in bone thinning in postmenopausal women.

CARRY A PERSONAL FAN.

Many women find relief from hot flashes by using a small personal fan. Inexpensive wood and paper fans or battery-powered personal fans are small enough to be carried in a purse and used anywhere.

TAKE YOUR TIME WITH LOVEMAKING.

Hormonal changes associated with menopause often cause a woman's vaginal mucous membranes to become thin and secrete less moisture. The result can be painful sexual intercourse. Some of this lack of moisture can be overcome by taking more time to make love, according to Lonnie Barbach, Ph.D., a nationally recognized sex expert and author of numerous books on the topic. Barbach also suggests exploring other ways of pleasuring one another in addition to intercourse.

USE CREAMS OR LUBRICANTS.

If patient lovemaking doesn't produce enough lubrication for the woman, Clark suggests using lubricating jellies (available in pharmacies), plain vegetable oil, or unscented cold cream. "One of the best lubricants is a product called Astroglide, because it's most like natural secretions," she says. "Jellies like K-Y Jelly are good, but Vaseline tends to be messy and gummy."

EXERCISE REGULARLY.

Menopause has been erroneously linked with depression. Several studies have found that women between the ages of 45 and 55 have no increase in susceptibility to depression. Mood swings during this time may have more to do with a woman's changing role and her self-concept and the physical changes of aging she's experiencing. "For many women," says Clark, "menopause is a milestone, a negative milestone, in their lives. They find the idea of menopause depressing. We need to discard those old ideas." Regular, aerobic exercise such as brisk walking does much to increase general health and raise spirits. It also appears to slow changes like loss of strength that many believe to be age related, but are actually more associated with a sedentary lifestyle.

Regular, weight-bearing exercises such as walking or jogging can also help stave off the bone thinning of osteoporosis, a problem for many menopausal women. Clark says bones get stronger with regular exercise no matter what your age. "Any weight-bearing exercise is good," says Clark. "But it has to be a weight-bearing exercise, not like swimming, to increase bone density."

GET SUPPORT.

"Another term for menopause is 'climacteric,'" says Susan Woodruff, B.S.N., childbirth and parenting education coordinator at Tuality Community Hospital in Hillsboro, Oregon. "That word applies because it is a really big change. You're closing one chapter in your life and moving on. You may notice body changes—new aches, pains, wrinkles. Menopause is one of life's major change signals. It's helpful to talk to other women about these changes."

Woodruff recommends joining a menopause support group sponsored by a local hospital, community college, or professional group. Or you might want to form your own support group with friends who are experiencing menopause. "Menopause affects how you see yourself, your self-concept, because your roles in life are changing at this time," says Woodruff. "A support group of other women who understand can really help you see yourself as a strong person experiencing a natural life change."

GET PLENTY OF CALCIUM.

"Everyone loses calcium as they get older," says Clark. "But in women, as estrogen levels decline, the rate of bone loss increases."

Sonja Connor, M.S., R.D., research associate professor in the School of Medicine at Oregon Health Sciences University in Portland, says, "At menopause, there's an outpouring of calcium in response to the lower estrogen levels. Unless you have really good stores of calcium already, during this time you're going to have an increased need for calcium."

Clark says postmenopausal women taking hormone replacement need 1,000 milligrams of elemental calcium daily; women not taking hormones need 1,500 milligrams of elemental calcium.

Dairy products are good sources of calcium, although you'll be doing yourself an even bigger favor if you choose those that are low in fat, such as skim milk, non-fat yogurt, and low-fat cheeses. For example, an eight-ounce glass of whole milk and an eight-ounce glass of skim milk contain the same amount of elemental calcium (350 milligrams), but the whole milk contains about

CALCIUM-RICH FOODS

Calcium is important at any age, but it becomes even more important for menopausal women in order to prevent the bone thinning of osteoporosis. Include these calcium-rich foods in your diet to ensure you're getting enough of this important mineral:

Almonds
Brewer's yeast
Cheese (opt for nonfat or low-fat varieties)
Dandelion greens
Ice milk or ice cream (opt for lower-fat varieties)
Kelp
Mackerel, canned
Milk (opt for skim or low-fat)
Mustard greens
Oysters
Salmon, canned with bones
Sardines, canned with bones
Soybean curd (tofu)
Yogurt (opt for nonfat or low-fat)

70 calories more from fat. To add to your calcium stores, eat a diet that is also rich in vegetables, fruits, and complex carbohydrates (see "Calcium-Rich Foods").

If your diet isn't calcium rich or if your stores of calcium are seriously depleted from a lifetime of poor eating habits, Clark suggests taking calcium supplements.

ESTROGEN REPLACEMENT THERAPY

Many physicians recommend that women take hormones to make up for the decrease in estrogen levels that occurs during menopause. Estrogen replacement therapy, or ERT (also called hormone replacement therapy or HRT), can reduce or eliminate the hot flashes and vaginal soreness and, in some women, decrease the risk of osteoporosis, says Sadja Greenwood, M.D.

However, ERT isn't without risk. Some studies have shown ERT may increase the risk of cancer of the breast and uterus. Amanda Clark, M.D., says studies have shown the increased risk of breast cancer is small and that the increased risk of uterine cancer can be eliminated by adding the hormone progestin. Women who have had any of the following are generally not recommended for ERT: cancer of the breast, uterus, or ovaries; clots in the legs, pelvis, or lungs; high blood pressure; diabetes; gallstones or gallbladder disease; or large uterine fibroids.

Clark believes that the benefits of ERT generally outweigh the risks. "Fourteen studies have shown that hormone replacement therapy helps prevent heart disease," she says. "Estrogen also helps maintain calcium uptake, which helps prevent osteoporosis."

Greenwood says women should thoroughly discuss the pros and cons of ERT with their physicians. If a woman opts for ERT, Greenwood says, she should take the lowest dose possible and be sure it combines estrogen and progestin to reduce the risk of uterine cancer.

Keep in mind that the number of milligrams of calcium listed on the label of a supplement may not reflect the amount of elemental calcium in the product. For example, it takes 1,200 milligrams of calcium carbonate to get 500 milligrams of elemental calcium. Ask your doctor or pharmacist for advice on choosing a calcium supplement.

EAT A BALANCED, LOW-FAT DIET.

Women at menopause not only have an increased risk of osteoporosis, they may also be at risk for heart disease. "At menopause, women's levels of LDL, or so-called 'bad' cholesterol, go up," explains Connor. "Within about ten years, they have the same risk for heart disease as men."

Connor says diet can go a long way toward preventing serious health problems like osteoporosis, cancer, and heart disease in menopausal women. "Diets high in animal products and salt cause the body to excrete more calcium, which contributes to osteoporosis," she says. "Menopausal women should eat less animal protein and less salt. If they switch to more foods from the vegetable kingdom and more complex carbohydrates, they'll be getting less fat [high-fat diets are related to some cancers and heart disease], more calcium, and more of the anticancer elements like beta carotene."

PLAN FOR MENOPAUSE.

"The problem," says Connor, "is that most women eat the typical American diet: 40 percent of calories from fat, 20 percent from sugar, and 5 percent from alcohol—essentially empty calories. That means they're getting nutrients from only 35 percent of their calories. On top of that, they don't do any regular exercise. When menopause comes, they need medical intervention in the form of hormone therapy just to catch up with what they've done to their bodies all these years."

Connor believes only a small percentage of women would need hormone therapy if they'd anticipate menopause by eating right and exercising regularly for at least 20 years before the onset of menopause. "Prevention is the best thing," she says. "A lifelong lifestyle of low-fat eating, not smoking, and exercising regularly will usually get you ready to face menopausal changes without any problems." And, of course, no matter what stage of life you're in, it's never too late to benefit from switching to a healthier lifestyle.

Menstrual cramps

6 Ways to Tackle Them

Three weeks out of each month you feel great. But then comes your period, and with it, those awful cramps. For most women, menstrual cramps last no more than one or two days each month. But this can seem endless when you're trying to function normally. And the congestive, bloating-type symptoms that frequently accompany these cramps may only compound the problem.

HELLO, DOCTOR?

All of these experts agree that if you notice your cramps getting more severe, or if you've never had menstrual cramps before and suddenly develop them, it is time to visit your doctor. "Women with primary menstrual cramps start having them when they first begin menstruating or within one to two years of the onset of menstruation," says Harold Zimmer, M.D. "So if you notice a significant change, you should be evaluated to see if there is some secondary cause for the cramps," he continues.

"Secondary cramps also tend to be pretty mean cramps that are often accompanied by nausea, vomiting, and even diarrhea," says Phyllis Frey, A.R.N.P. "They can also occur with backache and pain down the thighs."

"Primary menstrual cramps are hereditary," says Phyllis Frey, A.R.N.P., a nurse practitioner at Bellegrove OB-GYN, Inc., in Bellevue, Washington. "There is no specific cause determined. It just seems that during your period, your uterus cramps up and your sensitivity to that cramping is pretty acute," she explains.

"Sometimes, primary cramps will lessen after giving birth," says Harold Zimmer, M.D., an obstetrician and gynecologist in Bellevue, Washington. "We are not sure why this is, but it could be that the stretching out of the cervix during delivery reduces the pulling against it that can occur when the uterus contracts or cramps up," he adds.

The causes for secondary cramps could include endometriosis (the presence of endometrial tissue in places where it is not usually found), pelvic congestion, pelvic varicose veins, pelvic infection, or fibroids (benign tumors in the uterine wall). "Secondary cramps caused by fibroids tend to occur during actual ovulation, while those caused by endometriosis may be present throughout the month," says Zimmer. "With pelvic congestion or pelvic veins, the cramps tend to occur four or five days before the menstrual flow itself," he adds. While you may get some relief from secondary cramps with self-treatment, the underlying conditions that cause them really need to be treated by a physician. And Zimmer warns that exercising may actually worsen secondary cramps.

"Secondary menstrual cramps, on the other hand, are caused by some underlying condition, such as pelvic infection, pelvic lesions, fibroids, endometriosis, bad pelvic congestion, or pelvic varicose veins," says Zimmer. "They are usually a little worse than primary cramps, depending on how significant the underlying condition is."

In either case, menstrual cramps are usually the result of a prostaglandin excess. Prostaglandin is a hormone produced by the uterine lining that mediates many processes within the body. It can bring on headaches, intestinal cramps, and labor, according to Zimmer. While secondary cramps are usually treated by curing the underlying condition, primary cramps can be self-treated with over-the-counter medications and some basic comfort measures. Here are some suggestions:

TAKE IBUPROFEN OR ASPIRIN.

"These medications help to lower the level of prostaglandins, which can lessen or alleviate the cramps," says Zimmer. "These drugs also cost much less than those that a doctor would prescribe for cramps," adds Frey.

HOLD A HEATING PAD TO THE CRAMPED AREA.

"The heat will relax the muscles and soften the pain of the cramping," says Frey. "It works best if you can lie down at the same time," she says.

TAKE A HOT BATH.

"Just as with a heating pad, a hot bath relaxes the muscles and increases circulation to the pelvic area," says Zimmer. It can also relieve lower back pain.

MAINTAIN A REGULAR AEROBIC EXERCISE PROGRAM.

"This doesn't mean you have to exercise through an episode of cramps. Keeping up a regular exercise or fitness program the rest of the month seems to make these episodes less intense when they do occur," says Frey. "Exercising also increases pelvic circulation, which helps to clear out the excess prostaglandins a little faster," adds Zimmer.

DO SOME PELVIC-TILT EXERCISES.

"Getting down on all fours, bringing the elbows to the ground, and rocking back and forth tends to help some women," says Zimmer. "It works especially well for women with a retroverted uterus [one that is more swollen and puts more pressure on the back]," he adds.

TALK TO YOUR DOCTOR ABOUT BIRTH CONTROL PILLS.

"Birth control pills help to suppress ovulation, which lessens the severity of menstrual cramps," says Zimmer. "It is really not certain why they help so much," adds Frey. "It could be that by lessening the flow and length of a woman's period, the cramps are lessened as well," she continues. Birth control pills are not without side effects, however, and certain women should not use them, so be sure to discuss them thoroughly with your doctor.

Morning sickness

13 Ways to Ease the Queasiness

The nausea and vomiting of early pregnancy were written about as early as 2000 B.C. Unfortunately, the ancient Egyptians didn't have a cure for the condition, either.

Some 50 to 70 percent of American women will suffer from nausea or vomiting, or both, during the first three months (also known as the first trimester) of their pregnancies. The severity and even occurrence vary not only from woman to woman, but from pregnancy to pregnancy in the same individual.

Some women never have even the slightest touch of queasiness. Some are ill in the morning and recover by lunch. And some stay sick all day for days on end, wondering why it's called "morning sickness" when it lasts 24 hours.

No one knows what causes morning sickness. It is less common among Eskimos and native African tribes than in Western civilizations. But today's doctors emphasize it's not psychological, as was once believed. "Morning sickness is not a psychological rejection of the pregnancy," says Donald R. Coustan, M.D., professor and chair of obstetrics-gynecology at Brown University School of Medicine and chief of obstetrics-gynecology at Women and Infants Hospital of Rhode Island in Providence. "It is not a symbolic attempt to vomit up the baby."

Since hormones run amok during early pregnancy, researchers theorize that these abnormal hormone levels contribute somehow to the existence of morning sickness. A suspected culprit is human chorionic gonadotropin (HCG), the hormone tested in home pregnancy kits, which hits an all-time high in those first months. But other hormones may play a role as well. High levels of progesterone, for example, result in smooth-muscle relaxation, slowing down the digestive process, says Cheryl Coleman, R.N., B.S.N., I.C.C.E., a childbirth educator at Hillcrest Medical Center in Tulsa, Oklahoma, and director of public relations for the International Childbirth Education Association.

"There are a lot of changes going on in the pregnant woman's body," points out Kermit E. Krantz, M.D., university distinguished professor, professor of gynecology and obstetrics, and professor of anatomy at the Univer-

THE BRIGHT SIDE

The good news about morning sickness? (You doubt that there's anything good to say about this subject?) Studies have shown that women who experience nausea and vomiting early in their pregnancies are more likely to deliver full-term, healthy babies.

Researchers in Colorado Springs, Colorado, and Albany, New York, studied 414 pregnant women. Nearly 90 percent said they had some of the symptoms of morning sickness. But these women were more likely to carry their pregnancies to full term and deliver a live baby than the women who had no morning sickness at all. On the other hand, don't panic if you don't experience morning sickness. Plenty of women sail through pregnancy without nausea and deliver healthy babies.

sity of Kansas Medical Center in Kansas City. "Your kidneys increase their activity by 100 percent. Your blood volume will increase by 50 percent."

If you're suffering from morning sickness, you probably don't care what causes it. You just want relief. Time will eventually take care of it; the condition usually subsides after the third month. (Scant words of comfort.) While you're waiting for the second trimester to arrive, however, here's what the experts suggest that you try for relief:

HELLO, DOCTOR?

If morning sickness persists past the third month or you find yourself so ill that you're losing weight, see your physician. Watch out, too, for becoming dehydrated; you'll feel dizzy when you stand, or your urine output will be scanty and dark colored.

DON'T WORRY ABOUT CRUMBS IN THE SHEETS.
Keep crackers by the bed. Eating a few low-sodium crackers as soon as you wake up—and before you get out of bed—is the first line of defense against morning sickness.

GRAZE.
Eat frequent, small meals. You may want to eat five to six times a day. Sometimes, hunger pangs bring on the feelings of nausea. That's because acids in the stomach have nothing to digest when there's no food around.

DON'T DRINK AND EAT AT THE SAME TIME.
Drink your fluids between meals, instead of during meals, to avoid too much bulk in the stomach, says Krantz.

FILL UP ON FLUIDS.
You need at least eight glasses a day, says Krantz. "Avoiding dehydration is most important, especially in the summertime."

GO FOR A LIQUID DIET.

Your tummy may prefer liquids to solids, says Coustan. Get nutrients from bouillon, juices, and other liquids.

STICK TO BLAND FOODS.

This isn't the time to try that new Thai restaurant. Spicy foods just don't cut it right now.

CHOOSE COMPLEX CARBOHYDRATES.

Pasta, bread, potatoes—the foods you think of as starches—are easier to digest and they're soothing, says Coleman.

AVOID FATTY FOODS.

Fats are harder to digest than carbohydrates or proteins, explains Coleman.

DON'T SNIFF.

Certain odors often trigger the feelings of nausea. "Pay attention to what these triggers are and avoid them," suggests Coustan. "Let someone else do the cooking if that bothers you, for example."

AVOID SUDDEN MOVES.

Don't change your posture quickly. "Don't sit up in bed too suddenly," advises Krantz. "Get up easily."

TAKE VITAMIN B$_6$.

A number of physicians recommend this vitamin for morning sickness because of its ability to fight nausea. Talk to your doctor before trying a supplement, however, and be sure not to exceed 25 milligrams of the vitamin each day.

TAKE A HIKE.

OK, go for a walk outside every day. "It's a positive thing you can do for yourself," says Coleman. "And the exercise and fresh air may make you feel better." Be sure to check with your doctor before trying anything more strenuous than a stroll, however.

DON'T FORGET TO BRUSH.

If you do succumb to vomiting, take good care of your teeth and brush afterward. Otherwise, the frequent contact with the harsh acids in what you throw up can eat away at tooth enamel.

Motion sickness

13 Ways to Still the Savage Beast

O h that queasy sensation, when the world just won't stop swaying, bobbing, or just plain moving. No matter what the mode of movement—in the air, on the ground, or on the water—the result can be motion sickness. While many experts believe there may be a genetic tendency involved, they aren't exactly sure why some people get sick from riding in a car, boat, plane, or train. If you do, you're not alone. Motion sickness caused some pilots to drop out of training during World War II. And to this day, NASA astronauts are constantly combating this side effect brought on by weightlessness and space.

Motion sickness is believed to occur when the balancing system gets overloaded by the messages it's re-

PATCH UP THE PROBLEM

Another option for preventing motion sickness is to use a transdermal (skin) patch. Available with a prescription from your doctor, the patch adheres to the skin behind the ear or on the neck or forehead and dispenses small amounts of scopolamine, a drug that suppresses the body's balancing mechanisms. In order to be effective, however, you must take care to use the patch properly. If you are prescribed patches, the first one must be applied at least 12 hours before departure. Do not dispense them to anyone else, warns John Youngblood, M.D. Children and the elderly, in particular, are more likely to be sensitive to the medication in the patch. Children, for example, can become hyperactive as a result of wearing the patch.

ceiving from the eyes and inner ears. The brain responds to the conflicting messages by creating some of its own. "The first signs are usually sweating, hyperventilation, and light-headedness," says Michael S. Morris, M.D., an otolaryngologist and assistant professor at Georgetown University School of Medicine in Washington, D.C.

For some people, these reactions and the others associated with motion sickness, such as nausea, can be brought on merely by walking down the aisles in a supermarket or watching telephone poles whipping by a car window, says John Youngblood, M.D., associate professor at the University of Texas Health Science Center in San Antonio and president of the Austin Ear Clinic. And some people can get "motion" sickness from the sounds they hear, says Herbert Silverstein, M.D., president of the Ear Research Foundation and Florida Otologic Center in Sarasota.

No matter what the cause, once the symptoms set in, it's virtually impossible to stop motion sickness from running its course, says Silverstein. That's why it's important to try to prevent the symptoms from occuring before they have a chance to take hold. Here are some techniques you can try to keep motion sickness from setting in:

LOOK OFF INTO THE DISTANCE.

Not to daydream, but to focus on a steady point away from the rocky boat, plane, or car, to help you get your bearings. "Look as far to the horizon as you can," says Silverstein. This helps counteract the conflicting messages the brain is receiving from the topsy-turvy surroundings.

STAY ON DECK.

If you're on a boat, going inside or below deck will only intensify the symptoms. Instead, stay on deck so you can look at the horizon to help your body cope.

SIT OVER THE WING OF THE AIRPLANE.

"The wing is the most stable part of the plane, since the plane's body pivots on it," says Youngblood. And if you can get a window seat in this midsection, all the better. Then you can look out and set your sights far from the plane if you should get queasy.

FACE FORWARD ON THE BUS OR TRAIN.

This is so you can see the road ahead of you instead of concentrating on the busy movement taking place to the sides. And if you can, take a seat, because standing can also bring on motion sickness.

VOLUNTEER TO DRIVE.

Drivers are so busy watching the road that they're less apt to get carsick. If you haven't got a license, your next best bet is to "sit in the front seat so you can also anticipate the upcoming bumps and turns and, as a result, be less likely to get sick," says John W. House, M.D., associate clinical professor in the Department of Otolaryngology, Head and Neck Surgery at the University of Southern California at Los Angeles.

EAT A LITTLE OR DON'T EAT AT ALL.

About an hour before you leave, eat some plain crackers or a piece of bread or toast, some experts suggest. Others, such as Silverstein, recommend not eating at all before a trip to help keep your stomach calm and empty, in case you should start to get nauseated.

AVOID "HEAVY" FOODS AND ODORS.

For some unknown reason, the smell of spicy or greasy foods and strong odors can prompt motion sickness before or during a trip, reports the American Academy of Otolaryngology–Head and Neck Surgery in Alexandria, Virginia.

SAY NO TO ALCOHOL.

Avoid alcoholic beverages before and during a trip. "Alcohol goes through the bloodstream and into the inner ear, stimulating it and making a case of motion sickness even worse," explains Silverstein.

TAKE IT EASY.

After the first signs of illness, close your eyes and stay still until the queasy sensations pass, says Silverstein.

STAY CALM, COOL, AND COLLECTED.

"For anyone who's had motion sickness, just the thought of being in the same situation again can cause fear and anxiety, which can bring on a bout of motion sickness," says Silverstein. The same goes for those who are anxious about what they're about to do, like flying in a plane or riding in a boat. Try to stay as calm and relaxed as possible. Take a few deep breaths, close your eyes, and tell yourself that you will not get sick.

LEAVE YOUR READING AT HOME.

Reading causes your eyes to move back and forth, so they are not fixed on a single point. At the same time, your body is sensing, and reacting to, the movement from your ride. The result: sensation overload and motion sickness. For the same reason, an action-packed movie on a plane may cause you to feel ill. On the other hand, "if the movie is not too visually demanding, it just may do the trick to help you relax, forget your fear, and prevent you from becoming sick," says Silverstein.

TRY OVER-THE-COUNTER REMEDIES.

Antihistamines, such as Dramamine, Bonine, and Marezine, should be taken at least an hour before the trip for maximum effectiveness. "This gives the medication enough time to be absorbed into the bloodstream," says Youngblood. Always check the label for possible side effects, such as drowsiness or blurred vision, and take necessary precautions, such as not driving a car.

STAY AWAY FROM OTHERS WHO ARE SICK.
The power of suggestion is very strong, especially if you have a tendency to get a bit "green" yourself. As callous as it may sound, let someone with a sturdier stomach tend to the sick; you should be looking at the horizon or at another steady point in the distance.

Muscle pain

23 Steps to Relief

I t was a pickup game of basketball with the guys. Nothing too serious. But a day and a half later, you can barely move. You're so stiff, it feels like you've aged 100 years nearly overnight. Every time you try to move, your muscles cry out, "Stop! It hurts!" What's going on?

Well, weekend jock, you've overdone it, and your body is letting you know. Overworking muscles causes the muscle fibers to actually break down, says sports-medicine expert and world-class runner Joan Ullyot, M.D., author of *Women's Running* and *Running Free*. "Ideally, you should be able to get into shape without getting stiff and sore," she says. "But most of us believe we have to overdo it so we feel like we've done something."

In addition to the tiny tears that occur in muscle fibers, the muscles swell slightly, and the accumulation of muscle breakdown products like enzymes contribute to the feeling of stiffness and soreness.

Another common source of muscle pain is a cramp, an acute spasm of the muscle that can send you to the ground clutching the offending muscle and howling in pain. Muscle cramps can be caused by anything that interferes with the mechanisms that cause muscles to contract and relax. "Muscle cramping means not enough blood is getting to the area," explains Ellen Nona Hoyven, P.T., physical therapist and owner and director of Ortho Sport Physical Therapy P.C. in Clackamas, Oregon. "The muscle objects with pain."

Knowing how muscles contract and relax can help you understand why muscle cramps occur and how to prevent them. To cause muscles to contract, the brain sends an electric "contract" message via nerves to muscles. When this signal reaches the muscle, the minerals sodium and calcium inside the muscle and potassium outside the muscle move and cause the signal to flow along the muscle, making it contract. For muscles to contract and relax properly, they need the right concentrations of minerals as well as adequate supplies of fat, sugar, and oxygen.

Michael Martindale, L.P.T., a physical therapist at the Sports Medicine Center of Portland Adventist Medical Center in Oregon, says, "A muscle goes into spasm because you've traumatized it somehow. Often, it's a sign the muscle has depleted its glycogen, its energy supply, and that there are too many waste products in the area. In response, the muscle goes into spasm. The spasms, in turn, decrease the blood flow, which causes pain. The pain then causes more spasm, which causes even more pain."

While muscle soreness and cramps aren't life threatening, they can be very bothersome. Here are some tips to ease the pain and prevent the problem from recurring.

STOP THE ACTIVITY PRONTO.

If your muscle cramps up while you're exercising, STOP the activity. Don't try to "run through" a muscle cramp. "If you try to keep going while you have a cramp," says Ullyot, "you're likely to really injure the muscle by pulling or tearing it."

GIVE IT A STRETCH AND SQUEEZE.

When you get a cramp, stretch the cramped muscle with one hand while you gently knead and squeeze the center of the muscle (you can feel a knot) with the fingers of the other hand. "You want to stretch the cramped muscle in the opposite direction from the way it's contracted," explains Hoyven. "For example, if you have a cramp in the calf muscle, put your foot flat on the ground and lean forward. If you can't stand on your leg, sit on the ground and stretch the toes up toward the knee."

WALK IT OUT.

Once an acute cramp passes, don't start exercising heavily right away. Instead, walk for a few minutes to get the blood flowing back into the muscles.

SIP QUININE TONIC.

Ullyot says many competitive swimmers drink quinine tonic water to prevent cramps. Quinine was once used

MUSCLES THAT GO CRAMP IN THE NIGHT

You're sleeping peacefully when suddenly your leg is seized with a painful cramp. You're no longer sleeping and you're certainly no longer peaceful. What happened? You weren't even dreaming about exercise.

Cramps that occur during the night are usually due to a pinched nerve or an exaggeration of a normal muscle-tendon reflex. When you turn over in your sleep, nerves can get pinched, causing muscles to cramp. Other times, when you turn over, you contract muscles, and the tendons attached to the muscles stretch. The stretched tendon sends a message to the spinal cord, which, in turn, sends a message to the muscle, causing it to contract.

No matter what the cause of the cramping, the bottom line is that muscles that cramp at night have somehow gotten "stuck." The key is to short-circuit this cramping before it happens and disturbs your rest. Here's how:

Stretch before bed. Take a few minutes before retiring to

to treat malarial cramping. While there may not be scientific studies to support drinking quinine tonic for muscle cramps, Ullyot says, "If it's a placebo, it's one that really seems to work." You might want to give it a try and see if it works for you.

GO BANANAS.

Chrissy Kane, L.P.T., a physical therapist in the Outpatient Physical Therapy Department at Providence stretch the muscles that are subject to cramping. Calves are often culprits of nighttime cramping. Try the "runner's stretch"—stand two to three feet from the wall and lean your chest against the wall, keeping your heels touching the floor. You should feel a stretch in your calves.

Be sure you get enough calcium. Nighttime cramps are often associated with a lack of calcium in the diet. Eat plenty of calcium-rich foods like broccoli, leafy greens, and low-fat dairy products. If cramping is still a problem, consider taking a calcium supplement.

Lighten the load. Sometimes, cramps in the legs and feet can be caused from a pile of heavy blankets. Toss off a few blankets and keep your muscles warm with an electric blanket set on warm.

Massage the muscle. If you develop a cramp despite using preventive tips, massage the cramped muscle with long strokes toward the heart. Sometimes a massage before you go to sleep can keep those muscles loose and free of cramps.

Medical Center in Portland, Oregon, says, "Sometimes a lack of potassium in the muscles can cause muscle cramps." If you're plagued by frequent cramping, Kane recommends that you eat a banana a day to increase your potassium intake and keep the cramps at bay.

CHILL OUT.

If you know you've overexercised, immediately take a cold shower or a cold bath to reduce the trauma to muscles, says Martindale. World-class Australian runner Jack Foster used to hose off his legs with cold water after a hard run. He told skeptics if it was good enough for race horses, it was good enough for him! Several Olympic runners are known for taking icy plunges after a tough workout, insisting that it prevents muscle soreness and stiffness. If an icy dip seems too much for you, Hoyven recommends applying cold packs for 20 to 30 minutes at a time every hour. "Cold constricts the blood vessels and shunts blood away from the injured muscles, which reduces inflammation," she explains. "The cold numbs the surface skin and superficial structures in the area, which reduces pain. It also causes what we call a 'reflex inhibition' of the muscles, causing them to relax."

AVOID HEAT.

Cold can reduce muscle trauma, but heat can increase muscle soreness and stiffness, says Hoyven, especially during the first 24 hours after overdoing it. "Heat may feel good," she says, "but it increases circulation to the area, causing blood vessels to dilate and fluid to accumulate. If you use it too long, it causes congestion in the area and more soreness and stiffness." If you absolutely can't resist using heat on those sore muscles, Hoyven suggests that you don't use it for more than 20 minutes every hour. Or, better yet, try contrast therapy—apply a hot pad for four minutes and an ice pack for one minute. After three or four days, when the swelling has subsided, Martindale says you can resume hot baths.

TAKE AN ANTI-INFLAMMATORY.

Aspirin and ibuprofen are great for reducing muscle inflammation, says Ullyot. If aspirin upsets your stomach, try the coated variety. Aspirin creams can also reduce pain and inflammation.

DO EASY STRETCHES.

When you're feeling sore and stiff, the last thing you want to do is move, but it's the first thing you *should* do, says Martindale. "Studies have shown that light exercise the day after overexercising really helps," he says. "Stretch gently and do only 20 minutes or so of easy walking."

TAKE A SWIM.

Ullyot says one of the best remedies for sore muscles is swimming. "The cold water helps the muscle inflammation, and the stretching helps take out the kinks."

ANTICIPATE SECOND-DAY SORENESS.

You may feel a little stiff or sore a few hours after overexercising, but you'll probably feel even worse two days afterward. Don't panic. It's perfectly normal. "We call it delayed-onset muscle soreness," explains Martindale.

DRINK PLENTY OF FLUIDS.

One cause of acute cramps, especially when you're exercising during hot weather for an hour or longer, is dehydration. Be sure to drink plenty of fluids before, during, and after exercising. Ullyot recommends drinking at least half a cup of water every couple of miles.

THINK TWICE ABOUT SPORTS DRINKS.

Ullyot says you really don't need them unless you're exercising for longer than an hour at a time. "Water is best absorbed by the body," she says. "For most people, drinking water is better than drinking sports drinks."

Martindale also says it's important to replace lost fluids if you've overexercised. So drink up.

PASS THE BOUILLON.

If you know you're going to be exercising for longer than an hour in the heat, Ullyot says you can prevent muscle cramps by drinking a cup of bouillon before exercising. "You can drink bouillon instead of sports drinks to replace the sodium you'll lose through sweating."

MASSAGE IT.

Gentle massage, done a day or two after a hard workout, can help ease sore, stiff muscles, says Ullyot. "Massage is wonderful for bringing circulation to the area," she says. However, if done too forcefully or too soon after a workout, it can increase soreness and cause injury.

AVOID "HOT" AND "COLD" CREAMS.

The pharmacy and supermarket shelves are loaded with topical "sports" creams designed to ease sore, stiff muscles. Unfortunately, they don't do much, according to Martindale. "They just cause a chemical reaction on the skin that gives the feeling of warm or cold, but they don't actually heat or cool the tissues." If you do use the topical sports creams, test a small patch of skin first to make sure you're not allergic, and never use them with hot pads, because they can cause serious burns.

WRAP UP.

In cold weather, you can often prevent muscle cramping by keeping the muscles warm with adequate clothing. Layered clothing offers the best insulating value by trapping air between the layers. Some people like the compression and warmth offered by running tights.

WARM UP YOUR MUSCLES.

One way to prevent muscle cramping and injuries is to warm up muscles before exercise. Instead of stretching first, walk a little or bike slowly to "prewarm" the muscles. Then do a series of stretches appropriate for the exercise you're going to be doing. Even if you're only chopping wood or working in the garden, stretching before the activity will get your muscles ready for work and help prevent muscle cramping.

LEARN YOUR LIMITS.

The key to preventing muscle pain, soreness, and stiffness, says Martindale, is to learn your limits. "You don't have to overdo it to exercise," he says. "If you're feeling sore and stiff afterwards, you know you're doing too much. Take your time. Build up over several weeks. Learn what your body can and can't do, and pay attention to those limits."

Nausea and vomiting

9 Soothing Strategies

Perhaps it's the 24-hour bug or something you ate. Whatever, now you're feeling queasy and sick.

The tips that follow are designed to reduce your discomfort and to help your symptoms go away as quickly as possible. If vomiting is violent or persists for more than 24 hours or if your vomit contains blood, see a physician without delay.

EVALUATE THE CAUSE AND TREAT THE SYMPTOMS ACCORDINGLY.

Nausea and vomiting are two vague symptoms that can be caused by many illnesses, says Albert B. Knapp, M.D., an adjunct assistant attending physician at Lenox Hill Hospital in New York. If you suspect that your nausea and vomiting are due to a headache, motion sickness, morning sickness, or a case of food poisoning, see the corresponding section in this book.

STICK TO CLEAR LIQUIDS.

Your stomach probably doesn't need the added burden of digesting food, says Knapp. He recommends sticking to fluids until you feel a little better. "If you are vomiting, do not start fluids until the vomiting has stopped," he says. "Then start with warm fluids, since cold ones can irritate the stomach. The fluid should have sugar in it. The sugar helps absorption." Liquids are easier to digest and are necessary to prevent the dehydration that may occur from vomiting, according to Cornelius P. Dooley, M.D., a gastroenterologist in Santa Fe, New Mexico. He recommends diluted, noncitrus fruit juices.

LET IT RUN ITS COURSE.

The best cure for the 24-hour stomach flu is bed rest mixed with a tincture of time. "You'll feel miserable, but you've got to let it run its course," says Dooley.

DON'T DRINK ALCOHOL.

Alcohol can irritate the stomach. The same goes for fatty foods, highly seasoned foods, caffeine, and cigarettes.

STICK TO EASY-TO-DIGEST FOODS.

When you are ready to start eating again, start with soft foods, such as bread, unbuttered toast, steamed fish, or bananas, says Neville R. Pimstone, M.D., chief of hepatology in the Division of Gastroenterology at the University of California at Davis. "Avoid fats, and stick to a low-fiber diet," he says. What about chicken soup? "Chicken soup probably has too much fat," Pimstone says. Start with very small amounts of food and slowly build up to larger meals, says Steven C. Fiske, M.D., assistant clinical professor of medicine and gastroenterology at the University of Medicine and Dentistry of New Jersey in Newark.

LET IT FLOW.

The worst thing you can do for vomiting is to fight it, says Knapp. Trying to hold back the urge can actually cause tears in your esophagus.

TAKE PEPTO-BISMOL.

Over-the-counter stomach medications that contain bismuth, such as Pepto-Bismol, may coat the stomach and relieve discomfort, says Pimstone. However, he advises against taking Alka-Seltzer, which contains aspirin and may irritate the stomach.

TRY A COLD COMPRESS.

A cold compress on your head can be very comforting when you are vomiting, says Knapp.

MAINTAIN YOUR ELECTROLYTE BALANCE.
Along with replacing fluids, it is also important to maintain the balance of sodium and potassium (known as electrolytes) in your system, says Fiske. He recommends a sports drink, such as Gatorade, which is easy on the stomach and is designed to replace both fluids and electrolytes.

Nosebleeds

15 Ways to Get Out of the Red

"The nose is the most vascular area of the body," says H. Christopher Moore III, M.D., assistant professor of the Department of Otolaryngology/Head and Neck Surgery at the University of California at Irvine. This means that the nasal passages are packed with veins and capillaries, many lying just below the thin lining of the nostrils, practically waiting for the right conditions— very dry air, a picky finger, some dust or dirt—to get the blood flow started. Here's how to stop it:

CLOSE YOUR NOSE AND OPEN YOUR MOUTH.
Sit up, bend your head forward slightly, and pinch the soft part of the nose below the bony bridge, recommends Moore. At the same time, keep your mouth open to help you breathe.

Having your head tilted forward keeps blood from going down the back of the throat, which can cause you to cough, choke, or spit up blood. "Only a slight tilt of

YOU SHOULD'VE SEEN THE OTHER GUY!

Any trauma to the nose—an errant snowball, a fight in the schoolyard, a fall—can make the nose bleed, possibly break, and almost always, swell. And it's more difficult to stop a swollen nose from bleeding, because you can't pinch the nostrils too well, and it's probably bleeding from passages that are so far back that you can't pinch them effectively anyway.

"Place gauze in each nostril to help stop the bleeding," recommends H. Christopher Moore III, M.D. "And don't lie down unless you absolutely have to. By sitting up, you'll keep your head above your heart, and by doing that, less blood will flow to the nose." Gauze is preferred to cotton because it won't shed particles in the nose.

Zeb Koran, R.N., C.E.N., C.C.R.N., suggests applying ice directly to the nose as quickly as possible to decrease the swelling and bruising.

Is the nose broken? "A nose doesn't have to be broken to swell," says Koran. "But if it is crooked or dimpled, you probably have a break."

On the other hand, "a fracture in the nose may be undetectable, especially if the nose is swollen," according to James A. Stankiewicz, M.D. "You might not be able to tell until the swelling goes down." If you've taken a blow to the nose, it may be wise to have it checked by a physician just to be safe.

the head is enough, because otherwise you're causing too much pressure in the head and nose," says Zeb Koran, R.N., C.E.N., C.C.R.N., director of Educational Services for the Emergency Nurses Association in Chicago. In addition, "you can monitor how much blood you're losing," says Moore. That's why the old wives' tale that says that lying down is best is not only old but untrue. "They were under the mistaken belief, I guess, that if you couldn't see the blood coming out that it must be stopping," says Moore. If the bleeding hasn't stopped after about 20 minutes, apply pressure for another 20 minutes or so. If the bleeding hasn't ceased at that point, go to the doctor or emergency room.

MAKE YOUR NOSE COLD.

If your nosebleed is persistent, ice may stop the flow quicker. "Studies have shown that sucking on ice can constrict the blood vessels," says James A. Stankiewicz, M.D., vice-chairman and professor of the Department of Otolaryngology—Head and Neck Surgery at Loyola University Medical School in Maywood, Illinois. Moore recommends a cold compress of ice wrapped in a towel or washcloth and placed on the forehead and bridge of the nose. He also says "a bag of frozen peas smashed up like a beanbag and wrapped up in a towel can be very effective." (Frozen, unpopped popcorn in a sealable plastic bag can also be wrapped in a thin towel and used as an ice pack.)

SPRAY THE BLEEDING AWAY.

Over-the-counter nasal decongestant sprays may help stop a nosebleed. "Spray the nostrils every 10 to 15 minutes for about an hour to constrict the blood vessels," says Moore. If the bleeding does not stop after this time, stop using the spray and see a doctor.

KEEP A CHILD CALM.

Crying and sniffles will only prolong the bleeding.

LEAVE YOUR NOSE ALONE.

Resist the temptation to blow your nose, cough, sneeze, or sniffle after you've gotten the bleeding to stop. "If you do, you may dislodge the clot and start the bleeding all over again," says Koran. Also, try not to bend over for a while, as this creates pressure in the nasal passages. And if you must blow your nose, do it gently.

MOISTURIZE.

Dryness, especially the kind caused by forced-air heating in the winter, is one of the most common causes of nosebleed. "The elderly are particularly susceptible, since they are more likely to spend more time indoors in the winter," says Moore. To moisten the nose, Stankiewicz suggests applying a petroleum or water-based jelly just inside the front portion of the nostrils. He adds that the new over-the-counter saline sprays may be helpful, but they have yet to be studied by the American Academy of Otolaryngology–Head and Neck Surgery. Koran prefers a timeless remedy for at-home relief: "Place pans of water on the radiators," she advises. She also suggests steaming up the bathroom during a shower for a blast of humidity.

TURN ON A NEBULIZER.

This type of humidifying unit "can deliver slightly warm or cool air in big droplets," says Moore. Humidifiers, which produce a cool mist, and vaporizers, which distribute warm air, can also help combat dryness in the home. Moore recommends cool mist as most effective in helping a dry nose. Some experts, including Moore, believe that these units should be filled only with distilled water to combat the growth of bacteria, which reportedly can irritate the nasal passages and the entire respiratory system. Other experts, however, say that tap water is fine, as long as the unit is cleaned frequently.

AVOID ASPIRIN.

Aspirin is an anticoagulant, or so-called "blood thinner," which can aggravate a sensitive nose and cause it to bleed. Prescription anticoagulants, often used in the treatment of blood clots, can do the same. However, if you are on a prescription anticoagulant, do not stop taking it before discussing it with your doctor.

GET ENOUGH VITAMIN C AND ZINC.

Vitamin C, a component in the production of collagen, and zinc, helpful in the use of protein, are both important to the maintenance of body tissues, including the blood vessels. Be sure to eat a variety of foods in order to get enough of these nutrients. Good sources of vitamin C include citrus fruits and vegetables, including potatoes. Good sources of zinc include beef, liver, fish, whole-wheat products, brown rice, and popcorn.

CHECK YOUR IRON.

"If you're prone to frequent nosebleeds, you may want to increase your iron intake," suggests Stankiewicz. He recommends seeing your doctor first for a blood count and analysis. Iron-rich foods include liver, most lean red

HELLO, DOCTOR?

Angiofibromas are benign (noncancerous) tumors that, for an unknown reason, primarily afflict teenage males, says H. Christopher Moore III, M.D. These bumps lie in the back of the nasal passages and are difficult to diagnose. However, one symptom is frequent nose bleeding. If your teen has numerous nosebleeds with no identifiable cause, a visit to the doctor is in order.

meats, dark-meat poultry, spinach, and beans (such as kidney and lima).

CONTROL YOUR HYPERTENSION.

People with hypertension, or high blood pressure, may also suffer from arteriosclerosis, or hardening of the arteries, which can make blood vessels stiff and noncompliant. Some experts believe that such vessels in the nose may be more prone to bleed. If you find yourself with frequent nosebleeds and no explanation, and hypertension runs in your family, see your doctor. Only your physician can diagnose high blood pressure and recommend the proper course of therapy to control it.

DON'T SMOKE.

Here's yet another reason not to puff. "Smoking can irritate and dry out the nasal passages," says Stankiewicz. Smoking is also a factor in hypertension.

CONSIDER YOUR HORMONES.

Estrogen, especially in women, plays a part in the production of nasal mucus. The estrogen level in women ebbs and flows during the menstrual cycle and all but disappears in postmenopausal women. "As we age, the mucous membranes begin to atrophy in both women and men," says Moore. This atrophy can make nosebleeds likely. Postmenopausal women can consider estrogen replacement therapy. Keeping the nasal passages moist can also help reduce nosebleeds.

STOP THE PICKING.

If you can't seem to keep your child from picking his or her nose, you may want to try this: "Tape a single layer of half-inch gauze over the nostrils," says Stankiewicz. "The child will be able to breathe but will not be able to get his finger through the gauze."

TEACH YOUR CHILD TO USE TISSUES.

"Children imitate what their parents do," says Koran. "So showing your child how to use tissues may keep him or her from picking." This, may help prevent nosebleeds.

Oily hair

5 Tips for Cutting the Grease.

You wash and style your hair every morning, but within a few short hours, it looks stringy and dirty. You, like millions of others, have oily hair.

A certain amount of oil secretion from oil glands on the scalp is healthy and necessary. Sebum, the natural oil produced by the oil glands, is secreted to protect your hair shafts from breaking. Oil also gives your hair luster and shine. But, let's face it, with oily hair, you've got too much of a good thing.

Oily hair is a second cousin to oily skin, according to Nelson Lee Novick, M.D., associate clinical professor of dermatology at the Mount Sinai School of Medicine in New York. "The oil is just coming up on a different part of the skin," he says. "It's usually a genetic problem. But at certain times, most people have oilier hair due to fluctuations in hormones."

Women often complain of oilier hair at the beginning and end of the menstrual cycle. Paul Contorer, M.D., chief of dermatology for Kaiser Permanente and clinical professor of dermatology at Oregon Health Sciences University in Portland, says that for many people, oily hair begins at puberty. "We often see teenagers with oily hair because the androgen hormones stimulate the sebaceous glands to produce more oil," he explains.

While you can't change your family background or your hormones, there is plenty you can do to get your oily locks under control.

SHAMPOO OFTEN.

"People with oily hair can shampoo every day," says Contorer. "Keep in mind that hair is just dead protein. Washing often won't hurt it."

USE A "NO-NONSENSE" SHAMPOO.

Often, shampoos have all kinds of additives and conditioners in them. People with oily hair should use a good solvent-type shampoo, one that will cut the grease, says Contorer. "I tell my patients to add a couple of drops of Ivory Liquid to their shampoo," he says. If you don't like the idea of putting dishwashing liquid on your head, there are plenty of commercial shampoos that will cut through the excess oil, says Rose Dygart, owner of Le Rose Salon of Beauty in Lake Oswego, Oregon, and a cosmetologist and barber who has been teaching and practicing hair care for 35 years. "Look for a castile-type soap without conditioning additives," she advises. "Commercial products like Prell and Suave do a good job on oily hair." Dygart says normal hair needs a shampoo with a pH between 4.5 and 6.7, but oily hair requires a more alkaline product. Look for shampoos with a pH higher than 6.7, she says.

RINSE THOROUGHLY.

Whatever shampoo you use, be sure you rinse thoroughly. Soap residue will only collect dirt and oil more quickly, says Novick.

FORGET CONDITIONERS.

Conditioners coat the hair, something oily hair doesn't need, says Dygart. Apply a small amount of conditioner only to the ends if they've become dried out.

TRY AN ACIDIC RINSE.

One way to decrease the oil is to rinse with diluted vinegar or lemon juice after shampooing. Dygart says to use two tablespoons of white vinegar to one cup of water or use the juice of one lemon (strained) to one cup of water. Rinse the mixture through your hair, then rinse your hair with warm water.

Oily skin

10 Ways to Cope

You may welcome the shine from the sun, but, if you have oily skin, you probably dread the shine on your cheeks and forehead. Just as some people are born with dry skin, others are born with overly oily skin. "Oily skin is basically a genetic problem," says Margaret Robertson, M.D., a dermatologist in private practice in Lake Oswego, Oregon. "If your mother or father had oily skin, chances are good that you will, too."

Hormones also play a part. "We often see people with oily skin who are in their teens or early 20s, people who are undergoing hormonal changes," says Nelson Lee Novick, M.D., associate clinical professor of dermatology at Mount Sinai School of Medicine in New York.

But oily skin doesn't just affect teenagers and young adults. Many women notice oily skin problems during pregnancy, around the time of their menstrual periods, or at menopause. Even some types of birth control pills can increase skin oiliness.

One myth about oily skin is that it causes acne. "Acne is caused when oil becomes trapped below the skin's pores and becomes contaminated with bacteria," explains Novick. "When you have oily skin, the oil isn't blocked because it's coming to the skin's surface."

The good news about oily skin is that it keeps the skin younger looking. Over time, people with oily skin tend to wrinkle less than people with dry or normal skin.

455

HELLO, DOCTOR?

In most cases, oily skin can be treated at home. However, you'll want to call a doctor if:
- You develop acne.
- You notice any sudden change in your skin (if it suddenly goes from dry to oily, for example).

While you can't alter your genetics or completely control your hormones, there are plenty of things you can do to cope with your oily skin.

KEEP YOUR SKIN SQUEAKY CLEAN.

As anyone with oily skin knows, the oilier the skin, the dirtier the skin looks and feels. To help combat this feeling, it's important to keep the skin clean. Vera Brown, skin expert to many of Hollywood's stars and author of *Vera Brown's Natural Beauty Book*, says oily-skinned people should wash the skin at least twice a day.

Dermatologist Paul Contorer, M.D., chief of dermatology at Kaiser Permanente and clinical professor of dermatology at Oregon Health Sciences University in Portland, recommends a detergent-type soap. "I tell my patients with oily skin to mix a couple of drops of dishwashing detergent like Ivory Liquid in with their regular soap," he says. "It's a great solvent for the oil."

Brown thinks detergent soaps are too harsh for even oily skin and recommends twice-daily cleansing with a glycerine soap instead. If you find detergent soap too irritating for your skin, try the glycerine variety.

TRY ALOE VERA.

Brown likes to follow a thorough facial cleansing with pure aloe vera gel (available in health-food stores). "The aloe vera helps absorb oil," she says, "and it helps cleanse the pores." She recommends dabbing the face two to three times a day with cool aloe vera gel (keep it in the refrigerator) and letting it dry.

WIPE WITH ASTRINGENTS.

Contorer says that wiping the oily parts of the face with rubbing alcohol or a combination of alcohol and acetone (such as is found in Seba-Nil Liquid Cleanser) can help dry oiliness. "It's as good and less expensive than those astringents with perfumes in them," he says.

Frank Parker, M.D., professor and chairman of the Department of Dermatology at Oregon Health Sciences University in Portland, says oily-skinned people should wipe the face between washings with alcohol wipes. You can buy premoistened alcohol wipes in the cosmetic department of most stores. Novick recommends using alcohol, too, but he prefers the convenience of individually wrapped towelettes. "You can carry these with you and wipe the oil off every few hours," he says. "The alcohol acts as a degreaser."

CARRY TISSUES.

Novick says if you don't have towelettes, paper facial tissues can wipe away excess oils. You can also purchase oil-absorbing tissues from cosmetics companies that remove excess oil between cleansings, says Robertson.

CHILL OUT WITH COLD WATER RINSES.

Robertson advises splashing the face a couple of times a day with cold water. "The water is good for getting rid of excess oils, and I prefer it to adding more chemicals to the skin," she says.

BAN MOISTURIZERS.

While people with dry skin are forever smearing on moisturizers, oily-skinned people shouldn't use them, says Robertson.

Brown agrees. "In all my years of dealing with skin care, I've never seen a moisturizer that's good for oily skin," she says. "Oily-skinned people should never go to bed with cream on their faces."

Novick suggests avoiding the application of oils, too. "Never put mineral oil or petroleum jelly on oily skin," he says. "Applying external oils to oily skin can clog the pores and cause acne."

MIST IT.

With all the cleansing and wiping, you might be concerned about overdrying the skin. But if you shouldn't use moisturizers, what should you do? Brown says to use a facial mist. "You can buy facial mists in health-food stores," she says. "They're mineral water with herbs and vitamins added. You just spray them onto the face. They add moisture without adding oil or chemicals."

MAKE A SCRUB.

Brown says scrubs are excellent for removing excess surface oil. She recommends this almond-honey scrub: Mix a small amount of almond meal (ground almonds) with honey. Then *gently* massage the paste onto your skin with a hot washcloth. Rinse thoroughly. You can also make a scrub from oatmeal mixed with aloe vera, says Brown. Rub gently onto the skin, leave on for 15 minutes, then wash off thoroughly. If you suffer from acne on your face, however, you should probably skip the scrub, since it can aggravate already irritated skin.

MASQUE IT.

Masques applied to the face can reduce oiliness. Brown says you can purchase clay masques or mix Fuller's Earth (available at pharmacies) with a little water to make a paste. Apply to the face and leave on for about 20 minutes before rinsing off.

USE WATER-BASED COSMETICS.

Brown says oily-skinned people should stay away from cosmetics as much as possible. "Try and go without makeup as much as you can," she advises. When you do use makeup, Novick recommends water-based rather than oil-based types. "Go with the powder or gel blushers," he says. "And stay away from cream foundations that add oil."

Osteoporosis

17 Ways to Combat Brittle Bones

Sometimes it may seem like a losing battle. We're responsible for giving the body all the calcium it needs.

When we don't, it takes the bone-building mineral right from the reserves in the bones, "which leads to the breakdown of the bone structure," says Robert P. Heaney, M.D., John A. Creighton University Professor at Creighton University in Omaha, Nebraska.

Osteoporosis, or porous bones, affects many more women than men. This is so because after puberty, males have more bone at most sites than females do, explains Conrad Johnston, M.D., chief of the Division of Endocrinology and Metabolism at Indiana University School of Medicine in Indianapolis. So at peak bone mass, men are at an advantage. What's more, while both men and women begin to lose bone mass as they age, this loss becomes accelerated in women at menopause, when estrogen levels drop. Bone loss in women eventually levels off to about one percent per year, says Johnston. Men begin to lose bone mass sometime around age 45 or 50, he says, but they lose only about half a percent per year. Why men lose bone mass is unclear.

The best prevention: building strong bones now to prevent fractures and other complications later. Here's how to win the war against brittle bones.

MAKE LIKE ARNOLD SCHWARZENEGGER.

Well, not exactly. But weight lifting is a good way not only to build muscle but bone. "It stimulates the activation of new bone cells," says Richard C. Bozian, M.D., professor of medicine, assistant professor of biochemistry, and director of the Division of Nutrition at the University of Cincinnati. However, before beginning any weight-lifting program, consult your doctor. In general, always start with lighter weights and progress to heavier ones as you become stronger.

USE RESISTANCE TO MAKE YOUR BONES MORE RESISTANT.

"The skeleton is sensitive to mechanical load," says Johnston. Mechanical load is the amount of force you use against your skeleton, and certain activities that use the body's own weight as a force against gravity are the best way to "load up." The result: increased bone-cell production. You can actually see the results of loading in the significantly developed swinging arm of avid tennis and baseball players. "Exercise is one of the most positive things a woman can do to fight osteoporosis," asserts Bozian. While running is a top bone builder, some people find that it packs too much of a punch for their joints. Walking, besides being less stressful to the body, can be done by almost anyone, almost anywhere, without expensive equipment. And "the motion of walking helps the entire body," says Victor G. Ettinger, M.D., medical director of Bone Diagnostic Centres in Torrance and Long Beach, California. As for lower-impact activities, such as swimming and bicycling: "These are helpful, too," says Bozian. No matter which exercise you choose, Johnston recommends that it be performed one hour a day, three days a week for best results. Irony lies in the fact that those who exercise exhaustively, like professional athletes, can suffer from malnutrition. This can lead to a decrease in calcium intake. In women, it can also lead to amenorrhea, or no menstrual cycle, putting them at increased risk for osteoporosis.

MAINTAIN A HEALTHY WEIGHT.

If you are underweight (say, more than ten percent lighter than the average weight for your age and height), you are at higher risk for a deficiency of calcium and

FOR DAIRY LOVERS: HOW TO USE EVEN MORE

• Use milk instead of water to mix up hot cereals, hot chocolate, and soups.
• Substitute plain yogurt for half the mayonnaise in dressings.
• Top casseroles, omelets, toast, and baked potatoes with low-fat grated or shredded cheese.
• Add skim milk to coffee instead of adding fattening cream or nondairy creamer.
• Try low-fat and nonfat varieties of milk, cheese, sour cream, ice cream, and cottage cheese.

other important vitamins and minerals, which can affect your bones' health. If you are overweight, you may have stronger bones than someone thinner; however, you also may be less active and less likely to follow an exercise routine, which is also important to keeping bones healthy.

START DRINKING MILK AGAIN.
You may not have relished it, but Mom was right when she made you drink milk at every meal and sometimes in between. In addition to its calcium content, milk is fortified with vitamin D, and "vitamin D facilitates the absorption of calcium," says Bozian.

GET SOME SUN.

Rays of sunshine activate the vitamin D in the body. Studies have shown that women in Northern Europe and England, for instance, where the weather can be cold and dreary more often than not, have a higher rate of osteoporosis than women who are from warmer, sunnier climates. That doesn't mean you should go out and bake yourself in the sun, however. Fifteen minutes of sun exposure on the hands, arms, and face each day may be all that you need and should not be enough to greatly increase your risk of skin cancer. (Sunscreen, by the way, blocks out the light rays that are responsible for activating vitamin D.) On the other hand, if you are at increased risk of getting skin cancer, keep your skin protected from sunlight (see "Protect Yourself" in SUNBURN PAIN for tips on shielding your skin from the sun's damaging ultraviolet rays) and emphasize dietary sources of vitamin D, such as fortified milk, instead.

CUT DOWN ON CAFFEINE.

"Caffeine stimulates the loss of calcium through the urine," says Bozian. One study found that drinking more than two cups of average brewed coffee or four cups of average brewed tea per day can increase calcium loss.

PASS UP THE SALT SHAKER.

Salt can also increase the amount of calcium lost through the urine. "The more sodium you excrete, the more calcium you excrete," says Rose Hust, osteoporosis coordinator at the Knoxville Orthopedic Clinic in Tennessee. High-sodium diets may also contribute to osteoporosis in a less direct way, she adds. If you take a diuretic to pull excess salt out of the body, it will also pull out calcium.

HOW TO GET CALCIUM WITHOUT DRINKING MILK

For a variety of reasons, some people don't consume enough dairy products every day to get enough calcium. Dieters, for example, often shun dairy's high fat. Some individuals simply don't like the taste of milk and milk products. And yet others are lactose intolerant, which means their bodies have a hard time digesting dairy foods (see LACTOSE INTOLERANCE). Are these "dairy deserters" destined to a life of brittle bones? Not necessarily. There are many other sources of dietary calcium. To get the most calcium, eat foods in the raw; as foods are cooked, calcium can leach into the cooking water. Here are some nondairy, calcium-rich options:

Orange juice: The calcium-fortified variety, that is. "This is a wonderful alternative for people who simply don't like milk, because it is fortified to the same extent," says Robert P. Heaney, M.D.

Beans: Kidney and pinto head the list, and for the adventurous, tofu (soybean curd) is rich in both calcium and protein.

DON'T WORRY ABOUT PHOSPHORUS.

There has been some concern that consuming high levels of phosphorus can influence bone loss and risk of osteoporosis. The Food and Drug Administration addressed the issue, however, and found no evidence to substantiate this worry.

Broccoli: Yet another good reason to munch a few stalks—preferably in the raw.

Nuts: Hazelnuts, Brazil nuts, and almonds are among the best choices.

Fruit: Figs and prunes are very high in calcium.

Leafy greens: Romaine lettuce, collards, and kale are good choices. The exception: spinach. "The calcium in spinach is not readily available to the body," explains Heaney.

Salmon and sardines: Salmon is also a good source of vitamin D.

For those who are lactose intolerant, more and more dairy products, made with easily digestible lactic acid, are on the market. Lactic acid tablets are also available. And, you shouldn't have a problem with these two dairy products:

Yogurt: The lactose, or sugar, in yogurt, has already been broken down, so your digestive system won't have to do it. You can substitute yogurt for sour cream in recipes and as a topping for baked potatoes.

Hard cheeses: The lactose breaks down during the aging process.

BE WISE ABOUT PROTEIN.

For healthy bones, protein is a double-edged sword. "Too much protein in the diet can increase calcium excretion," says Hust. However, protein is needed to help maintain a component of bone called collagen, which is made up of proteins. It's not so much a question of eating

THE FACTS ON FLUORIDE

"Fluoride is the only substance we know that actually builds up bones," says Victor G. Ettinger, M.D. "But the problem is, we just don't know how much to give." While fluoride is a bone builder, it is generally believed that too much of it can actually make bones brittle. But even scientific studies have not yielded that same conclusion every time. "Some studies have found that fluoride had no effect on bone-fracture rate," says Conrad Johnston, M.D. "Others have shown a decrease in the amount of fractures suffered by patients." Inconclusive studies are one reason why "the use of fluoride therapeutically, especially in large doses, remains very controversial," Johnston adds.

Through similar tests, drugs containing fluoride have been studied but not approved by the U.S. Food and Drug Administration. Others, like Didronel, are considered experimental. Didronel was initially developed for those with Paget's disease, a condition in which the bones thicken and soften. The drug was found to build bone, so it is used on a very limited basis to treat osteoporosis. A study coordinated through Emory University in Atlanta has shown a reduction in the rate of fractures in patients who have taken Didronel. However, the drug has been administered over a short time and to only a few patients. As typified by this study, the testing of fluoride drugs continues, so final recommendations about the use of fluoride in treating osteoporosis cannot yet be made by the medical community.

too much protein, but of not getting enough calcium to balance out the amount of protein in the diet. If you have an adequate calcium intake, you probably don't need to worry about getting too much protein. However, if you don't get much calcium in your diet, you'd be wise to avoid consuming an excess amount of protein.

SCHEDULE YOUR FIBER INTAKE.

"Fiber can decrease calcium absorption by combining with calcium in the intestine, and at the same time, by increasing the rate at which food is passed through the intestinal tract," explains Hust. But don't eliminate fiber from your diet altogether. Just try to have calcium-rich foods or calcium supplements between—not during—fiber-rich meals.

MAKE YOUR OWN SOUP.

When preparing stock from bones, add a little vinegar to leach the calcium out of the bones. "The amount of calcium in a single pint of homemade soup is equal to the calcium found in a quart or more of milk," says Hust.

SAY NO TO ALCOHOL.

It interferes with the body's ability to absorb calcium.

PUT OUT THAT CIGARETTE.

"Smoking has been shown to be associated with lower bone mass," says Johnston, since nicotine interferes with calcium absorption.

CHECK YOUR MEDICINES.

Antacids that contain aluminum can interfere with calcium absorption. And some prescription drugs can increase the amount of calcium lost in the urine. For instance, diuretics, which are used to treat hypertension; tetracycline, an antibiotic often used to treat severe cases of acne; and high doses of cortisone drugs or steroids, such as those used to treat arthritis, are a few of the offenders.

REPLACE YOUR ESTROGEN IN MENOPAUSE.

The hormone estrogen is vital to the maintenance of bone. When estrogen levels decrease after menopause, bone loss is "dramatically accelerated," says Ettinger. Estrogen replacement therapy can help slow that calcium drain. Estrogen replacement therapy is not for every woman, however, so be sure to discuss it thoroughly with your doctor.

CAREFULLY CONSIDER CALCIUM SUPPLEMENTS.

"Chances are, if you are a candidate for supplements, your diet is not only low in calcium but in other nutrients the body needs," says Heaney. "Your best bet is to primarily get calcium from the foods you eat." If your doctor recommends that you take a supplement, never exceed 2,500 milligrams per day; excessive calcium can lead to kidney stones. The supplement should be taken between meals with juice instead of water, says Hust. The reason: The vitamin C in fruit juices helps the body absorb calcium.

GET THE RIGHT AMOUNT OF CALCIUM.

Women, especially, need different amounts of calcium at different times of their lives. The Recommended Daily Allowance (RDA) for females age 11 to 25—the big bone-building years—is 1,200 milligrams. After age 25, the

RDA is 800 milligrams; however, the National Institutes of Health recommends 1,000 milligrams after age 25. The RDA for postmenopausal women is 1,500 milligrams, and for pregnant women, it's 2,000 milligrams daily. Men should increase their calcium intake as they age, from 800 milligrams to 1,000 milligrams a day. For both men and women, consuming close to 3,000 milligrams a day can be toxic, says Bozian, and can interfere with the absorption of the vital minerals copper and zinc.

Poison ivy, oak, and sumac

11 Prevention and Treatment Tips

The itching can drive you absolutely crazy. All you want to do is scratch like a maniac. Getting a rash from poison ivy, oak, or sumac is maddening. It's almost enough to make you want to give up going outside ever again. Fortunately, you don't have to. You simply need to know how to take steps to avoid these foes and what to do to get relief if your preventive steps fail.

When you get a rash from poison ivy, oak, or sumac, you've had an allergic reaction to the oil, or sap, found inside the plant. This oil, which is clear to slightly yellow, is called urushiol. It oozes from any cut or crushed part of the leaves and stem, so just brushing a plant may not elicit a reaction. Oil content in the plants runs highest in the spring and summer, but cases are reported even in the winter, according to William Epstein, M.D., a professor of dermatology at the University of California at San Francisco.

Poison ivy, oak, and sumac are hardy weeds that can be found throughout the United States, except in Hawaii, Alaska, and some desert areas of Nevada, says Epstein. Poison ivy is found east of the Rockies, poison oak grows in the West and Southwest, and poison sumac thrives east of the Mississippi River. All three produce similar reactions, and if you're allergic to one, you'll probably react to the others as well.

Cases of poison ivy, oak, and sumac affect 10 to 50 million people in the United States each year, Epstein says. In fact, these plants constitute the single most common cause of allergic reactions. A lucky 10 to 15 percent of Americans are tolerant of these plants, but another 10 to 15 percent are quite sensitive. The rest of us fall in between, with varying levels of sensitivity.

What muddies the waters is that a person's sensitivity can change over time, even from season to season. You could be quite sensitive to poison ivy as a child and carry no allergy to the weed as an adult. "Some people will never get poison ivy, and others may get it at any age," says William Dvorine, M.D., chief of dermatology at St. Agnes Hospital in Baltimore. "It [a reaction to one of these plants] can appear early in childhood, or sometimes it can appear late in life," Dvorine says. So it's not safe to assume that you will always be immune if you are now. But on average, says Epstein, a person's sensitivity tends to decline with age.

Your level of sensitivity determines how bad a reaction you'll have. Once the oil touches the skin, it starts to penetrate in minutes. Within 12 to 48 hours, a red, itchy rash appears, followed by blisters that may weep and later get crusty. The area usually heals in about ten days. Among the very sensitive population, affected areas will quickly swell up, the rash can be severe and painful, and the reaction may take up to three weeks to clear up if left untreated. For those in this category, Epstein says it's important to see a doctor as soon as they realize they've been in contact with the plant.

Even for people who are not that sensitive, a rash from poison ivy, oak, or sumac is no fun. So here are some tips for preventing the problem in the first place and some simple ways to treat the rash if it does occur. (While the remedies often refer to poison ivy, the steps are generally appropriate for poison oak and poison sumac as well.)

KNOW THE PLANT SO YOU CAN AVOID IT.

Find out what the plant looks like in your area, because appearance will vary. "Poison oak in Northern California doesn't look like poison oak in Southern California," says Epstein. Typically, poison ivy is a vine or a low shrub with grayish white berries and smooth, pointed leaves usually in groups of three. The reddish leaves turn green in the summer and redden again by autumn, according to Charlie Nardozzi, an horticulturist with the National Gardening Association in Burlington, Vermont. Poison oak is a shrub or small tree with greenish white berries and oaklike leaves usually in groups of three. Poison sumac is a woody shrub found in swampy, boggy areas that has smooth-edged leaves and cream-colored berries. The leaves of poison sumac retain their reddish color and aren't grouped in threes. Spotting the plants isn't al-

POISON-IVY MYTHS

A number of widely held beliefs about poison ivy just simply aren't true. William Epstein, M.D., offers the real story on some long-standing myths:

Scratching poison ivy blisters will spread the rash. The oil in the plant spreads the rash, not the fluid in the blisters. If you get the oil on your hands, for instance, and you touch different parts of your body, it will spread to them. This happens long before the blisters have even formed. It is true that you should avoid scratching the blisters, but only because your fingernails may have germs on them that could start an infection.

The old saying "Leaves of three, let them be" always holds true. This is usually the case for poison ivy and oak—but not every time. Leaflets may come in groups of five, seven, or even nine.

You can catch poison ivy from someone else. The rash can't travel from person to person through the blister fluid or any other way. Only the oil can be spread by contact.

ways easy. Poison ivy can mimic other plants, such as Virginia creeper, and can twine itself around English ivy. "I've tried to make myself an expert, yet I'm fooled all the time," says Hillard H. Pearlstein, M.D., assistant clinical professor of dermatology at Mount Sinai School of Medicine in New York. You'll decrease your chance of being exposed to one of these plants, however, if you become familiar with their typical appearance.

Dead poison-ivy plants can do you no harm. This may seem logical, but it's not true. The oil from the leaves and stem can remain an active allergenic chemical for up to several years. "That's a very well-known syndrome now, because a lot of people are outdoors in the wintertime. They see sticks in the snow, collect them to make a fire, and it turns out they've picked up poison ivy," says Epstein.

The juice from crushed plantain leaves will prevent a case of poison-ivy rash. There's no scientific proof to back this claim, although hikers often try this as a preventive strategy.

You can't be immunized against poison ivy. You can, but Epstein doesn't recommend it. The procedure requires a great deal of time, effort, and commitment from both the patient and doctor, and there are side effects. If you're considering immunization, talk to an expert and get the facts. "The worst thing is to get started and then find out the treatment is worse than the allergy," says Epstein. In his opinion, immunization should only be used as a last resort.

COVER UP.

Long pants, long-sleeved shirts, boots, and gloves provide a barrier between you and the plant's oil. This is especially important if you're sensitive and you know you're going to be in an area that might contain poison ivy. "My wife, who is a gardener, is exquisitely sensitive. She's learned to cover up or suffer the consequences," says Pearlstein.

DON'T LET YOUR PETS ROMP IN WOODED AREAS.

If you get a rash from poison ivy but can't remember being near the plant, you may have your pet to thank. "A common way to get poison ivy is to pet a cat or dog that's run through the stuff," says Pearlstein. The oil gets on the animal's fur and can get transferred to you. Epstein also suggests that you be careful with gardening tools, bicycle tires, golf balls, and anything else you use outside that might come in contact with the oil. Once there, the oil can remain active for a long time, so you can get poison ivy again and again without touching the plant itself if you don't use care when handling these outdoor items and rinse them after each use.

RINSE YOUR CLOTHES OUTSIDE.

If you think you've had a close encounter with poison ivy, the oil may be all over your clothes. If you walk inside your home without rinsing your clothes, you may transfer the oil to rugs or furniture. Water deactivates the oil, so once your clothes are soaked, they're safe. Epstein also recommends rinsing camping, hunting, and fishing gear so you don't start off your next vacation with a case of poison ivy. Don't forget your shoes. "Many times, people will step on twigs or pieces of the vine and the oil will get on their shoes," says Dvorine. At night, if you take your shoes off by grabbing the sole or the heel, you may grab onto more than you bargained for and end up with a nasty case of poison ivy.

HEAD FOR WATER FAST.

This should be your first step if you suspect you've gotten into poison ivy. Whether it's a stream, lake, garden hose, or faucet, if you can get to water within five to ten minutes after contact, you may be able to wash the oil off before all of it sinks in. "The sooner you get wet, the better effect you're going to get," says Epstein.

CARRY RUBBING ALCOHOL WITH YOU.

The oil from poison ivy isn't absorbed into the skin all at once; it sinks in fairly gradually. If you move quickly enough, you may be able to use rubbing alcohol to extract some oil from the skin, suggests Epstein. If you think you've been exposed to the weed and you're heading back inside for the day, wash down the exposed areas with rubbing alcohol and then rinse well with water. Don't use a cloth wipe, Epstein cautions, because that may just pick up the oil and put it somewhere else. And don't use the alcohol near your eyes.

COOL OFF THE ITCH.

If preventive steps failed and you've got a rash, cool water may help ease the itch. "A cool bath or cool shower is wonderful," says Pearlstein. Placing ice-cold compresses on the rash may also provide relief.

SMOOTH ON SOME CALAMINE LOTION.

"People typically cover themselves with calamine lotion," says Pearlstein. "That's the time-honored solution." Indeed, calamine lotion can be mildly soothing and help to dry the rash. Apply it in a thin layer, however, so that the pores are not sealed.

APPLY BUROW'S SOLUTION.

This lesser-known product (sold without a prescription) can soothe and relieve mild rashes when put on compress-style. It's often sold under the name Domeboro, in a tablet or powder form that you mix with water (according to package directions). Ask your pharmacist if you're having trouble locating it.

GO SOAK YOURSELF.

Bathing in lukewarm water mixed with oatmeal or baking soda may help to dry oozing blisters and soothe irritated skin, says Epstein.

TRY HYDROCORTISONE CREAMS.

Sold without a prescription, these creams may offer some relief for mild rashes. Epstein says that for anything but the mildest cases, however, these over-the-counter creams are not strong enough to help. If you have a rash that is severe enough to take you to the doctor, he or she may prescribe more potent steroids.

Postnasal drip

9 Ways to Slow the Flow

Hrmphh. Haack. Those sounds you make every morning to clear your throat could mean you're suffering from postnasal drip. That's a polite term for the feeling that there's an accumulation of mucus in the back of your throat. What you probably don't realize is that your sinuses normally produce one to two quarts of thin, clear mucus each day. "It's usually nonirritating and you don't notice it going from your nose to your throat," explains James A. Stankiewicz, M.D., professor and vice-chairman of the Department of Otolaryngology–Head and Neck Surgery at Loyola University Medical School in Maywood, Illinois. The mucus helps moisturize and cleanse the air you breathe and it keeps the tissues in your nose and sinuses lubricated so they can do a better job.

But when your nose runs amok and doubles up on production—or makes less, which ends up being thicker and stickier—the problems can start. "Sometimes patients think they're making too much mucus when it's thicker because they notice it then," says Stankiewicz.

And sometimes you may not even notice the drip but may complain instead of a chronic sore throat, hoarseness, or the need to constantly clear your throat, says Gary Y. Shaw, M.D., associate professor of otolaryngology, head and neck surgery at the University of Kansas Medical Center in Kansas City. "If you control the postnasal drip, then these other symptoms improve."

What causes the sinuses to make this shift in production?

• **Allergies.** "That's one of the most common causes," points out Sally Wenzel, M.D., assistant professor of medicine at National Jewish Center for Immunology and Respiratory Medicine in Denver.

• **Colds.** A runny nose is probably the most noticeable symptom of a cold. Wait it out a week and you should start feeling better.

• **Obstructions.** Polyps, small tumorlike growths in the mucous membranes, or a deviated septum can block the flow of mucus or cause it to change by affecting the flow of air.

• **Sinus infection.** You'll probably need to see a physician for a prescription for antibiotics to clear up this one. If mucus is yellow or green and thick, you've probably got an infection.

• **Environment.** If you're exposed to a dry, dusty environment or to such irritants as cigarette smoke or pollutants, your mucous membranes will dry out and you'll end up with thicker, reduced amounts of mucus. Sometimes, switching from hot to cold temperatures suddenly, or vice versa, can turn on mucus-producing glands, says Shaw. "You go from hot, humid air outside in the summertime to dry, cool air indoors."

• **Pregnancy.** Stankiewicz suspects hormones are to blame.

• **Age.** The older you are, the less mucus your body makes. In addition, high blood pressure drugs and other medications may change mucus production, points out Stankiewicz.

If you're suffering from postnasal drip, here's how you can help clear up the problem:

IRRIGATE YOUR NOSE AND SINUSES.

It takes practice to get the hang of this, but some doctors swear by it. Take one cup of water at body temperature and add one-half teaspoon of salt and a pinch of baking soda. Use a nasal syringe and inject a bulbful of the saline solution into one nostril while you close off the back of your palate and throat. Tilt your head back, then forward, and then to the sides for about eight to ten seconds in each position. (You have four sinuses on each side, so you're trying to reach all of them.) Then forcibly blow out the solution. "It's not a pretty sight," Wenzel warns. Do three to four bulbfuls on each side.

Be sure to keep your syringe clean; use rubbing alcohol and rinse with water after each use. If you don't have a bulb syringe, you can cup the salt solution in your hands and inhale. You can irrigate up to four to six times a day when you're suffering from problems, or twice a day "for maintenance," says Wenzel.

USE A SALINE SPRAY.

If you're a little squeamish about using a syringe, you can buy an over-the-counter saline nasal spray, such as Ayr, NaSal, or Ocean. Be sure you're getting a saline spray, however, and not a decongestant nasal spray that can have a rebound effect after prolonged use. You can also "package" your own spray, according to Shaw's recipe: Bring one liter of water to boil, add one table-spoon of salt, boil, then let cool. Keep the solution in a closed container in the refrigerator and use it at room temperature in a spray bottle that provides a fine mist, or inhale it, cupped in your hands.

HUMIDIFY THE AIR.

If you live in a dry climate or you're inside with artifi-cially heated air during the winter, your sinuses can use some help. A home or room humidifier can help, as can placing open containers of water on the radiators in your home. "If you see a very light film of moisture on win-dows, then your indoor humidity is high enough," says Stankiewicz.

DRINK FLUIDS.

In other words, keep your body well hydrated by drink-ing eight glasses of fluid a day. Don't rely totally on milk, coffee, or tea, and avoid alcoholic beverages. "Kids who

LOOK TO YOUR STOMACH

Sometimes, what you're trying to clear out of your throat in the morning isn't mucus after all. It may be the contents of your stomach.

Gastroesophageal reflux, the medical name for heartburn, can result in the acid-rich contents of the stomach coming back up in the throat during the night. And it may not necessarily cause a burning sensation, the telltale sign of heartburn.

If you wake up with a bad taste in your mouth, do a lot of throat clearing, and have hoarseness that improves as the day goes on, your problem may not be postnasal drip at all, says Gary Y. Shaw, M.D.

Try elevating the head of your bed six to eight inches, avoiding meals or snacks within two hours of bedtime, and cutting out caffeine and alcohol, which relax the muscle that keeps the esophagus closed. You can also try over-the-counter antacids.

Other swallowing problems may also be to blame. The muscles used in the complicated process of swallowing become weaker with age. And you tend to swallow less frequently while sleeping. Plus stress can cause muscle spasms anywhere in the body—including the throat.

drink a lot of milk aren't getting that much fluid," warns Stankiewicz. "Milk is more of a solid than a liquid." Caffeinated coffee, tea, and sodas—as well as alcohol—

can actually have a diuretic effect and pull fluid from your system.

AVOID THE ALLERGENS.

That's the best—and probably most difficult—way to treat allergies, if they're responsible for your postnasal-drip woes. If you're allergic to cats, you can try to stay away from them. Allergies to ragweed pollen or house dust are harder (see ALLERGIES for suggestions).

TREAT YOUR ALLERGIES.

You can also keep allergies under control with medications like antihistamines, decongestants, and prescription topical inhaled steroids. To fight drowsiness, a common side effect of nonprescription antihistamines, Stankiewicz recommends cutting an over-the-counter

HELLO, DOCTOR?

If you suspect that you have a sinus infection, especially if your nasal mucus is thick and yellow or green, see your doctor. You may need a prescription for an antibiotic.

In addition, if you have postnasal drip that just won't go away, you may want to have an ear, nose, and throat specialist (an otolaryngologist) examine you. He or she can determine if a mechanical problem, like polyps, is to blame.

WHEN THE CURE BECOMES THE PROBLEM

Over-the-counter nasal sprays offer temporary relief from a stuffy nose and clogged sinuses. But overuse of such products can leave you worse off than ever.

Sprays that contain phenylephrine hydrochloride, oxymetazoline hydrochloride, and xylometazoline hydrochloride have a rebound effect. They're vasoconstrictors; that is, they reduce inflammation or swelling of the nasal passages by preventing blood flow. But after using them for three or four days, constricted blood vessels rebel—they rebound and swell. So limit your use of such sprays to a few days at a time, recommend the experts.

product in half and taking it every four to six hours instead of taking a whole one every eight hours. You could also try a combination antihistamine and decongestant, since the latter tends to be stimulating and may balance out the drowsiness caused by the antihistamine. If you find that an antihistamine quits working after a couple of months, try another one. "Your body becomes tolerant of one type and it won't be effective anymore," Stankiewicz says. Remember that antihistamines have a drying effect and tend to decrease and thicken mucous secretions.

TAKE A DECONGESTANT.

Over-the-counter products like Sudafed help the sinuses drain. Don't rely on decongestant nasal sprays, however; they can have a rebound effect (see "When the Cure Becomes the Problem"). And men over 60 who tend to suffer from urinary tract obstructions will have problems taking a decongestant, Shaw says.

STAY AWAY FROM IRRITANTS.

If you know that cigarette smoke triggers your sinuses, stay away from smoky areas. Ditto for anything else that causes trouble.

GARGLE.

It's no cure, but it may bring some relief for a sore throat, says Stankiewicz. Add one-half teaspoon of salt to a cup of warm water, says Wenzel.

Premenstrual syndrome

11 Ways to Ease the Discomforts

You've heard the joke before. A woman flies off the handle at work or at home and everyone around her chimes in with, "It must be that time of the month again."

The joke, of course, misses the point that women, at times, actually do get upset by their demanding husbands, whiny kids, and stressful jobs. For some women, however, the joke holds more truth than they'd like to believe. For these women, "that time of the month" really is a period of emotional imbalance, anger, depression, and anxiety. Situations that they normally cope with well suddenly become insurmountable. And the energy and health they enjoy most of the time give way to fatigue, achiness, and weight gain almost overnight.

These women have what is known as premenstrual syndrome, or PMS, a condition that has no known cause and no complete cure. But research into the topic has brought about several theories as to what may make some women more vulnerable to PMS.

"The two most widely held theories, neither of which has huge support, include an ovarian hormone imbalance of either estrogen or progesterone and a brain hormone change or deficiency," says Harold Zimmer, M.D., an obstetrician and gynecologist in private practice in Bellevue, Washington. Zimmer stresses that no single cause of PMS has ever been proven and that much of the research is contradictory.

Whatever the cause, the symptoms can include anxiety, irritability, mood swings, and anger; indeed, these symptoms occur in more than 80 percent of women who suffer from PMS. Other symptoms may include sugar cravings, fatigue, headaches, dizziness, shakiness, abdominal bloating, breast tenderness, and overall swelling. Much less common are depression, memory loss, and feelings of isolation. The symptoms, and their severity, vary from woman to woman.

"Symptoms are definitely cyclic, and that is one of the main criteria for diagnosing this condition. And the symptoms generally disappear with the onset of the woman's period," says Phyllis Frey, A.R.N.P., a nurse practitioner at Bellegrove OB-GYN, Inc., in Bellevue, Washington. "It's often the emotional symptoms that bring people in to the doctor," she adds.

As for what you can do to relieve the discomfort of PMS, there are several home remedies. And according to Zimmer, the home remedies probably work as well as, or better than, the medical remedies available. Here's what you can try:

MAINTAIN A WELL-BALANCED DIET.

Include lots of fresh fruits and vegetables, starches, raw seeds and nuts, fish, poultry, and whole grains. "It is just sort of common sense dietary measures," says Zimmer.

GO EASY ON SUGAR.

Your cravings for sugar may be strong during this time, but giving in to them may make you feel even worse. To make fending off your sugar cravings a little easier, try keeping healthy snacks readily available and keeping sugary foods out of the house—or at least out of your reach. If you can't give up the sweets completely, try eating only small amounts at a time, and opt for things like fruits or apple juice that can help satisfy your sugar craving *and* provide nutrients.

EAT SMALL, FREQUENT MEALS.

Don't go long without food because that can intensify your premenstrual symptoms, says Zimmer.

AVOID ALCOHOL.

Both Zimmer and Frey stress that alcohol will only make you feel more depressed and fatigued. Alcohol also depletes the body's stores of B vitamins and minerals and disrupts carbohydrate metabolism. It also disrupts the liver's ability to metabolize hormones, which can lead to higher-than-normal estrogen levels. So if you need to be holding a beverage at that party, try a nonalcoholic cocktail, such as mineral water with a twist of lime or lemon or a dash of bitters.

CUT DOWN ON CAFFEINATED BEVERAGES.

These include coffee, tea, and colas. Caffeine can intensify anxiety, irritability, and mood swings. It may also increase breast tenderness. Try substituting water-processed decaffeinated coffee; grain-based coffee substitutes such as Pero, Postum, and Caffix; and ginger tea.

CUT THE FAT.

Eating too much dietary fat can interfere with liver efficiency. And some beef contains small amounts of synthetic estrogens. Too much protein can also increase the body's demand for minerals. Opt for smaller servings of lean meats, fish or seafood, beans, peas, seeds, and nuts. Use more whole grains, rice, vegetables, and fruits to fill out your meals.

PUT DOWN THE SALT SHAKER.

Table salt and high-sodium foods such as bouillon, commercial salad dressings, catsup, and hot dogs can worsen fluid retention, bloating, and breast tenderness.

PRACTICE STRESS MANAGEMENT.

"Learning to control and reduce your level of stress has a great effect on reducing the symptoms of PMS," says Zimmer. Try joining a stress-management or stress-reduction program at your local hospital or community college; learning biofeedback techniques; meditating; exercising; or doing anything that helps you to relax and cope with stress.

TRY NOT TO PLAN BIG EVENTS DURING YOUR PMS TIME.

"I don't like to encourage my patients to plan their lives around their menstrual cycle, but if they have the option of planning a big social event at some time other than their PMS time, it would help them out to do so," says Zimmer. "The increased stress of the event will only make the PMS symptoms worse," he adds.

EXERCISE AEROBICALLY.

"Besides being a great stress reducer, aerobic exercise triggers the release of endorphins (the natural brain opiates) and produces a 'runner's high,'" says Zimmer. "Good forms of aerobic exercise include running, stairstepping, bicycling, or taking an aerobics class," he continues. "The social environment of a health club can also make you feel better by encouraging you to interact with other people," he adds. He also goes on to say that increasing the pelvic circulation can help to rid the body of some of the bloating associated with PMS. Try to exercise for 20 to 30 minutes at least three times a week. If you are too fatigued to exercise during the actual PMS period, don't. Doing so the rest of the month should help in itself.

TALK IT OVER.

Try to explain to your loved ones and close friends the reason for your erratic behavior. "One of the biggest stresses on a woman during this time is family. And it's not only the stress of feeling bad when she flies off the handle at someone, but also of having to apologize for her behavior later on," says Zimmer. He recommends enlisting the aid of your family and close friends by asking them to understand what the problem is and to realize that when you lash out at them you are not as in control as you would like to be. "If your child is really acting out and yelling at you for something during your PMS time, you might remind him that this is not the best time for him to be getting you angry. Hopefully, he'll see this as his cue to go outside and play," Zimmer explains. "You have to walk a fine line, though, and not begin using PMS as an excuse to be nasty to people," he adds.

If the emotional symptoms are causing problems in your relationships, consider getting some counseling from a mental-health professional. Ask your physician to refer you to someone.

Psoriasis

25 Coping Techniques

Psoriasis is a noncontagious, chronic skin condition that produces round, dry, scaly patches of different sizes covered with white, gray, or silvery white scales. If you suffer from this incurable disease, you're certainly not alone. According to the National Psoriasis Foundation, between three and four million Americans have the disease. Approximately 150,000 new cases are diagnosed every year.

Not only is psoriasis common, but it's also very mysterious because there seem to be few "absolutes" about it. Doctors aren't sure what causes it, although they believe it tends to run in families. However, you may have psoriasis and have no family history of the disease. It can appear at any age, but most often it strikes between the ages of 20 and 50. It's also been diagnosed in children and infants.

Psoriasis even behaves mysteriously. Sometimes, it can be very mild, with only a few patches. The next day, however, great patches of it may cover the body. Treatment is difficult because what works for one person may not work for another, and treatments that were effective often become ineffective or vice versa.

Doctors do know that whatever causes psoriasis somehow shifts production of replacement skin cells into overdrive. "Something is causing the upper layer of the skin to overgrow," explains Jon M. Hanifin, M.D., professor of dermatology at Oregon Health Sciences University in Portland. "Normally, it takes about 30 days for skin cells to migrate up to the surface. With psoriasis, it takes three to four days."

This speeded-up cell growth is what causes the scaly patches, called plaques. There are several types of psoriasis, but the plaque-forming type (called plaque psoriasis) is the most common. The plaques can appear anywhere on the body. However, they most commonly occur on the scalp and lower back and over the elbows, knees, and knuckles. When psoriasis affects the fingernails and toenails, it causes pitting and brownish discoloration and sometimes cracking and lifting of the nail.

While there currently isn't a cure for psoriasis, there are ways to make living with psoriasis easier. Follow these simple strategies:

DON'T GIVE UP.

Psoriasis isn't life threatening, but it can be terribly frustrating. Skin experts say a positive, never-say-die attitude can help people with psoriasis find relief. "At one time, the National Psoriasis Foundation conducted a survey and found that 75 percent of its members had given up trying to treat their psoriasis," says Hanifin. "Medicine is coming up with new treatments every day, and some old treatments that might not have worked in the past for you may work now."

MOISTURIZE.

"If the skin becomes too dry, it can crack and bleed. It also makes the skin susceptible to secondary infections," explains Diane Baker, M.D., a clinical professor of dermatology at Oregon Health Sciences University in Portland who serves as an advisor to the National Psoriasis Foundation. The solution is to never let your skin become dry, says Baker. Moisturizing also reduces inflammation, helps maintain flexibility (dried plaques can make moving certain parts of the body difficult), keeps the psoriasis from getting worse, and makes the scales less noticeable. The heaviest, or greasiest, moisturizers work best at locking water into the skin. Thick moisturizers like Eucerin, Aquaphor, and Neutrogena Norwegian Formula Hand Cream are all effective. But you can also use inexpensive cooking oils, lard, or petrolatum. "I tell my patients that Vaseline works as well as anything," says Mark Lebwohl, M.D., director of clinical dermatology at Mount Sinai School of Medicine in New York and medical advisor to the National Psoriasis Foundation. "It helps prevent drying and fissuring."

GET OUT IN THE SUN.

"A high proportion of people with psoriasis clear their lesions with exposure to sunlight," says Lebwohl. "I advise people to go to the seashore."

Although doctors aren't sure exactly what ultraviolet light does, it seems to slow skin cell replication. For many years, people have flocked to the Dead Sea to treat their psoriasis. "At 1,300 feet below sea level, the sunlight at the Dead Sea is like none other in the world," says Lebwohl. "Some people thought the psoriasis improvement might be due to the Dead Sea water, but they've tried taking the water to other places and it doesn't work. It's the sunlight."

While you may not be able to schedule your next vacation at the Dead Sea, you can take advantage of the healing effects of the sun. However, be careful not to burn, because this damages the skin. And Hanifin suggests "greasing up the scale with Vaseline or mineral oil before going in the sun."

LIGHT UP YOUR LIFE.

Ultraviolet light B (UVB) therapy can be administered at home. The National Psoriasis Foundation says 80 percent of psoriasis sufferers have good results with it. Home light units are similar to those used in a doctor's office. *Don't use a home UVB unit, however, without first talking with your physician.*

Be very careful to avoid burning, and have your skin checked regularly by a physician who can recognize skin cancer. When purchasing a UVB home unit, the National Psoriasis Foundation suggests these guidelines:

• Look for safety features like key switches or disabling switches that keep the machine from being used when the owner is not around.

• Make sure the unit has a reliable and accurate timer.

• Check to ensure there are safety guards or grids over the lamps.

• Look for equipment that is both stable and durable.

• Ask about replacement bulbs and their cost.

TAKE A SOAK.

Showering, swimming, soaking in a tub, and applying wet compresses all can rehydrate very dry skin and help remove thick, scaly psoriasis without damaging the skin, says Hanifin. Since thick scaling can act as a barrier to both medications and ultraviolet light, it's important to gently remove as much scale as possible. Regular soaking also helps reduce itching and redness of lesions. Keep the bathwater tepid rather than hot (hot water can increase itching), and add a little oil (mineral oil is inexpensive and works well) to the bath to help seal in the water.

While soaking helps remove plaque scales, Lebwohl warns that it also removes the skin's oils, its natural protection against moisture loss. To prevent overdrying the skin, he recommends moisturizing with a heavy emollient immediately (within three minutes) after your soak.

BEAT THE TAR OUT OF IT.

Tar-containing shampoos, creams, and bath additives have been successful psoriasis treatments for many years. "Tar products are old standbys," says Hanifin.

"There are effective over-the-counter lotions and tar shampoos like Baker's PNS that loosen scale."

Baker says tar-containing bath oils are especially helpful for psoriasis that is widespread on the body.

BRING ON THE SALICYLIC ACID.

Lebwohl says over-the-counter salicylic acid shampoos and creams literally "eat scale."

TRY OVER-THE-COUNTER CORTISONE.

Hanifin says, "Cortisone creams can bring dramatic relief for psoriasis. They're especially helpful for psoriasis in body folds or on the face." Stronger, one percent cortisone creams are now available over the counter in pharmacies.

PASS THE PLASTIC WRAP.

Doctors have known for years that covering psoriasis lesions helps them go away. "Covering lesions also helps force medication into the skin and keeps moisture in the skin," explains Baker. You can use plastic wrap or you can buy over-the-counter patches (Actiderm). Apply the medication or moisturizer, and cover the area. Be careful, however, that the skin doesn't become too soggy and subject to secondary infection.

CHOOSE SOAPS CAREFULLY.

Harsh soaps can dry and irritate the skin and increase itching. Baker suggests using a mild, unscented soap. Many mild, "superfatted" soaps that contain moisturizers are available, such as Basis, Alpha Keri, Purpose, Nivea Cream Bar, and Oilatum. You can also choose one of the many soap-free cleansers such as Lowilla Cake,

KITCHEN SOLUTIONS

Many anti-itch remedies can be made up right in your own kitchen. The National Psoriasis Foundation suggests the following do-it-yourself recipes:

• Dissolve 1½ cups of baking soda in three gallons of water to use as an anti-itch compress.

• Add a handful of Epsom salts or Dead Sea salts to your bath water. You can also add a squirt of mineral oil or baby oil to the water with the salts.

• Put three tablespoons of boric acid (available in pharmacies) in 16 ounces of water and use as a compress.

• Add two teaspoons of olive oil to a large glass of milk and use it as a soothing bath oil.

• Add a cup of white vinegar to the bath to ease itching.

Aveeno Cleansing Bar, and pHisoDerm Dry Skin Formula if your skin is dry and irritated. No matter what product you choose, Hanifin says to be sure to rinse off well to prevent drying and itching.

PASS THE WARM OLIVE OIL.
If psoriasis scale is a problem on your scalp, Lebwohl suggests that you warm a little olive oil and gently massage it into the scale to help soften and remove it.

WIPE OUT THE ITCH WITH ANTIHISTAMINES.

Scratching can damage the skin, something you don't want to do with psoriasis, says Hanifin. He suggests trying over-the-counter antihistamines when the itch is more than you can handle.

TRY FISH OIL.

Recent research from the University of California at Davis and the University of Michigan at Ann Arbor suggests that large oral doses of fish-oil supplements may help control psoriasis. Doctors have long known that Greenland Eskimos, who eat large quantities of cold-water fish, rarely suffer from psoriasis. Some believe the Eskimos' consumption of fish-oil may be the reason. Participants in the fish-oil studies had to consume unusually large quantities of the oil to achieve positive results. Before you try fish oil yourself, talk with your physician.

HUMIDIFY.

Dry indoor air is associated with dry skin, which is bad news for psoriasis sufferers. Hanifin suggests using room humidifiers to raise the humidity in your home or office. Even setting out pans of water on your radiators may help to increase indoor humidity somewhat.

AVOID INJURING YOUR SKIN.

Robert Matheson, M.D., a dermatologist in private practice in Portland, Oregon, who frequently works with the National Psoriasis Foundation, says it's important to avoid injuring your skin. Even mild injuries like sunburn, scratches, and irritation from tight clothing can make psoriasis worse in some people. "Skin injuries often cause psoriasis to appear in the injury area," explains Matheson. "It's called the Koebner phenomenon."

USE SKIN PRODUCTS CAREFULLY.
Lebwohl says that the skin of people with psoriasis is more susceptible to irritating substances. He advises caution in using products, such as hair dyes and straighteners, that can irritate the skin. "Make sure your skin is in very good shape before you use these types of products," he says. "Don't use them if you have open wounds."

TREAT INFECTIONS PRONTO.
Systemic infections like strep throat (streptococcal infections) can trigger psoriasis flares in some people. "If you suspect you have an infection like strep," says Matheson, "have it treated by a doctor right away."

STAY TRIM.
For reasons doctors haven't been able to identify, psoriasis tends to be worse and harder to control among people who are obese, says Baker. While a weight cause-and-effect hasn't been established, it's a good idea to stay trim. If you're already overweight, try eating a low-fat diet and getting regular exercise to shed excess pounds.

BE CAREFUL WITH MEDICATIONS.
Certain medications such as antimalarials, beta blockers (Inderal), lithium, and other drugs can worsen psoriasis in some people. Be sure your physician knows about your skin condition and discuss the possibility of reduced dosages or alternative medications.

RELAX.

Baker says stress is definitely a factor in psoriasis. "Stress can really make psoriasis flare up," she says. "Recognize that everybody's life has stress and learn to relax."

Sensitive teeth

5 Tips to Keep You Smiling

You take a drink of iced tea, bite down on a candy bar, or slurp some hot soup and the electric stinging sensation in one or more of your teeth sends you flying out of your seat. You've got "sensitive teeth," a rather mild name for what can be a wildly uncomfortable condition.

So what's going on? Why do your teeth react to hot, cold, sweet, or sour, and sometimes even to pressure? Well, it could be many things, according to Jack W. Clinton, D.M.D., associate dean of patient services at Oregon Health Sciences University School of Dentistry in Portland. "The difficulty with sensitive teeth is there is a wide variety of problems that can cause the teeth to become sensitive," he says. "It can be as simple as a 'bruised' tooth from biting down too hard on something, to as complicated as necrotic, or dead, tooth pulp that requires root-canal work."

One or more teeth can become sensitive to pressure, even to mild chewing, when a tooth is "bruised" or traumatized from biting down too hard or from having a tooth worked on at the dentist's office. Often, teeth feel sensitive after they've been cleaned or filled. Sometimes this kind of sensitivity can take weeks or even months to go away. In other cases, people can cause tooth sensitivity by habitual tooth grinding or clamping the jaws tightly. This type of sensitivity to pressure isn't something to worry about if it happens once or twice and goes away in a day or two. The tooth or teeth simply need time to recover from the trauma. It's when the pressure sensitivity is persistent that you should suspect something like a break, crack, or decayed tooth and should see your dentist.

Sensitivity to temperature usually means that teeth have been compromised in some way, says Clinton. Sometimes it means one or more teeth are hitting too soon or too hard and the "bite" must be readjusted by a dentist. "Teeth may be hard," explains Clinton, "but they move around. Bone is reabsorbed or, sometimes, habits like thumb sucking can move teeth around and change how the teeth come together."

By far, the most common cause of sensitivity to temperature and sweet or sour foods is exposed dentin, according to Sandra Hazard, D.M.D., managing dentist for Willamette Dental Group, Inc., in Oregon. Exposed dentin can be the result of dental decay, food or toothbrush abrasion, or gum recession. "Dentin is the material underneath the enamel and what the roots are made of," Hazard explains. "The dentin has microscopic nerve fibers that, when exposed, cause the sensitivity."

If you develop sensitivity in one or more teeth, first see your dentist to determine the cause. Then, if your sensitivity is caused by simple enamel abrasion or by normal gum recession, you can try these strategies for relief:

BRING ON THE DESENSITIZING TOOTHPASTE.

Unfortunately, widespread tooth sensitivity due to enamel abrasion or gum-line recession can't be treated with dental fillings. One of the best home remedies for overall sensitivity, says Hazard, are the desensitizing toothpastes available over the counter. "They contain a special ingredient that fills up the tubules in the dentin and decreases sensitivity," she says. In addition to brushing with desensitizing toothpaste, Ken Waddell, D.M.D., a dentist in private practice in Tigard, Oregon, suggests putting some of the toothpaste on your finger or on a cotton swab and spreading it over the sensitive spots before you go to bed. Spit, but don't rinse. "You should see considerable relief in two or three weeks," he says.

TRY A FLUORIDE RINSE.

Fluoride rinses, available without a prescription at your local pharmacy or in the dental section of grocery stores, can help decrease sensitivity, especially for people with decay problems, says Hazard. Use it once a day. Swish it around in your mouth, then spit it out.

Sometimes, people with sensitive teeth need a stronger fluoride rinse or gel than the ones available over the counter, says Ronald Wismer, D.M.D., a dentist in private practice in Beaverton, Oregon, who sees many patients with sensitive teeth. "If you've had a periodontal procedure like root planing to get rid of plaque," he says, "your dentist can apply a fluoride that can help decrease sensitivity."

KEEP YOUR TEETH CLEAN.

It's particularly important to keep plaque, the white gummy substance that forms on teeth, off areas that are

HELLO, DOCTOR?

While you can often self-treat generalized tooth sensitivity, see your dentist if:

• Your teeth are persistently sensitive to pressure.

• A single tooth is persistently sensitive. "This often indicates the pulp of the tooth is dead," explains Ronald Wismer, D.M.D. "You need to see a dentist as soon as possible."

• Sensitivity doesn't decrease after two weeks of using desensitizing toothpaste.

• You have prolonged pain. "Any pain that lasts longer than one hour indicates you should see a dentist," says Sandra Hazard, D.M.D.

• The gums around a sensitive tooth change color.

• You have any obvious decay.

sensitive. "As plaque metabolizes, it produces acid, which irritates the teeth," explains Hazard. "It can cause sensitive teeth to react even more strongly when stimulated." Brush at least twice a day, preferably right after eating, and floss at least once a day.

USE A SOFT TOOTHBRUSH.

Often, people actually cause tooth sensitivity by brushing incorrectly with a hard-bristled brush. "Before I knew much about brushing, I brushed too hard with the wrong toothbrush and caused enamel abrasion on the right side of my mouth," admits Hazard.

When the gum line recedes (often as a natural part of the aging process), exposed dentin becomes even more vulnerable to toothbrush abrasion. "Enamel is very hard," says Wismer, "but dentin isn't and is much more subject to abrasion by things like brushing." Use a brush with the softest bristles you can find, and apply only a small amount of pressure when brushing. Avoid using a "scrubbing" action to clean the teeth.

SAY ENOUGH TO SNUFF.

Chewing tobacco, also known as "dip" or "snuff," has become a popular habit, especially among many teenagers. They mistakenly believe it's less harmful than smoking cigarettes. However, in addition to causing mouth cancers, chewing tobacco causes the gums to recede, a major cause of gum sensitivity and decay. Habits like sucking on hard candy, while safer than snuff, can also cause enamel abrasion and tooth sensitivity.

Shaving discomfort

13 Ways to Nip the Nicks

You have probably seen those men who have little wads of toilet paper stuck to their face. In fact, you may be one of them. Therefore, you know perfectly well that those wads are not the latest fashion statement, designed to complement your tie or handkerchief. Those wads are there because you missed getting that most elusive of worldly things—the perfect shave.

You just missed it, too, didn't you? You missed it by a nick.

Nicks, scrapes, burns. It may sound like the inventory of an emergency ward, but most men encounter these discomforts on a regular basis in their own bathrooms.

So here are some tips on how to avoid turning your morning ritual into a nightmare and keep the toilet paper off your face. (Of course, women who shave their legs are not immune to these discomforts, either. So while this article is primarily geared toward men, the advice can help women get a softer, gentler shave as well.)

BE PREPARED.

Proper preparation is the key to a good shave, says Gordon Scarbrough, owner of Moler Barber College in Portland, Oregon. That means moistening and softening your face before you even apply the soap. For the best results, do it with a warm, moist towel or washcloth held to your face. At the very least, splash warm tap water on your face.

FOLLOW THE GRAIN.

Shave with the grain; that is, move the razor in the direction that the hair grows, advises Andrew Lazar, M.D., assistant professor of clinical dermatology at Northwestern University School of Medicine in Chicago. Generally, that means shaving down on the face and neck and up on the lower neck.

SHAVE IN THE SHOWER.

The shower is the perfect place to shave, according to Scarbrough, because the steam and the hot water soften and moisten your skin and beard. Shaving your face as your final duty in the shower makes good sense for your skin.

CUT UP YOUR CREDIT CARDS.

Well, at least don't use them as a measure of proper shaving. Joseph P. Bark, M.D., chairman of dermatology at St. Joseph Hospital in Lexington, Kentucky, says men have been trying to live up to an old shaving commercial that showed a credit card being rubbed against a shaved face. "If it made a lot of scraping sounds, you didn't pass the credit-card test," says Bark. He says to cash in that tired idea, and instead invest in the notion that shaving less closely will save you a lot of discomfort.

STOP PLAYING DOUBLES.

"The bad actor in all this is the double-track razor," says Bark. He says the first blade pulls up the skin around hairs, then the second blade shaves off the nubbin of skin. "It's like using a nuclear weapon to mow your lawn," says Bark. Try a single-blade, disposable razor instead.

FROTH YOUR FOAM.

Many men think that foam out of a can is moist enough to apply directly to dry skin. Wrong, says Scarbrough. You need added moisture, or it will almost be like shaving dry skin. Splash water on your face liberally before adding the foam.

BUMPING OFF RAZOR BUMPS

Razor bumps, usually found on the neck and caused by ingrown hairs, are a common shaving problem encountered by curly-haired men. The problem often can be solved by not shaving so close, and by shaving with the grain of the whiskers. For more tips on how to rid your face and neck of these painful, unsightly bumps, refer to INGROWN HAIR.

BE SHARP.

A dull blade can scrape your skin, so don't try to get too many shaves out of one razor. Some men's beards are so coarse that a razor will be effective for only one shave.

TRY AN ELECTRIC.

Electric razors don't shave as closely as a double-track razor and may be less irritating to the skin, says Bark.

USE A QUALITY AFTERSHAVE.

Cheaper brands are just plain alcohol, says Scarbrough. A good aftershave should refresh the skin, cleanse it of bacteria, plus heal it from the shaving. He looks for aloe vera or other natural healers as ingredients.

TRY A SUNSCREEN.

"Use a sunscreen as an aftershave every day and you can look younger and not have skin cancer," says Bark.

HEAL THYSELF.

While your face is healing from razor burn, use an over-the-counter hydrocortisone lotion as your aftershave, Bark suggests. It will speed the healing.

QUIT SHAVING.

If you need to be clean shaven at work, try giving up shaving for the weekend. Bark says growing just a quarter-inch beard will cure razor burn. When it's time to shave again, don't shave too close.

SAY STYPTIC.

Ask for it at the drugstore and keep it handy in the bathroom so you can use it when you nick yourself. You can get a styptic pencil or styptic powder. Dab it on the nick, press down momentarily with your finger, and the bleeding should stop. Alum contained in the pencil or powder draws the skin up to seal the wound, says Scarbrough. Rinse off any residue, and you're ready to face the world—without that snippet of toilet paper.

Shinsplints

10 Ways to Say Goodbye to the Pain for Good

Perhaps you were in the middle of your morning run or your evening aerobics class and it came on like gangbusters: shooting pain starting in the front of your ankle and continuing up almost to your kneecap. Now, when you touch the area on either side of your shinbone, it feels sore and tender. Could it be shinsplints?

"'Shinsplints' is a garbage-basket term used to describe any kind of shin pain that comes from exercise," says Michael J. Henehan, D.O., director of the Sports Medicine Department at Stanford/San Jose Family Practice Residency Program in San Jose, California. "It is an injury that comes from overuse."

Most shin pain, although annoying, is minor and can be treated with the guidelines that follow. However, if the pain persists or recurs, see a doctor. You may be suffering from a stress fracture—a tiny chip or crack in the bone. Stress fractures won't go away on their own and, without treatment, may become serious.

DON'T WORK THROUGH THE PAIN.

You won't earn points in athlete's heaven for trying to tough out the pain of shinsplints, says Henehan. At best, the pain won't get better and at worst, you'll be setting the stage for a more serious injury. "Stay off it until you're pain free," Henehan says. "You can also cut back your mileage if you're a runner, but you ought not to run at all if the pain is severe."

ICE IT.

Ice is the treatment of choice for reducing the inflammation of any sports injury, and shinsplints is no exception, according to William E. Straw, M.D., a clinical associate professor of medicine at Stanford University School of Medicine in California and team physician for the San Francisco Giants. He recommends using water that's been frozen in a Styrofoam (or paper) cup; massage the area with the ice for ten minutes at a time, up to four times a day for a week or two. You can also try icing the area with a bag of frozen vegetables, such as peas or corn kernels, suggests Jeffrey L. Tanji, M.D., an associate professor of family practice and director of the Sports Medicine Program at the University of California at Davis Medical Center. Better yet, ice the area with a bag of frozen unpopped popcorn kernels.

TAPE IT.

Taping up your shin with an Ace bandage or with a neo-prene sleeve that fits over the lower leg may be comforting for shinsplints, says Henehan. "Compression seems to relieve the discomfort, perhaps by decreasing the amount of pull on the muscles."

TAKE TWO ASPIRIN.

Over-the-counter analgesics, such as aspirin and ibuprofen, are very effective in relieving the pain of shinsplints, according to Straw. These medications serve as anti-inflammatories, bringing down the swelling and inflammation that may come with these injuries. Acetaminophen may ease the pain but probably won't do much for inflammation. Women who are pregnant or nursing a baby, as well as aspirin-sensitive individuals, should check with their physicians before taking any medications.

TRY AN ATHLETIC INSOLE.

Since shinsplints often arises as a result of excessive pounding, a padded insole placed inside the shoe may help, according to Henehan. These insoles help soften the blow of your foot's landing on hard ground. You can

CHOOSING A SNEAKER

A good sneaker is an important investment for anyone who runs or does aerobics, doctors agree. Wearing shoes with worn-out or poorly cushioned insoles only paves the way for overuse injuries. When shopping for athletic shoes, look for a good fit (with at least a thumb's width of room at the toe and with the heel held firmly), good cushioning (especially in the forefoot, for an aerobics shoe) and extra-supportive material on the inside heel-edge of the sole, says Spencer White, director of research engineering at Reebok International Ltd. in Stoughton, Massachusetts.

Runners should replace their shoes approximately every 500 miles; aerobicizers every four to five months, White says.

purchase them at an athletic shoe store, sports supply store, or even some grocery stores. They range in price from about $7 to $20.

TUNE IN TO YOUR BODY.

The biggest reason that people get overuse injuries is because they don't pay attention to the signals their bodies give them, says Tanji. "When you're running and you start to feel pain, you need to back off on the pace or the distance," he says.

STAY OFF THE CEMENT.

Another way to lower the impact of your routine is to be sure you exercise on forgiving surfaces, according to Henehan. "For running, the best surface is a track where you have a material that is somewhat shock-absorbent," he says. "Crushed gravel and finely trimmed grass [without holes in the ground] are good choices. Asphalt is better than concrete. Also, rubberized, indoor track surfaces are good." If you do aerobics, stay away from cement floors, even carpeted ones, Henehan says. Suspended wood floors are best.

CROSS TRAIN.

One way to give rest to shinsplints without cutting out exercise altogether is to switch to another type of activity, according to Straw. "Stationary bicycling and swimming are good replacements for running or aerobics," he says. "You need to do something without the pounding."

DON'T RUN ON HILLS.

Running up and down hills may contribute to shinsplints, says Tanji. He suggests avoiding hills until the pain goes away.

PREVENT THE INJURY FROM OCCURRING IN THE FIRST PLACE.

Warming up before exercise may help prevent injury, according to Frank Spano, M.D., an internist at Bridgeport Medical Group in Connecticut. "When you warm up, you increase your heart's supply of blood to your tissues," he says. "You also relax your muscles so that they don't start out so tight. This lowers the likelihood of injury." Spano recommends gentle stretching exercises and starting off slowly before building speed. Tanji tells his patients to do ankle circles before they begin their run.

Side stitch

9 Ways to Stop It

You're running, biking, or walking briskly along when suddenly you're gripped with a sharp pain in your side. With each breath, the pain becomes more intense. You've developed a "side stitch," a sudden, sharp pain in the upper part of your diaphragm.

No one is actually sure what causes side stitch, according to fitness expert Covert Bailey, author of the bestsellers *Fit or Fat* and *The New Fit or Fat*. "No research has ever been able to demonstrate what's really going on with a side stitch," he says. "It remains one of the body's mysteries."

Most authorities believe a side stitch is a cramp in the diaphragm, the "breathing muscle," a large, flat, muscular membrane that separates the chest and abdominal organs and helps force air into and out of the lungs. Exactly why the diaphragm cramps, however, remains unclear. Some believe that exercise like running decreases blood flow to the diaphragm, causing it to go into spasm. Raising the knees to run contracts the belly muscles, which increases pressure inside the belly and presses on the diaphragm from below. During exercise, air tends to get into the lungs more easily than it gets out, so the lungs fill with air and press on the diaphragm from above. The dual pressure, says the theory, squeezes the diaphragm and shuts off its blood flow, resulting in cramping.

Another theory suggests that side-stitch pain results from gas trapped in the large intestine. Exercise, like running, speeds up intestinal contractions and pushes gas toward the end of the colon, or large intestine. If the colon is blocked by a hardened stool, cramping can result.

Some experts believe that, in some people, side stitch may be related to an intolerance to wheat or dairy products. People with such allergies, they say, who exercise within 24 hours of eating these foods may develop cramping or even diarrhea. Others suggest side stitch can be brought on by any food in the stomach and exercising too soon after eating.

While the experts haggle about what causes side stitch, you can learn to prevent it and, if it does occur, make it stop quickly. Here's how:

BELLY BREATHE.

Competitive distance runner and sports medicine expert Joan Ullyot, M.D., author of *Women's Running* and *Running Free*, says most side stitches come from improper breathing. "Many people, especially beginning runners, don't breathe properly when they're exercising," she says. "They breathe too shallowly."

Michael Martindale, L.P.T., a physical therapist at the Sports Medicine Center at Portland Adventist Medical Center in Oregon, agrees. "People often learn to breathe using only their upper chest muscles rather than the diaphragm muscles," he explains. "During exercise, when they need more air, they breathe faster and even more shallowly."

Ullyot says the key to side-stitch prevention is deep belly breathing. To help people learn how to breathe, Ullyot has people lie on their back with a book on their abdomen. "I have them breathe in all the way into the belly," she says. "The book must move up when breathing in and down when exhaling."

TRY THE "GRUNT" EXHALE.
Because it's much more difficult to empty the lungs than fill them during exercise, it's important to exhale all the way into your belly. Force air out while exhaling by pushing your abdomen out while making a grunting sound.

SLOW DOWN.
Being out of condition and exercising too intensely causes you to breathe quickly—and more shallowly. Martindale suggests cutting back on the intensity of your activity. "Slow down," he says. "Build your endurance over several weeks."

STOP.
Some people, particularly competitive runners, believe you should "run through" a side stitch. However, unless you're in a race, Ullyot says the best idea is to stop completely until the pain subsides.

USE THE "ONE HOUR" RULE.
If you've eaten, wait at least an hour before exercising, says Ullyot. "Food in the stomach doesn't bother some people, but for others it can cause cramping," she says.

HELLO, DOCTOR?

Sometimes, angina pectoris, a serious pain caused by lack of oxygen to the heart, is mistaken for side stitch. See a doctor immediately if you have pain that:

• Emanates from beneath the breastbone or from the neck or radiates down the left arm

• Is accompanied by shortness of breath

• Is brought on by emotional tension and/or physical exertion

MASSAGE IT.
"Anytime a muscle is denied blood, it will go into spasm and cause pain," says physical therapist Ellen Nona Hoyven, P.T., owner and director of Ortho Sport Physical Therapy P.C. in Clackamas, Oregon. "Massage increases circulation and relaxes muscles." If you develop a stitch, gently massage the area with your hands.

USE THE "POKE AND BLOW" TECHNIQUE.
One way to relieve diaphragm pressure is to reach deeply with your fingers into your belly just below your ribs on the right side. At the same time, purse your lips tightly and blow out as hard as you can, advises Martindale.

PRACTICE RUNNING FAST.
One of the possible causes of side stitch is weak abdominal and diaphragm muscles. To increase endurance

and strengthen the diaphragm, try running fast a couple of times a week.

STRENGTHEN ABDOMINAL MUSCLES.

Strong abdominal muscles can help prevent side stitch. Try doing bent-leg partial sit-ups in which you raise the shoulders about six inches off the ground. Or lie on your back and lift your straight legs a few inches off the ground and hold for 20 to 30 seconds at a time.

Slivers

5 Ways to Remove Them Safely

It's cold and you're hauling in firewood. But you forgot to wear gloves. Suddenly, you feel a sharp pain in your hand—yep, you've got a sliver.

Essentially, a sliver (or splinter) is a puncture wound with debris in it. You can also get slivers of glass, metal, or plastic, but wood slivers are the most common.

While a cut is a vertical slice and a scrape is the horizontal removal of the outer skin, a puncture wound is a stab deep into the tissue. In the case of a sliver, it's the foreign object—the sliver—that causes the puncture and stays in the tissue. Most slivers aren't serious and can be treated at home. Here's how:

TWEEZE IT.

"If the sliver is sticking above the skin, it's pretty easy to remove it with tweezers. Sterilize the tweezers with alcohol, grasp the sliver as close to the skin as possible, and gently pull it out," says Louisa Silva, M.D., a general practitioner who sees plenty of slivers in her private practice in Salem, Oregon.

NEEDLE IT.

When slivers don't stick out of the skin, sterilize a needle with alcohol and use it to push the sliver out from the bottom, says Paul Contorer, M.D., chief of dermatology for Kaiser Permanente and clinical professor of dermatology at Oregon Health Sciences University in Portland. "It's important to push the sliver out from the bottom," he says, "or it's likely to break up and leave parts of the sliver in the skin."

SLICE IT.

Too often, slivers are deep and people poke and prod with tweezers and end up bruising the tissue all around the sliver site, according to Robert Matheson, M.D., a dermatologist in private practice in Portland, Oregon. "Use a new, clean razor blade," he advises, "and make an incision parallel to the sliver, right above it. Then gently spread the incision and pick out the sliver." While slicing into your skin may sound gruesome, Contorer says it shouldn't hurt. "The top layer of skin is dead tissue," he explains. "As long as you use a sharp razor or knife and don't cut too deeply, you won't even feel it." Be sure to sterilize the instrument with alcohol first.

CLEAN IT.

Once you've got the sliver out, clean the wound thoroughly with soap and water. "Clean it really well," advises Silva. "There's a much higher rate of infection with puncture wounds that are deep and dirty." After cleaning with soap and water, Contorer likes to use hydrogen peroxide to make sure all the debris has been cleaned out. "The hydrogen peroxide releases oxygen, kills bacteria, and speeds healing," he says.

SQUEEZE ON THE ANTIBACTERIAL OINTMENT.

If the wound hasn't immediately closed up or if you've used the slice technique to remove the sliver, apply an antibacterial ointment like Polysporin or Neosporin and cover with a bandage. Contorer says he prefers Polysporin because fewer people have allergic reactions to it.

Snoring
9 Ways to Turn Down the Volume

Snoring is a problem that, it would seem, hardly needs an introduction. However, as a definition, snoring is "a harsh and noisy sound made by the nose and mouth during sleep," according to Philip R. Westbrook, M.D., F.C.C.P., director of the Sleep Disorders Center at Cedars–Sinai Medical Center in Los Angeles and past president of the American Sleep Disorders Association. It is a common affliction, affecting 20 percent of men and 5 percent of women between the ages of 30 and 35, and 60 percent of men and 40 percent of women at age 60. Despite its frequency, however, snoring is a sleep disorder that can have serious medical and social consequences. The tips that follow may help you sleep more peacefully. Pleasant dreams!

SLEEP ON YOUR SIDE.

"Much of the reason for snoring is positional," says Westbrook. "It occurs when the individual is on his back, not on his side. This clearly suggests that one should avoid sleeping on one's back. Rather than use your bed partner's elbows to help you accomplish that, place two tennis balls in a sock and pin the sock to the back of your pajama top. Make it so uncomfortable to sleep on your back that you sleep on your side."

AVOID ALCOHOL AND TRANQUILIZERS.

Alcohol and sleeping pills can depress your central nervous system and relax the muscles of your throat and jaw, making snoring more likely, according to Karl Doghramji, M.D., director of the Sleep Disorders Center at Jefferson Medical College of Thomas Jefferson University in Philadelphia. These substances are also known to cause sleep apnea, a dangerous condition that has been linked with cardiovascular disease, he says.

LOSE WEIGHT.

Excess body weight, especially around the neck, puts pressure on the airway, causing it to partially collapse, Westbrook says. "It becomes like trying to suck air through a wet [paper] straw. It limits the amount of air that comes in. Turbulence is created, and the soft tissues flap in the breeze, so to speak, creating the noise." It usually takes a significant weight loss, about ten percent of total body weight, to make an improvement.

GET YOUR ALLERGIES TREATED.

Chronic respiratory allergies may cause snoring by forcing sufferers to breathe through their mouths while they sleep, says Doghramji. A decongestant or antihistamine before bedtime may help, he says. Another help for a blocked nose is saline spray, which may be purchased at any drugstore, says German Nino-Murcia, M.D., founder and medical director of the Sleep Medicine and Neuroscience Institute in Palo Alto, California. (You can make your own saline solution by mixing a cup of water at body temperature, a half teaspoon of salt, and a pinch of baking soda. Then put the solution in a clean nasal spray bottle or nasal syringe and squirt it into your nose.) "An ultrasonic humidifier is also a good idea," he adds (see ALLERGIES).

BUY A MOUTH GUARD.

Your dentist or doctor may be able to prescribe an antisnoring mouth guard, says Doghramji. "The guards fit into the mouth and make sure that the upper and lower teeth are held together," he says. "It prevents the lower jaw from sagging backwards." This, in turn, may help quiet the snoring.

STOP SMOKING.

"Smoking can be very irritating to the lining of the upper airway, including the nose," says Westbrook. "Your snoring may improve if you quit." Of course, kicking the habit is beneficial to your health in other ways, too.

KEEP A REGULAR SCHEDULE.

"People who are sleep deprived will tend to snore," says Thomas Roth, Ph.D., chief of the Division of Sleep

WHAT'S WRONG WITH SNORING, ANYWAY?

We have come to think of snoring as a normal phenomenon in our society. However, there are serious problems associated with it. Medically, the biggest danger is an association with sleep apnea, a disorder linked to cardiovascular disease. Apnea should be suspected if snoring is excessively loud or if there are gaps in breathing, says German Nino-Murcia, M.D. Other symptoms are extreme daytime sleepiness (although most snorers, not just those with apnea, are sleepier than nonsnorers during the day) and uncontrollable weight gain, says Karl Doghramji, M.D. If any of these symptoms accompanies your snoring, see a doctor without delay.

There are also serious social consequences of snoring, which should not be trivialized, according to Philip R. Westbrook, M.D., F.C.C.P. "Although snoring has been an object of derision and humor, it certainly is not very funny for the person who has to listen to it," he says. "And a lot of wives have moved out of bedrooms and houses because of snoring. People may refuse to take trips because they snore. While some of the complaints are not always justified [they may serve as an excuse for other underlying problems], snoring can be loud enough to harm the hearing."

If snoring has not improved after a month of trying these suggestions, your doctor may be able to help.

Disorders Medicine at Henry Ford Hospital in Detroit. "If you find that you are sleepy during the day, you may not be getting enough sleep." Sleep deprivation also increases the volume of the snoring, says Nino-Murcia, and may cause sleep apnea, although physicians aren't sure why. "Keeping a regular sleep-wake cycle is also helpful," Nino-Murcia says.

SEE A DOCTOR IF YOU ARE PREGNANT AND SNORING.

Sometimes, women who are pregnant will begin to snore, according to William C. Dement, M.D., a professor of psychiatry and behavioral sciences in the School of Medicine at Stanford University and director of Stanford University's Sleep Disorders Center in California. The snoring may begin because of the increased body weight and because the hormonal changes of pregnancy cause muscles to relax. Whatever the cause, snoring during pregnancy may be a sign of sleep apnea, which can decrease the oxygen supply to the fetus, Dement says. "Snoring during pregnancy is a serious problem that people haven't paid much attention to," he says. "During pregnancy, sleep is already disturbed by the need to urinate and by discomfort, which may mask other problems." So if you are pregnant and you or your partner notice that you've begun to snore, bring it to the attention of your doctor.

ELEVATE YOUR HEAD.

Sleeping with your head raised may take some of the pressure off of the airway, making breathing easier, according to Roth. "Sleep halfway sitting up," he says. "Prop yourself up with pillows."

Sore throat

10 Steps for Quick Relief

A sore throat can be a minor, but annoying, ailment, or it can be a symptom of a serious illness. Causes range from a stuffy nose or a cold to strep throat. Since untreated strep throat can lead to rheumatic fever and scarlet fever, it's important to get medical help as early as possible into the illness. Symptoms of strep throat include fever, body aches and pains, malaise, and severe sore throat. If you have these symptoms, or if you have a sore throat lasting more than two or three days, it makes good sense to see a doctor. For mild sore throats that accompany a cold or an allergy, the tips below may help ease your discomfort.

GARGLE WITH WARM SALT WATER.

"If you are a good gargler, do it with very warm, normal saline solution," says V. E. Mikkelson, M.D., a recently retired general practitioner in Hayward, California. "Use one-half teaspoon of salt to a cup of water. It is an extremely comforting fluid and won't do any harm."

GARGLE WITH LISTERINE.

Another good gargling fluid is the mouthwash Listerine, according to Robert S. Robinson, M.D., a general practitioner in Metter, Georgia. "Take it straight from the bottle [but don't share the bottle with anyone else] and do it frequently," he says.

DR. MIKKELSON'S SORE THROAT TONIC

What do good, old-fashioned general practitioners prescribe for a sore throat? Besides the tips described here, mixed with a little tincture of time, some advise special brews guaranteed to soothe both body and soul. The following is a favorite of V.E. Mikkelson, M.D.; it was extracted from a book of home remedies published more than 130 years ago. He says he's tried it and swears that it is surprisingly palatable and works wonders.

> 1 tablespoon honey, any kind
> 1 tablespoon vinegar, preferably
>   apple-cider vinegar
> 8 ounces hot water

Mix all the ingredients together in a mug and sip slowly (but don't let it get cold). Use as often as desired.

DRINK HOT LIQUIDS.

If you're not good at gargling, drink hot fluids, be they coffee, tea, or hot lemonade, Mikkelson says. "The act of swallowing will bathe most of the tissue involved with heat," he explains. "There is something almost mysterious about moist heat. I think microorganisms find it very noxious. I have seen so much benefit in applying hot packs to the skin to fight infection. The same principle holds for the inside of the throat. But since you can't put a hot pack down there, the next best thing is sloshing hot water on it frequently."

TAKE AN ANALGESIC.

Plain old aspirin, acetaminophen, or ibuprofen can do wonders for sore-throat pain, according to Stephen Kriebel, M.D., a family physician in Forks, Washington. However, aspirin should not be given to children under the age of 21 years because of the risk of Reye's syndrome, a potentially fatal condition. Pregnant and nursing women should check with their doctor before taking any medication.

REST AND TAKE IT EASY.

Common sense dictates staying in bed and resting when a sore throat's got you down. Taking it easy leaves more energy to fight the infection, Mikkelson says.

SUCK ON HARD CANDY.

"Hard candy and lozenges help the pain get better," according to Kriebel. "The sugar itself helps as much as anything. It has a soothing effect. It also helps with tickly coughs. And you don't have to go with brand names."

KEEP YOUR NASAL PASSAGES CLEAR.

Doctors agree that two of the most common causes of sore-throat pain are postnasal drip and a dry throat that results from sleeping with your mouth open when your nasal passages are blocked. Decongestants, especially those containing pseudoephedrine (read package labels), may be helpful in stopping the flow, according to Alvin J. Ciccone, M.D., F.A.A.F.P., a family physician and an associate professor in the Department of Family Medicine at Eastern Virginia Medical School in Norfolk. Kriebel recommends using a nasal saline spray. He also says that investing in a humidifier for use at night would be beneficial.

SPRAY IT.

Analgesic sprays, such as Chloraseptic, may be effective in temporarily relieving sore-throat pain, according to Kriebel. The only problem with this remedy is that the effect is not terribly long lasting. You may have to spray several times an hour. However, the sprays won't harm you and may take the edge off of an extremely painful throat.

STEAM IT OUT.

One old-fashioned remedy for a cold or sore throat is a steam tent—sitting with your face over a bowl of steaming hot water. And if you drape a towel over your head, this will serve to keep the steam in. The effectiveness of this remedy is more than an old wives' tale, according to Kriebel. "There have been a couple of scientific studies done on steaming," he says. "They show that it may shorten the length of time it takes for the infection to go away."

KEEP THE FLUIDS COMING.

Ciccone advises his patients who have a sore throat to drink as much fluid as they possibly can—at least eight to ten eight-ounce glasses per day. "Fluids lubricate the throat and prevent it from drying out," he says. They also soothe the throat and help to prevent further irritation. "They may even help to shorten the course of the illness," Ciccone says.

Stings

14 Ways to Avoid and Treat Them

You hear the buzz, you see the bee, but before you know it—zap, you're stung. Almost all of us have had this experience at least once, and it's no fun. But if you know what to do, you can take the ouch out of being stung and perhaps prevent the attack from happening in the first place.

Bees, yellow jackets, hornets, wasps, and fire ants all have stingers that inject venom into their unfortunate victim. The normal reaction is redness, pain, itching, and perhaps some swelling around the sting area, which lasts for a few hours.

For the one to two million people who are highly allergic to the venom of stinging insects, the consequences can be much worse, according to the American Academy of Allergy and Immunology. "Some may have a local allergic swelling, which is usually larger than five inches and can encompass the entire arm or leg or face," says David Golden, M.D., assistant professor of medicine at Johns Hopkins University in Baltimore and chair of the Insect Committee at the American Academy of Allergy and Immunology. This swelling isn't immediate; it develops over a 12- to 24-hour period.

The most serious allergic reactions involve the whole body. Symptoms may include hives, wheezing, difficulty in breathing, dizziness, and nausea, after which shock and unconsciousness may occur. People suffering from these types of allergic reactions need emergency medical treatment. It's estimated that fifty people die every year from anaphylactic shock brought on by insect stings.

Thankfully, for most of us, a sting is little more than a minor nuisance you can do something about.

EASING THE PAIN

Here are some simple suggestions for minimizing a sting's pain quickly and easily. Be sure to keep an eye out for signs of a more severe reaction so that medical help can be sought immediately if necessary.

APPLY UNSEASONED MEAT TENDERIZER.

"Take a teaspoonful of meat tenderizer, mix it with a few drops of water, and put it right on the sting," says Jerome Z. Litt, M.D., assistant clinical professor of dermatology at Case Western Reserve University School of Medicine in Cleveland. "You can get almost instantaneous relief." This works thanks to an enzyme in the tenderizer called papain or bromelain, which dissolves the toxins the insect has just injected into you. Litt recommends carrying a bottle with you when you know you're going to be outdoors in areas where bees are likely to be present. That's probably a good idea, because if you don't put it on fairly soon after you've been stung, it won't work. "Once the venom proteins are really into the skin, then it's too late for the meat tenderizer to reach those proteins and degrade them," says Golden.

TRY A BAKING-SODA PASTE.

If you don't happen to have any meat tenderizer, try "plan B." "Baking soda will relieve some of the itching and swelling but won't neutralize the venom," says Litt.

SCRAPE THE STINGER OUT.

Bees and some yellow jackets have barbed stingers that anchor in your skin after you're stung. (Other stinging insects have smooth stingers that remain intact on the bug.) You should get the stinger out as soon as possible, because it will continue to release venom into your skin for several minutes after the initial sting. Resist the urge to squeeze, grab, or press the stinger, however. Doing that will just make matters worse by pumping more venom into your skin. "Instead, lift the stinger up gently with a clean fingernail or knife blade," says Litt. "Then scrape gently and the stinger will come out."

PUT IT ON ICE.

Rub ice over the sting site. This may help to reduce some of the inflammation and swelling, says Litt.

TAKE AN ANTIHISTAMINE.

If the itchiness from a sting is bugging you, you might try an over-the-counter antihistamine for relief, suggests Golden.

PREVENTING FUTURE STINGS

Even better than alleviating the discomfort of a sting is preventing one from happening in the first place. Here are some things that you can do to help protect yourself from getting stung.

KEEP YOUR COOL.

If a wasp, yellow jacket, or any stinging insect flies near you, stay calm. "You should move away very slowly and don't flap, wave, or swat," says Litt. Getting agitated like that may incite the insect to sting.

UNSWEETEN YOUR SWEAT.

Ever notice how certain people just seem to attract insects more than others? "What it is that attracts those insects is not clear," says Golden, but it may have to do with the smell of a person's sweat or his or her body odor. One theory, though so far unsubstantiated, is if you can change the smell of your sweat, insects may keep their distance. "I believe eating onions and garlic or taking high doses of vitamin B sometimes can prevent insect stings," says Litt. Don't take large doses of any vitamin without your doctor's OK.

DON'T WEAR BRIGHT, FLOWERY CLOTHES OR ROUGH FABRICS.

These seem to attract insects. Stick to smooth fabric and light-colored outfits in tones of white, tan, green, or khaki when you plan to spend time outdoors.

GO FRAGRANCE FREE.

Perfumes, colognes, after-shaves, hair sprays, and scented soaps will attract insects. You may feel a bit bland without your favorite fragrance, but it may be well worth it in terms of preventing painful stings.

LEAVE BRIGHT, SHINY JEWELRY AT HOME.

"Insects find bright jewelry and other metal objects alluring," says Litt. So, make less of a fashion statement.

KEEP YOUR SHOES ON.

Walking barefoot outside may feel great, but when you're in grassy areas, it's not such a wise idea. "Bees love clover, and the yellow jackets live in the ground, so bare feet are very vulnerable to insect attacks," says Litt.

KEEP FOOD COVERED WHEN OUTSIDE.

Picnics are a summer family favorite, but open food attracts stinging insects. Keep covers on food as much as possible and keep the lids on garbage cans as well. You're best off to steer clear of public trash cans that are partially open on top.

WATCH WHAT YOU DRINK FROM.

If you're downing a cold drink outdoors, use caution. "Never drink from a soda can or anything that you can't see inside," says Golden. "There's nothing worse than getting stung on your tongue or throat."

BE AWARE OF YOUR SURROUNDINGS.

When doing yard work or gardening, be on the lookout for hives. Nests can be found in the eaves and attic of your home and in trees, vines, shrubs, wood piles, and other protected places. Disturbing a nest, even by accident, can irritate the insects. The American Academy of Allergy and Immunology suggests using extreme care when operating power lawn mowers, hedge clippers, or tractors.

Stomach upset

23 Ways to Tame Your Tummy

If your tummy is bothering you, play detective with your symptoms. It's alimentary, my dear Watson.

First question: How long has this been going on? Chronic, long-term stomach upset is something you should be discussing with your doctor. But if your temperamental tummy is something that hit you after a big meal or a party, it's likely that it's just temporary.

"We try to separate out the temporary 'I ate too much pizza' from the long-term," says Sherman Hess, B.S., R.Ph., a pharmacist in Portland, Oregon, who has guided many a gastronomically upset customer to the antacid shelf.

Temporary stomach upset may be due to indigestion or flu. Often, it's the result of something you ate. Here are some tips that can help you.

TRY SOME SODA.
Soda pop, particularly 7-Up and other noncaffeinated varieties, helps to settle stomachs, says Hess.

TAKE FRUIT JUICE FOR FLU.
If you have the flu, with diarrhea and/or vomiting, fruit juice will help resupply the potassium and other nutrients your body has lost.

DON'T COUNT ON MILK.
Douglas C. Walta, M.D., a gastroenterologist in Portland, Oregon, says milk often hinders rather than helps stomachs because some people can't digest it easily. "Milk is probably the biggest contributor to gut upset that I see in the population over 30," he says.

EASE OFF ON COFFEE.
Coffee may irritate the stomach. "It's controversial whether it's the acid or the caffeine or both," says Walta.

WHAT'S IT TO YOU?

"What you consider indigestion and what I consider indigestion is very variable," says Douglas C. Walta, M.D.

The word can be tagged to a wide range of maladies, some of them simple, some of them serious. Walta says he tells patients to drop the word "indigestion" and to just describe to him their gut feelings. Also, it's helpful to him to know if patients feel better or worse after eating. They may be describing what could be a pre-ulcer disease or a gallbladder problem. In some cases, especially in older individuals, the symptoms may be tied to a cancerous condition.

That's why Walta is concerned about attaching the label "indigestion" to too many symptoms. The rule of thumb is, if the condition persists, see a doctor.

HOLD OFF ON THE BOOZE.

Alcohol also is an irritant to the stomach lining, Walta says.

LIGHTEN UP ON PEPPER.

Red and black pepper are frequently identified as gastrointestinal irritants, says Kimra Warren, R.D., a registered dietitian at St. Vincent Hospital and Medical Center in Portland, Oregon. Try cutting back to see if your symptoms improve. If you find that they don't, then pepper isn't your problem.

DON'T SMOKE.

Walta notes that smoking is often associated with ulcers. Cigarette smoke is a gastrointestinal irritant.

WATCH YOUR DIET.

Eat foods that are easy to digest. David M. Taylor, M.D., a gastroenterologist and assistant professor of medicine at Emory University in Atlanta and the Medical College of Georgia in Augusta, says the stomach has a tough time with fatty, fried foods. "A high-carbohydrate, low-fat, high-bulk diet is the best thing," he says.

INCREASE FIBER GRADUALLY.

A high-fiber diet is good for your health, but don't go too high too fast. A gradual change of diet, with a slow but continual addition of fiber, will help to offset tolerance problems.

CHOOSE VEGGIES CAREFULLY.

You may love broccoli, but if you have a problem with gas, perhaps you should cut back, suggests Warren. Too much of certain gassy vegetables, namely broccoli, cauliflower, and brussels sprouts, can be a problem.

LIMIT PROBLEMATIC FRUITS.

Some people get tummy problems from eating apples and melon. Pay attention to whether your stomach upset followed eating one of these. If so, skip it.

WORRY ABOUT THE QUANTITY, NOT QUALITY.

Walta says it's a myth that hot, spicy foods create stomach problems. So go ahead and eat spicy food. Just don't overload your stomach.

COOK GASLESS BEANS.

Warren says if you throw out the water in which you've soaked the beans overnight, and cook them in fresh water, you'll significantly decrease their gassiness.

THINK ABOUT YOUR DIET.

Problem foods can be very individualistic. Identify the foods that you are sensitive to, then avoid them.

EXERCISE YOUR BODY.

"Exercise is very helpful," says Taylor. Even a brief walk, particularly after meals, may aid in digestion and help you feel better.

DRINK PLENTY OF WATER.

Nutritionists recommend six to eight glasses of water a day to help with digestion.

AVOID LAXATIVES.

If you have constipation, it's better to avoid laxatives, says Taylor. Instead, go the more natural route and take bran or a commercial bulking agent such as Metamucil.

LAY OFF THE ASPIRIN.

Aspirin and nonsteroidal anti-inflammatory drugs, such as ibuprofen, can actually create ulcers. "What causes ulcers to bleed is aspirin," says Walta. If you have a sensitive stomach but you need pain relief, try acetaminophen or enteric-coated aspirin.

TAKE AN ANTACID.

Antacids are very effective in soothing stomachs, but they can have side effects. For example, magnesium-based antacids can cause diarrhea, while calcium-based antacids can cause constipation. Antacids with aluminum hydroxide also can cause constipation.

SWITCH BRANDS.
Sometimes, a different brand of antacid may prove to be more effective.

DON'T TAKE AN ANTACID FOR TOO LONG.
Side effects from antacid use usually don't appear unless a person has taken the medication for several days. But if the problem has persisted that long, it's time to call the doctor.

TRY AN ANTACID IN TABLET FORM.
Hess suggests taking an antacid in tablet form because the dose is lower than in liquid preparations and therefore may not contribute to constipation or diarrhea.

RELAX.
After disease is ruled out as the cause of stomach discomfort, the underlying culprit often turns out to be stress. Stress frequently translates into physical problems. Along the gastrointestinal tract, these problems can include indigestion, irritable bowel syndrome, constipation, and diarrhea.

The cure: Unwind. Relax. Taylor says he recommends "hobbies, running or tennis or hiking or karate, or communing with nature, or sex, or whatever" when stomach troubles seem to be stress related. He says one of the most effective prescriptions is to take a trip. "They come back and say, 'Gee, doc, it's remarkable. I went away skiing and now I don't have any trouble.'"

Sunburn pain

12 Ways to Soothe the Sizzle

The sun. People have worshipped it for thousands of years. But only in the last century have people worshipped the sun by baking themselves in it to a golden tan—or, as may be more often the case, to an angry red burn. But the sun can do much more damage than simply give you a painful sunburn. Dermatologists say that prolonged exposure to sunlight causes brown spots; red, scaly spots; and drying and wrinkling. Worst of all, it can cause skin cancer.

Although few things can penetrate the skin's outer layer (stratum corneum), the sun's ultraviolet rays easily pass through this layer and damage the cells and structures beneath. Ultraviolet light comes in two varieties: ultraviolet A (UVA), the so-called "tanning rays," which do not cause sunburn (except at very high doses), and ultraviolet B (UVB), the "burning rays." UVA rays can pass through window glass in cars, houses, and offices, while UVB cannot. Both types penetrate the outer layer of the skin and cause damage.

Ultraviolet rays that pass through the stratum corneum cause pigment-producing cells called melanocytes to produce brown pigment (melanin). This is the skin's effort to protect itself from the invading rays and prevent further damage to skin structures. How much and how quickly the melanocytes can produce pigment depends largely on genetics. Dark-skinned people more readily produce melanin, while light-skinned individuals, especially those of Northern European ancestry and Orientals, don't produce it well or produce it in blotches that appear as freckles. These people can't tan no matter how hard they try and tend to be "quick fryers," readily burning even with mild sun exposure.

If your skin doesn't produce the protective melanin pigment well, or if you're overexposed to the sun before the pigment can be manufactured and dispersed, the ultraviolet rays damage the epidermal cells. "The sun's rays actually cause the skin cells to die," says James Shaw, M.D., chief of the Division of Dermatology at Good Samaritan Hospital and Medical Center and associate clinical professor of medicine at Oregon Health Sciences University, both in Portland. "Even if you develop only a mild redness, you're killing the top layer of your skin just as you would with a thermal burn from touching something hot."

Damage to skin cells is more prevalent among fair-skinned people, and the immediate effect is a sunburn. Over time, the effects can be much more serious— blotchy brown spots and even skin cancer.

Ultraviolet light can even damage the dermis, the layer of skin that gives your skin its shape, texture, strength, and elasticity. Sunlight breaks down the thick, strong tissue structure of the dermis, rendering it weak, thin, and less elastic and making it appear wrinkled and saggy.

You'd probably never expose yourself to a sunburn again if you could see the dramatic damage to your skin under a microscope—cells are shriveled and dead; formerly thick, red bundles of connective tissue have been ground into a gray smudge; thin-walled, superficial blood vessels are dilated and may be leaking fluid; and DNA sequences, which tell the skin how to repair and replicate itself, are damaged, causing it to produce precancerous cells and even cancerous cells.

Many of us ignore doom-and-gloom sun-exposure warnings. After all, that bronze tan looks wonderful. If you've overexposed your skin to the sun and end up with a sunburn, the home remedies that follow can make you feel better until Mother Nature can heal the burn. Keep in mind, though, that the remedies given here cannot reverse the damage caused by the sun's rays. "Once you've been overexposed to the sun," says Shaw, "the damage to the skin is already done. But you can make yourself more comfortable while you wait for it to get better."

APPLY COOL COMPRESSES TO THE SKIN.

Shaw advises using cool compresses to help ease the pain of a sunburn. To do this, soak a washcloth in cool water and apply it directly to burned areas. Don't use ice on the sunburned skin. Rewet the compress often and reapply it several times a day. You can also add a soothing ingredient, such as baking soda or oatmeal, to the compress water. Simply shake a bit of baking soda into the water. Or wrap dry oatmeal in a cheesecloth or a piece of gauze and run water through it. Then toss out the oatmeal, soak the compress in the oatmeal water, and apply it to the skin.

STAY OUT OF THE SUN.

Skin that is sunburned is much more vulnerable to additional burning. "Stay indoors and out of the sun for several days after getting burned," says Margaret Robertson, M.D., a dermatologist in private practice in

(Continued on page 540)

PROTECT YOURSELF

For years, we've heard doctors warn us about the drying, wrinkling, burning, and cancer-causing effects of the sun. Many of us ignore those warnings because a golden-brown tan looks great. But scientists have found the danger may be worse than they thought. Evidence suggests that a hole in the ozone layer (a layer in the atmosphere that protects us from the damaging effects of the sun) may form over the northernmost parts of the United States, Canada, Europe, and Russia within the next decade.

The Skin Cancer Foundation says one in three cancers diagnosed this year will be skin cancer. One in six Americans will develop skin cancer in his or her lifetime. And 1 in 105 people developed melanoma, the most deadly form of skin cancer, in 1991; that's more than twice as many as were diagnosed in 1980.

Fortunately, there is plenty you can do to protect your skin from the damaging effects of the sun.

Cover up. The Skin Cancer Foundation says that hats and clothing made of dark, tightly woven materials absorb ultraviolet light better than cotton fabrics in lighter shades. Dry fabrics offer more protection than wet ones.

Spread on the sunscreen. Frank Parker, M.D., says people need a sunscreen with a sun protection factor (SPF) of at least 15. "Fair-skinned people should always wear a sunscreen with an SPF of 15 to 20," he says.

If you're fair-skinned, Margaret Robertson, M.D., suggests putting an extra layer of sunscreen on the night before sun exposure, for extra absorption.

Spread it on thick, too. Applying only a thin coat of sunscreen can reduce its effectiveness by as much as 50 percent. Apply the sunscreen 15 to 30 minutes before exposure. Reapply every two hours—more often if you're sweating or getting wet.

Protect your ears. Too often, people forget to protect sensitive spots like the tops of the ears, the hairline, the "V" of the chest, the nose, and the hands. The Skin Cancer Foundation says 80 percent of skin cancers occur on the head, neck, and hands.

Be careful between 10:00 A.M. and 3:00 P.M. The sun's rays are most intense during this time of the day, says Parker. Stay indoors during this time, or if you must be outdoors, cover up and wear sunscreen.

Take care on cool, cloudy days. Ultraviolet light can penetrate cloud cover. Take precautions even when the sun isn't shining brightly. And protect yourself from rays reflected from snow, concrete, or other surfaces.

Don't forget your lips. "The lips are very vulnerable to sunlight," says James Shaw, M.D. "A lot of skin cancers occur on the lips." Use a lip balm with an SPF of at least eight and reapply often.

Avoid sunbathing. "Most Caucasians shouldn't try to get tan," says Parker. "In fact, many light-skinned people won't tan no matter how hard they try."

If you feel you must sunbathe, take it slowly and let your skin gradually build up protective melanin. Don't use tanning oils. "They enhance the ultraviolet light and can make a burn even worse," says Shaw.

Lake Oswego, Oregon. Be aware that when you're out-doors during the day, even if you're in the shade, you're being exposed to ultraviolet light. While shade from a tree or an umbrella helps, much of the sunlight your skin is exposed to comes from light reflected off surfaces such as concrete, sand, and boat decks. Ultraviolet rays can also penetrate clothing. As much as 50 percent of the sun's damaging rays can get through clothing. So if you're already sunburned, indoors is the best place for you to be.

In addition to staying out of the sun while you have a sunburn, Robertson says it's important to stay cool. A burn causes the skin's blood vessels to dilate and literally radiate heat from your skin. You'll be more comfortable if you drop the room temperature down and keep it cool inside. So turn on the air conditioner or switch on a fan.

COOL OFF WITH A SOAK.

A good way to cool the burn, says Shaw, especially if the burn is widespread, is to soak in a tub of cool water. Avoid using soap, which can irritate and dry the skin. If you feel you must use soap, use a mild one, such as Dove or Aveeno Bar, and rinse it off well. Definitely skip the washcloth and bath sponge. Afterward, pat your skin gently with a soft towel.

Robertson says she prefers cool showers to baths for treating sunburns. "If you soak too long in a tub," she explains, "you can dry out the skin and increase peel-ing."

TOSS IN SOME OATMEAL.

Frank Parker, M.D., professor and chairman of the Department of Dermatology at Oregon Health Sciences

University in Portland, likes the cool-soak idea, too, but he suggests adding skin soothers such as oatmeal or baking soda to the bath. Prepare the oatmeal like you would for an oatmeal compress—wrap the dry oatmeal in a cheesecloth or piece of gauze, run the water through it as it's coming out of the faucet, then throw out the oatmeal. Another way to do this is to buy Aveeno powder, an oatmeal powder, at your local pharmacy or health-food store; follow the package directions. If you use baking soda, sprinkle it liberally into the water. Keep the soak to 15 to 20 minutes in order to avoid overdrying the skin. When you get out, let the water dry naturally on your skin so that you don't wipe off the baking soda or oatmeal.

BRING ON THE ALOE VERA.

The thick, gel-like juice of the aloe vera plant can take the sting and redness out of a sunburn, says Shaw, especially if it's applied immediately to a new burn. "Aloe vera causes blood vessels to constrict and can take some of the redness and soreness out of your burn," he says. Aloe vera is available at nurseries in plant form. Simply slit open one of the broad leaves and apply the gel directly to the burn. Apply five to six times per day for several days.

TAKE AN OVER-THE-COUNTER PAIN RELIEVER.

Nonprescription pain relievers such as aspirin and ibuprofen can relieve pain and cut the inflammation of a sunburn, says Robertson. Take the medication with food as directed on the bottle. If you find that aspirin or ibuprofen upsets your stomach, try taking an enteric-coated form of aspirin. Another option that's easier on the stomach is acetaminophen. While it won't bring down inflammation, it will relieve pain from the sunburn.

DRINK UP.
You can easily become dehydrated when you've got a bad sunburn. Robertson says to drink plenty of fluids, especially water, like you would if you had a fever. "It's important to stay hydrated," she says. "Keep drinking until your urine is relatively clear. If your urine is cloudy, you may not be drinking enough."

TRY A TOPICAL ANESTHETIC.
Topical anesthetics like Solarcaine may offer some temporary relief from pain and itching, says Robertson. She recommends that you look for products that contain lidocaine, which is less likely than some of the other anesthetics to cause an allergic reaction. Because some people do have allergic reactions to such products, she advises testing a small area of skin before use.

Topical anesthetics come in both creams and sprays. The sprays are easier to apply to a sunburn. If you use one, avoid spraying it directly onto the face. Instead, spray some onto gauze and gently dab it on your face.

GET RELIEF WITH HYDROCORTISONE.
Over-the-counter hydrocortisone creams or sprays can bring temporary relief from sunburn pain and itching, says Parker. Look for those containing 0.5 percent or 1 percent hydrocortisone.

MOISTURIZE.
The sun dries out the skin's surface moisture and causes cells and blood vessels to leak, drying the skin out even

HELLO, DOCTOR?

While most sunburns can be effectively treated at home with the remedies described here, you should call the doctor if:

- You have extensive blistering.
- You have a total body burn.
- Your blisters break and become infected.
- You develop chills and a fever and feel shaky.
- You feel unwell, as if you have the flu.
- The pain and itching get worse after the first 24 hours.

further. In addition, while cool baths and compresses can make you feel better, they can also dry your injured skin. To prevent drying, apply moisturizer immediately after your soak, says Shaw. For even cooler relief, chill the moisturizer in the refrigerator before using.

WATCH THE BLISTERS.

If a sunburn is bad enough, the skin blisters. Robertson warns, "A bad sunburn with extensive blistering can be life threatening." If you have extensive blistering, see your doctor immediately.

If you have just a few blisters, watch that they don't become infected. Don't pop them and don't remove their protective skin covering, says Robertson.

TAKE A TINCTURE OF TIME.
Ultimately, the one thing that will heal your sunburn is time, says Robertson. No product can speed the process. Even when your sunburn is healed, be careful in the sun, because it'll take several months for your damaged skin to return to normal. If you overdo it in the sun while your skin is still healing, your skin will burn faster and be more damaged than before.

Swimmer's ear

5 Ways to Sidestep It

The water, the sun, plenty of swimming and splashing around—to many people, these are the ingredients for a perfect summer day spent by the pool or at the beach. Add a painful ear infection to the picture, and the scenario quickly slides downhill. That's what can happen to you if swimmer's ear strikes, unless you know how to prevent the problem.

Swimmer's ear, an infection of the outer ear canal, sometimes can be caused by a fungus, but common bacteria is usually the culprit. "It got the name swimmer's ear because it's quite prone to happen in the summer, when people are in the water a lot and they have water lying in the ear for a long period of time," says Donald B. Kamerer, M.D., F.A.C.S., a professor in the Department of Otolaryngology at the University of Pittsburgh School of Medicine and staff physician at the Pittsburgh Eye and Ear Hospital. Those are just the right conditions for the development of swimmer's ear, because bacteria thrive in a warm, moist environment. Also, exposure to large amounts of water tends to wash away the oily, waxy substance that normally lines and protects the ear canal. "Then the antibacterial protection is lost, bacteria begins to enter, and it can get out of hand," says Jay E. Caldwell, M.D., director of the Alaska Sports Medicine Clinic in Anchorage.

External ear infections don't just occur in swimmers or in the summertime. "We see them all year round," says Kamerer. Getting water in the ear from showers may cause them, but sometimes you don't need to be around water at all. "People who play inside their ear canals with bobby pins or all sorts of implements sometimes get infections started by scratching the very delicate skin in the ear canal," says Kamerer. Many people also use cotton swabs to clean their ears daily, which can actually hinder their efforts to keep their ears healthy. "The ear has a way of keeping itself clean," says Caldwell. "Q-tips or bobby pins or whatever you put in there just scrapes the surface and breaks down the fairly resilient barrier against bacteria."

Swimmer's ear usually starts with an itching or tingling in the ear. Resist the urge to scratch, though, which will only make the problem worse. After that, you may experience mild to severe pain. With more serious cases, discharge drains from the ear, and you may have some hearing loss from swelling of the ear canal. You should see your doctor right away if this occurs (see "Hello, Doctor?"). One way to help you determine if the infection is in the outer ear is to gently pull on your ear, wiggle it, and move it back and forth. If that hurts, it's likely to be an outer-ear infection such as swimmer's ear.

So that you won't have to suffer through this, here's what you can do to prevent swimmer's ear:

WATCH WHERE YOU SWIM.

Avoid jumping into pools, ponds, lakes, oceans, or any other body of water in which the water may not be clean. Dirty water means more bacteria.

GET THE WATER OUT.

A key to preventing swimmer's ear is to not let water sit in the ear. You can usually feel water swish around in your ear if there's still some in there after a shower or swim. "Shake the water out of your ear if you've been swimming or diving," says Alexander Schleuning, M.D., professor and chairman of the Department of Otolaryngology/Head and Neck Surgery at Oregon Health Sciences University in Portland.

ADD A FEW DROPS.

Over-the-counter antiseptic eardrops, such as Aqua Ear, Ear Magic, or Swim Ear, used after swimming may help to prevent or ease the problem for those who swim a lot and are already familiar with the symptoms of swimmer's ear. According to the Academy of Otolaryngology–Head & Neck Surgery, you can also whip up an antiseptic mixture of your own using equal amounts of rubbing alcohol and white vinegar, as long as you have normal eardrums and your doctor says it's safe (see "Hello, Doctor?"). White vinegar kills bacteria and fungus. The alcohol absorbs water and may kill bacteria and fungus as well. You can buy a dropper bottle at a pharmacy. Along the same lines, Kamerer recommends that people who swim a lot put a couple of drops of rubbing

HELLO, DOCTOR?

Mild cases of swimmer's ear may improve if you keep your ears dry and use antiseptic eardrops for a few days. But Alexander Schleuning, M.D., suggests that if you have persistent pain in your ear that lasts more than an hour or if there's discharge from the ear, you should see a physician. The Academy of Otolaryngology-Head & Neck Surgery cautions that if you have ever had a perforated, punctured, ruptured, or otherwise injured eardrum or have had ear surgery, you should consult an ear doctor before you go swimming and before you use any type of eardrops.

alcohol in their ears following swimming or drop in a mixture of half white vinegar, half water.

PULL ON A BATHING CAP.
While this may not afford much protection for a competitive swimmer who's constantly in the water, says Caldwell, it may keep water out for the casual swimmer. "If it's a tight bathing cap that fits over the ears, across the forehead, and around the back of the neck, it may help," says Kamerer.

DON'T POKE AROUND IN YOUR EARS.
"I always tell my patients not to put anything in their ear smaller than their elbow," says Caldwell. You can exac-

erbate a mild case of swimmer's ear or get an infection by poking, swabbing, or scratching inside the ear. Wax produced in the ear puts up a barrier that is antibacterial and protects against moisture. "If you undo nature's system, you set yourself up for trouble," says Kamerer.

Tartar and plaque

16 Tips to Control Them

Advertising claims have added the terms "tartar" and "plaque" to the vocabulary of the average American, as products promise to rid our mouths of these pesky substances. How true are these claims? And what roles do tartar and plaque play in our oral health?

For starters, let's define the two players. Plaque, which is actually by far the most villainous, is a soft, sticky, nearly invisible deposit that accumulates on teeth and dental restorations (fillings, crowns, and dentures, for example) and on the gums and the tongue. "It's an organized mass of oral bacteria," explains Erwin Barrington, D.D.S., professor of periodontics at the University of Illinois in Chicago. Some of those bacteria cause tooth decay, and some are responsible for periodontal, or gum, disease.

Plaque is always with us. A newborn's mouth is sterile, but only for the first ten hours or so of life, according to

Sebastian G. Ciancio, D.D.S., professor and chairman of the Department of Periodontology, clinical professor of pharmacology, and director of the Center for Clinical Dental Studies at the School of Dental Medicine at the State University of New York at Buffalo.

Tartar is a calcified material that often contains bacterial debris and sometimes plaque. It's a white, chalky substance. Although tartar (also called calculus) can make it easier for plaque to stick around, the stuff is generally considered to be primarily a cosmetic problem.

Plaque is the culprit in cavities and gum disease. "As plaque matures and gets older, it becomes even more dangerous because it changes," says Michael G. Newman, D.D.S., adjunct professor of periodontology at the University of California at Los Angeles School of Dentistry and president of the American Academy of Periodontology. As certain bacteria in plaque feed off fermentable carbohydrates (which include sugars, even those in fruit and milk, and starchy foods such as breads, pastas, and crackers), they produce an acid that eats away at tooth enamel, causing cavities. Other bacteria infect the gums, resulting in redness, inflammation, and bleeding. These are symptoms of gingivitis, the earliest stage of gum disease. If left untreated, gum disease may progress to the point that the infection literally destroys the bone that anchors the teeth roots. That's why gum disease is the major cause of tooth loss among adults over age 35.

Both plaque and tartar can form above and below the gum line. It takes a dentist or hygienist to remove tartar from anywhere in the mouth and to remove plaque from below the gum line. And regular professional cleanings—as often as your dentist recommends—will help make

THE FDA AND PLAQUE FIGHTERS

The Food and Drug Administration (FDA) has stepped into the plaque-fighting arena. In the last few years, some 40 products have claimed to reduce plaque and even treat gingivitis, the early stage of gum disease.

That has led to questions from the FDA, which convened a review panel in early 1992 to examine the safety and effectiveness of these products. An FDA spokesperson said there are no safety concerns in particular, but "there's not really a lot known about the safety and effectiveness of these products." The review should be completed in 1994 or 1995.

One reason for concern: Gingivitis, the early stage of gum disease, is not a condition that can be diagnosed by the consumer. And the use of some antibacterial products may disguise some of the obvious symptoms of gingivitis at the gum line while the disease continues to progress, says Michael G. Newman, D.D.S.

That can also result from the use of baking soda and peroxide, a mixture popularized in the early '80s as the Keyes Technique, which made dental headlines with the promise of no more periodontal surgery. Studies failed to back up those claims, but consumers still cling to the hope that they can treat their periodontal disease at home. By trying to do so, they may end up with worse problems.

"I've seen several cases where people stripped the surface of their gum tissue raw," says Newman. "They think a little's good so a lot's better."

your home care more effective, points out Christine Dumas, D.D.S., a Los Angeles dentist who is a consumer advisor and spokesperson for the American Dental Association (ADA) and an assistant professor of clinical dentistry at the University of Southern California. It's also important to have the condition of your gums checked through a periodontal probing. "It should be as routine as getting your blood pressure checked," she says.

You can, however, try to keep plaque under control. "It takes physical contact," says Barrington. "You can't rinse it away." Here's what you can do.

BRUSH.

"It's not how often but how well you brush," says Barrington. "You can brush ten times a day, but if you do a sloppy job, you're getting no benefits."

The ADA recommends the following method:

1. Hold the brush at a 45-degree angle against the gum line. "Most of us, when we brush in the morning, are worried about getting the cornflakes out from between our teeth," explains Dumas. "But we completely miss the gum line." Point the brush upward, or toward your nose, when you're cleaning the upper teeth; downward, or toward your chin, when you're doing the lower teeth.

2. Use a short (about the width of half a tooth) back-and-forth motion to clean the outer surfaces of your teeth. Focus on just one or two teeth at a time. And be gentle; you're not scrubbing the floor or the bathtub. "People try to use too much force, and that can injure the gums," says Marilyn C. Miller, D.D.S., F.A.G.D., codirector of the Princeton Dental Resource Center in New Jersey.

3. Use this same stroke on the inside surfaces of all the teeth, except the front ones. Remember to keep the brush angled (at 45 degrees) toward the gum line.

4. Scrub the chewing surfaces of your back teeth with the brush held flat in the same back-and-forth motion.

5. Tilt the brush vertically, and use the front part of the brush in short up-and-down strokes to clean the inside surfaces of the front teeth. "People tend to ignore the back sides of their front teeth," says Miller.

6. Don't forget to brush your tongue. It can harbor disease-causing plaque, too.

USE THE RIGHT TOOLS.

The ADA recommends a soft nylon brush with end-rounded, polished bristles. Hard bristles can wear away the enamel that protects your teeth and can form grooves in the teeth. Using such bristles, which Dumas calls "the Brillo pad philosophy of cleaning," can damage tender gums, too, causing them to recede, or pull away, from teeth. Get a brush that's small enough to reach all of your teeth, especially those in the back. Some adults may actually prefer using a child-sized brush. Don't be stingy with toothbrushes, either—replace your brush every three months, or sooner, if the bristles become frayed, splayed, or worn.

DON'T WORRY ABOUT GOING HI-TECH.

You can wield your old-fashioned manual toothbrush as effectively as any electric product. But if your manual dexterity's not up to par, or you're just plain lazy, one of the new electric brushes on the market may be just the product for you. "They can be a great motivator," says Dumas.

USE A FLUORIDATED TOOTHPASTE.

Choose a product with the ADA's seal of acceptance. What's so wonderful about fluoride? It combines with the minerals in saliva to "remineralize," or strengthen, the teeth, preventing cavities in both children and adults. You may think you don't get cavities anymore, but as you get older, your gums recede, exposing the roots of teeth, which lack the protective coating of enamel and are prone to a type of decay known as root caries.

TRY A TARTAR-CONTROL TOOTHPASTE.

If you're one of the people who tend to develop a lot of tartar, using such a product can help. "It doesn't stop tartar from forming, but it slows down the formation rate," points out Barrington. Chemicals such as pyrophosphate in the toothpaste interfere with the deposits of calcium salt. Ciancio says studies show up to a 30 to 40 percent reduction in the amount of tartar deposits.

FLOSS.

Too many people think of flossing simply as a way to get the roast beef or popcorn kernels out that are stuck between the teeth. "But it's really the best way to clean between the teeth and to clean under the gums," explains Miller.

Here's how to floss correctly:

1. Start with 18 to 24 inches of floss, and wind most of it around the middle or index finger on one hand (whichever finger is the most comfortable for you).

2. Wrap the rest of the floss around the same finger on the other hand. Think of this other finger as the take-up spool for the used floss. Don't scrimp. "Floss is cheap," says Miller. "And if you don't use enough, you're

THE FOODS YOU EAT

"Grazing" all day long can be cruel to your teeth. Every time you eat, you also feed the plaque in your mouth. Those bacteria like to feast on far more than the simple sugars we once learned cause cavities. They like all "fermentable carbohydrates"—that includes starches such as bread, crackers, and pasta. Natural sugars, such as honey and molasses, are tasty to the bacteria, too, as are the sugars found in fruits and even milk.

You can't stop eating these foods, but you can try to adopt some habits that are kinder and gentler to your teeth. Here's how, according to Carole Palmer, Ed.D., R.D., cochair of the Division of Nutrition and Preventive Dentistry at Tufts University School of Dental Medicine in Boston:

Limit how often you eat sugar-containing foods. "Have your cake with your meal if you brush afterward," Palmer suggests. Don't suck on hard candies all day long. "It's

just re-introducing the bacteria to another spot when you don't use a clean section of floss for each tooth."

3. Hold the floss taut with your thumbs and forefingers, leaving about an inch of floss between them.

4. Use a gentle "sawing" kind of motion as you pull the floss between the teeth. Be careful not to snap it into the tender gum tissue.

5. When you've reached the gum line, curve the floss into a "C" shape to fit snugly around the tooth, and slide it into the space between the gum and tooth gently.

really not the amount of sugar you eat but the patterns of usage."

Don't sip. "If you drink sweet drinks like soda or sugar-sweetened tea or coffee, drink it pronto—don't dillydally," she says. Using a straw may help limit the exposure to teeth.

Chew sugarless gum. Chewing the gum stimulates the flow of saliva, which helps to cleanse the mouth and protect the teeth.

Choose tooth-healthy snacks. Munch on raw vegetables, crunchy fruits like apples (which, though they contain natural sugars, are low on the list of foods that are dangerous to the teeth), plain peanuts, and cheeses. The French have the right idea, apparently, with ending a meal by eating cheese (although some varieties of cheese are high in fat and sodium). Drink plain club soda or unsweetened or artificially sweetened tea, coffee, or soda instead of sugar-containing beverages.

6. Bring the floss out from the gum and scrape the side of the tooth. "Remember, you're following the shape of the tooth to remove the plaque from that side," explains Virginia L. Woodward, R.D.H., past president of the American Dental Hygienists' Association. After you pull the floss out, be sure to use a fresh section of floss in order to clean the tooth on the other side of that space.

7. Be sure to clean the back side of the last tooth on each side.

RELAX ABOUT WAX.

Don't worry about choosing between waxed or unwaxed floss. Pick what's comfortable. Flavored flosses are fine, too, especially if you find yourself using them more frequently. If your fingers are too awkward, you suffer from arthritis, or you have a lot of bridgework, you may find floss threaders or floss holders helpful; they're available at drugstores. Ask your dentist or hygienist if you have questions about how to use these devices properly.

KNOW THAT THERE'S NO SUBSTITUTE FOR FLOSSING.

Flossing is your best bet. "Nothing can substitute for floss," says Woodward. "There's nothing available that can clean between the teeth as well." But if you absolutely, positively refuse to floss, ask your dentist or hygienist about alternatives. Barrington recommends soft wooden interproximal cleaners, like Stim-u-Dents. Interproximal brushes, which look like tiny bottle brushes, work, too, but won't always fit in tight spaces between teeth. Oral irrigators "can be a terrific adjunct," says Newman, but again, are no substitute for flossing.

Dumas warns against using Stim-u-Dents, the rubber tips on brushes, or oral irrigators until after you've brushed and flossed, because of the danger of pushing debris deeper into a pocket. "This is why it's important to know the state of your periodontal health," she stresses.

ESTABLISH A ROUTINE.

For both brushing and flossing, start at the same spot in your mouth each time and work your way around. By getting into this habit, you may be less likely to miss cleaning any tooth surfaces.

HELLO, DOCTOR?

Careful dental hygiene at home, along with regular professional cleanings and checkups, can help control tartar and plaque and prevent gum disease. In addition, you should keep an eye on the state of your mouth so that any problem that may develop can be taken care of promptly. The American Dental Association recommends calling your dentist if:

- You have persistent bad breath.
- There is pus between the teeth and gums.
- Your "bite," the way your teeth fit together, has changed.
- You have loose or separating teeth.
- Your gums consistently bleed.
- The gums at the gumline appear rolled instead of flat.
- Your partial dentures fit differently than they used to.

TEST YOURSELF.

Disclosing tablets or solution, available at drugstores, can reveal the plaque that's left after you've cleaned your mouth. "You may be aghast at what you see," warns Woodward. Don't get discouraged: "There's no way you can remove 100 percent of the plaque," says Barrington.

WET YOUR WHISTLE.

Saliva naturally cleanses the mouth and helps fight bacteria, says Irwin D. Mandel, D.D.S., professor emeritus of dentistry at Columbia University School of Dental and Oral Medicine in New York. But dry mouth is a side effect of some 300 to 400 different medications, including antidepressants, antihistamines, and drugs used to treat high blood pressure and Parkinson's disease. A disease called Sjogren's syndrome, which can accompany some rheumatoid conditions, also slows down the flow of saliva (and causes dry eyes, too). If you've had radiation therapy to the head and neck for cancer, your saliva glands may have been damaged.

You can fight dry mouth with sugarless gum or candy or with artificial saliva, available over the counter, suggests Mandel. Take frequent sips of water. Rinse with a mixture of one teaspoon of glycerine in a glass of water. Coat the lips, mouth, and tongue with mineral oil (then spit it out), especially at night when dry mouth tends to worsen.

DON'T RELY ON "MIRACLE" RINSES.

You can't rinse plaque and tartar away. The commercials on television look so appealing: A swig of this product, a few swishes in the mouth, and, like magic almost, all that nasty plaque is gone. If it were only that simple.

Only two products have the acceptance of the ADA's Council on Dental Therapeutics for reducing plaque: Peridex, available by prescription only, contains 0.12 percent chlorhexidine, a powerful germ-fighter, and over-the-counter Listerine, which relies on a combination of oils like menthol, eucalyptol, and thymol, along with alcohol. "These products are not substitutes for brushing and flossing," warns Barrington.

As for Plax, a prebrushing rinse, several studies have disputed its claims. And in 1989, the National Advertising

Division of the Council of Better Business Bureaus asked the company to discontinue its ads citing it was 300 percent more effective in removing plaque than brushing alone.

Newman looks at it another way. "Do you really want to use more chemicals in your body than you need to?" he asks, when thorough brushing and flossing can keep plaque and tartar under control for most people.

Teething

9 Tips to Ease Baby's Discomfort

Drooling. Gum inflammation. Irritation. Fussiness. Any parent who has cared for a baby knows well the symptoms of teething, the process of the first (primary) 12 teeth erupting through the surface of the gums. The teeth, which form before the baby is born, usually begin surfacing around six or seven months of age with a single lower central incisor. Most children have all of their primary teeth by age three. But, like many things in nature, teeth don't come in on a set schedule. "Parents often have the wrong idea about when their baby's teeth should come in," says Ken Waddell, D.M.D., who sees many children in his private practice in Tigard, Oregon. "The first tooth usually comes in at 6 or 7 months, but it's also normal to come in at 2 months or 12 months of age."

Although there can be a wide range of timing among children, generally, the central incisors, the teeth right in the middle of the jaw on the top and bottom, come in at 6 to 12 months; lateral incisors at 9 to 13 months; canine (cuspids) at 16 to 22 months; the first molars at 13 to 19 months; and the second molars at 25 to 33 months.

The process of teething, or "cutting" all of these baby teeth, can be painful for both the baby and the parents. When a tooth pushes through the sensitive gum mucosa, it hurts, and the baby is likely to become cranky and fussy. But each baby is individual, emphasizes Susan Woodruff, B.S.N., childbirth and parenting education coordinator at Tuality Community Hospital in Hillsboro, Oregon. "Every baby responds differently to the process of teething," she says.

Some babies seem to sail through cutting new teeth without so much as a whimper, while others are enraged and restless the entire time. How long teething lasts varies widely, too. Jack W. Clinton, D.M.D., associate dean of Patient Services at the Oregon Health Sciences University School of Dentistry in Portland, says, "Some babies can pop a new tooth through in a matter of a few hours. For others, it may take as long as a couple of days."

Teething symptoms often include crankiness, drooling, chewing, crying, gum redness, decreased appetite, and difficulty sleeping. In addition, some babies spit up and have mild diarrhea due to gastrointestinal reactions to changes in the character and amount of their own saliva. Other babies develop a red and slightly swollen rash on the cheeks, chin, neck, and chest from the saliva's contact with the skin. Sometimes, teething causes babies to develop a mild fever, congestion, and ear pulling that often mimics middle-ear infection. Relax. All of these symptoms are normal.

HELLO, DOCTOR?

Sometimes, teething symptoms can mimic other, more serious health problems. Call the doctor if the baby develops:

• A very severe rash that covers the back, arms, and legs. This may indicate a bacterial or viral infection.

• A sustained fever or pus in the eyes. The baby may have a respiratory infection.

• Fever, fussiness, vomiting/diarrhea, and pulling on or gesturing to the ear. The baby may have an ear infection.

With the helpful hints that follow, you can make your baby more comfortable during teething:

MASSAGE THOSE GUMS.
"Pressure often helps relieve the pain," says Clinton. He suggests gently rubbing baby's gums with a clean finger.

COOL IT.
Woodruff says giving the baby something cold to chew on helps soothe inflamed gums and distracts the child. She recommends a cold washcloth, chilled pacifiers, a frozen banana, or cold carrot. "Anything cold that is safe is great," says Woodruff. "Babies especially enjoy things like bananas that taste good."

Clinton suggests giving the baby an ice cube wrapped in a clean washcloth to suck on. You'll have to hold the washcloth for a very young child. Don't let the child chew directly on ice, because this can harm the gums. And, of course, keep an eye on the child at all times to make sure that he or she doesn't choke.

BABY-BOTTLE IT.

One of the tricks Woodruff teaches her new mothers is to fill a baby bottle with water or juice, tip it upside down so the liquid flows into the nipple, and freeze it. The baby then can happily chew on the bottle's frozen nipple.

LET 'EM CHEW.

"Anything the baby can chew on will help the tooth work through the gum," says Waddell. "Be imaginative and find things the baby will like." He suggests apple wedges, or for younger babies, apple wedges placed in a washcloth that the parent holds. Woodruff likes to let teething babies chew, too. She says commercial teething biscuits are good (though they can be messy), and slightly stale bagels make excellent baby chewies.

DISTRACT THEM.

Ronald Wismer, D.M.D., a general dentist in Beaverton, Oregon, says distracting teething babies may be the best solution. Try playing with them with a favorite toy or rocking or swinging them. Sometimes, a rousing game of peekaboo is all that's needed to distract baby.

TRY PAIN RELIEVERS.

Over-the-counter pain relievers like Children's Liquid Tylenol (not aspirin) can offer relief for up to four hours, says Woodruff. However, since you can't give children pain relievers around the clock, choose a time like bedtime when pain relief is most needed. Don't give more often than three times in 24 hours.

NUMB THOSE GUMS.

Commercial oral anesthetic teething gels (for example, Orajel and Anbesol) give temporary relief and can often get baby over a difficult time, Wismer says.

TRY TEETHING TABLETS.

Pharmacies carry so-called herbal "teething tablets" that dissolve almost instantly in the mouth, are safe for the baby, and provide temporary relief, says Woodruff.

KEEP A TOWEL HANDY.

Teething often causes plenty of drooling, and the saliva can cause skin irritation. Wismer advises carrying a soft towel to clean up baby often. If that isn't enough, protect the skin with petroleum jelly or zinc-oxide ointment.

Temporomandibular joint (TMJ) syndrome

6 Strategies to Ease TMJ Discomfort

If you experience headaches, bothersome clicking and popping in the jaw, or pain in the face, neck, or shoulders, the problem may literally be all in your head. You may suffer from a misalignment of the temporomandibular joint (TMJ), the joint that allows your mouth to open, close, and move sideways. The American Dental Association estimates that as many as ten million Americans may have TMJ syndrome or TMJ dysfunction. Unfortunately, it's a condition that often goes undiagnosed or misdiagnosed and untreated.

Five pairs of muscles and the temporomandibular joint that connects the upper and lower jaws allow you to open and close your mouth and control the forward, backward, and side-to-side movements of the lower jaw. Any problem that prevents this complex system of muscles, ligaments, bones, and joints from working together may result in what is known as TMJ syndrome.

The jaw joint can become misaligned from a variety of causes—teeth that don't fit together properly due to genetics, orthodontia, or tooth grinding (bruxism); habits like cradling the phone between the ear and shoulder; or injuries like whiplash or a blow to the jaw. Stress plays a major role, too, and people often experience their first TMJ discomfort during stressful times.

According to Ronald Wismer, D.M.D., former president of the Washington County Dental Association in Oregon, nearly half the patients in his Beaverton, Oregon, practice have misaligned jaw joints, but only half of those experience any symptoms. In some cases, he says, conservative home care can alleviate the pain and discomfort. In others, professional help is important.

The following are some tips for coping with your TMJ disorder. If the conservative treatments described here don't give you relief, seek help from a dentist, preferably one who is a TMJ specialist.

IS IT TMJ DISORDER?

The American Dental Association says that if you answer yes to any of the following questions, you may have a disorder of the temporomandibular joint (TMJ) and should seek help from a TMJ specialist:

• Do you have frequent headaches, especially in the morning?

• Do you clench or grind your teeth?

• Have you noticed any teeth, especially the eye teeth, wearing down?

• Do your jaw muscles feel tender?

• Does your jaw make popping or clicking sounds when you open your mouth?

• Do you ever have any difficulty trying to open your mouth?

• Do you have facial pain? Neck pain? Teeth pain? Shoulder pain?

• Is it painful or uncomfortable to chew, yawn, or open up your mouth widely?

• Does your jaw ever get stuck once you've opened or closed it?

• Do you have pain in or around the ear?

• Do your ears feel stuffy or itchy?

• Do you suffer from earaches without having ear infections?

• Do you have ringing, roaring, hissing, or buzzing in the ears?

• Do you often feel dizzy?

MASSAGE THOSE JAWS.

Ken Waddell, D.M.D., a TMJ specialist in Tigard, Oregon, recommends conservative treatment first. "Muscle spasms cause pain," he says. "To relax the muscles, try massaging the jaw joint just in front of the ears."

HEAT IT UP.

Heat is an excellent muscle relaxant, says Wismer. Use a hot pad or hot-water bottle to ease aching jaw, neck, and shoulder muscles. Keep the heat low enough not to cause burns.

COOL IT DOWN.

Ice packs are also excellent for relieving pain, says Waddell.

TAKE OVER-THE-COUNTER PAIN RELIEVERS.

Wismer says that over-the-counter products like aspirin, acetaminophen, and ibuprofen can relieve pain in the muscles. Aspirin and ibuprofen can also help bring down inflammation.

TEACH AN OLD DOG NEW TRICKS.

Become aware of and eliminate habits—such as resting your head on your hand, cradling the phone between your shoulder and cheek, or clenching your teeth—that tend to stress the jaw joint.

RELAX.

"Stress is a major player in TMJ problems," says Waddell. Gregg R. Morris, D.C., a chiropractor in private practice in Beaverton, Oregon, who has worked with TMJ patients for more than ten years, agrees. "Stress can cre-

FIND A TMJ PRO

Your TMJ symptoms may require professional help. A TMJ dental specialist may need to create a special mouthpiece, or "splint," to help the muscles relax. The jaw may need to be permanently realigned through subtle tooth grinding (equilibration), moving teeth (orthodontics), or moving bony structures (orthopedics). In a few cases, surgery may be required.

Successful treatment may also require the services of an orthopedist; a neurologist; an ear, nose, and throat specialist; and a physical therapist or chiropractor. Stress reduction may require the help of a mental-health professional. Look for professionals with whom you feel comfortable and who will take the time to explain things to you. TMJ specialist Ken Waddell, D.M.D., advises, "Look for someone who is honest and who doesn't promise you the moon." Here are some questions that you may want to ask:

• What is your experience in treating TMJ disorder?

• What special training, if any, have you received in treating TMJ disorder?

• How many TMJ patients have you treated? What is your success rate?

• How long does treatment usually last? How much does it cost?

• How do you feel about a team treatment approach? What specialists do you typically use when assembling a team?

ate a cycle of muscle tension and pain that needs to be broken." Both Waddell and Morris recommend relaxation techniques, such as progressive relaxation, in which you consciously relax muscles starting with the head and working down the body to the feet.

You might also try visualization exercises to let go of stress. Find a quiet, comfortable place where you won't be disturbed. Close your eyes and take a couple of deep breaths. Now, imagine yourself in one of your favorite places—a beach, a mountain meadow, a country lane. Let yourself feel the sights and sounds. Feel yourself relaxing in this special place. You have nothing you have to do, nowhere you have to go. After several minutes of enjoying this visualization, take a couple of deep breaths and slowly open your eyes. You may find that you feel amazingly relaxed and refreshed from this "mental vacation."

If neither of these works for you, find something that does help you relax when you feel tense.

Toothache

9 Ways to Ease the Pain

"**F**or there was never yet philosopher that could endure the toothache patiently." Shakespeare was right. The toothache isn't easy to endure. The good news: With improved dental care and regular checkups, the excruciating pain of a toothache is not as common as it once was. But when pain does occur in the mouth, it's an important signal that you should not ignore—even if it goes away on its own.

Tooth pain is varied. Perhaps most common is the minor pain caused by sensitive teeth. You eat or drink something hot, cold, or sweet and feel a momentary twinge. (See SENSITIVE TEETH for advice.) Some people suffer achy teeth because of sinus problems; that's probably the case if you notice that the pain is limited to your upper teeth and that several teeth are affected at one time. Recent dental work can cause a tooth to be sensitive to temperature changes for a few weeks.

Some types of pain deserve immediate attention from a dentist. If you feel a sharp pain when you bite down, you may have a cavity, a loose filling, a cracked tooth, or damaged pulp (the inner core of the tooth containing the blood vessels and nerves). Pain that sticks around for more than 30 minutes after eating hot or cold foods can also indicate pulp damage, either from a deep cavity or a blow to the tooth. And the stereotypical toothache with constant and severe pain, swelling, and sensitivity is definitely trouble. "If the pain wakes you up at night, it's serious," says Joseph Tenca, D.D.S., M.A., past president of the American Association of Endodontists and professor and chairman of the Department of Endodontics at Tufts University School of Dental Medicine in Boston. It may be an abscessed tooth where the pulp of the tooth has died, resulting in an infection that can spread to the gum and bone.

Pain associated with the pulp of the tooth is kind of tricky. It can let you know that damage has occurred. "But the degeneration of the nerves (in the pulp) can be very rapid," points out Alan H. Gluskin, D.D.S., associ-

TOOTHACHE MYTHS

Don't fall for these myths—you could end up causing more damage by believing in them.

Put an aspirin on the tooth. If you want to use aspirin to help relieve the pain of a toothache, swallow it with a glass of water. Do not place it on the tooth or surrounding gum. "That's a fallacy," says Joseph Tenca, D.D.S., M.A. "Aspirin does not work locally." What's worse, you may end up with a severe burn from the aspirin on your gum or cheek that can take four to five days to heal. "You're only adding to your problems," he says.

A toothache means you'll lose the tooth. Not so anymore. "Just because you have a bad toothache doesn't mean the tooth will have to be extracted," reassures Tenca. Root-canal therapy can save an abscessed tooth or one with damaged pulp. Root-canal therapy involves making a small opening in the tooth, removing the pulp in the root canal (that's where the name of the procedure comes from), filling the canal with a material called gutta percha, and then, usually, crowning the tooth. Sometimes, tiny metal posts are placed in the canal to help strengthen the tooth.

If the pain disappears, the problem's gone. "You don't have that kind of pain for no reason," says Alan H. Gluskin, D.D.S. He points out that coronary problems can cause pain in the lower jaw, while mouth pain can be referred to the ears, neck, or even shoulder. "Don't ever ignore pain in the head and neck."

ate professor and chairperson of the Department of Endodontics at the University of the Pacific School of Dentistry in San Francisco. "They can die within a 12-hour period." So the pain disappears. But the tooth hurts again as dead tissue becomes infected or abscessed.

That's why putting off dental attention for a toothache can mean bad news. But if it's 3:00 in the morning, you can take some temporary measures:

TAKE TWO ASPIRIN . . .

Or acetaminophen or ibuprofen, "whatever over-the-counter analgesic you use to relieve your headaches," says Tenca. Roland C. Duell, D.D.S., M.S., professor of endodontics with the Department of Oral Health Practice at the University of Kentucky College of Dentistry in Lexington, points out that ibuprofen is best at relieving inflammation, which may accompany a toothache.

APPLY OIL OF CLOVES.

You can pick this up at the pharmacy. Follow the directions for use, and be sure to put it only on the tooth and NOT on the gum. Otherwise, your burning gums may distract you from your toothache. And remember, oil of cloves won't cure the toothache; it just numbs the nerve.

COOL THE SWELLING.

Put a cold compress on the outside of your cheek if you've got swelling from the toothache.

CHILL THE PAIN.

Holding an ice cube or cold water in the mouth may relieve the pain, says Tenca. But if you find that it simply aggravates your sensitive tooth, skip it.

WHEN PULP GOES BAD

Most of us don't think of our teeth as being alive, but they are. Each tooth contains what's called the pulp, composed of nourishing blood vessels and nerves.

If that pulp is damaged or exposed, the nerves can die, and the tooth can become infected, or abscessed. What can cause this? A deep cavity, a cracked tooth, or a hard blow to the tooth (from biting down on a popcorn kernel, for example).

"Once the pulp has been damaged or exposed, it can't repair itself," says Roland C. Duell, D.D.S., M.S. "It will need treatment." That's why you need to pay attention to any pain you experience from your teeth.

KEEP YOUR HEAD UP.
Elevating your head can decrease the pressure in the area, says Duell.

RINSE.
You can't really rinse away the pain, but you can rinse with warm water to remove any food debris. Tenca suggests using one teaspoon of salt in a glass of warm water.

FLOSS.
No, it's not a cure, but flossing is another way to remove any food debris that could be trapped. The rubber tip on

your toothbrush or a toothpick (if used with caution) can help dislodge any stuck food. "Sometimes, food can get lodged in the gum, and the pain mimics that caused by pulpal problems," says Tenca.

BE CAREFUL WITH THE HOT, THE COLD, AND THE SWEET.

These foods and beverages may aggravate an already sore and sensitive situation.

PLUG IT.

If the tooth feels sensitive to air, cover it with gauze or even sugarless chewing gum until you can get to the dentist.

Traveler's diarrhea

20 Ways to Battle It

Montezuma's revenge, Delhi belly, Turkey trot, and Casablanca crud. Such colorful names give you a good idea of the misery to expect from traveler's diarrhea, a disease that can spoil an expensive and eagerly anticipated vacation.

It was once believed to be caused by a change in water, indulgence in spicy foods, or too much sun. Not so anymore. Researchers have found specific bacteria to blame. These bugs take up residence in the upper intestine and produce toxins that cause fluids and electrolytes (minerals like sodium and potassium that help regulate many body functions) to be secreted in a watery stool.

If you visit nearly any developing country in Latin America, Africa, or Asia, you've got a 30 to 50 percent chance of spending a few days in close contact with your bathroom. Less risky are countries such as southern Spain and Italy, Greece, Turkey, and Israel, where some 10 to 20 percent of tourists come down with traveler's diarrhea. Posing the lowest risk are Canada and northern Europe.

Your actions, however, can help influence that risk. If you really want to try food from the local street vendor or insist on drinking tap water, you're increasing your chances of coming down with traveler's diarrhea.

If you do get sick, it will probably last for two to four days, although some ten percent of cases can last for more than a week. And you may also experience—as if the diarrhea weren't enough—abdominal pain, cramps, gas, nausea, fatigue, loss of appetite, headache, vomiting, fever, and bloody stools.

Most common is watery diarrhea, sometimes accompanied by vomiting and a fever under 101 degrees Fahrenheit. If you actually get bacillary dysentery (caused by the Shigella bacteria), you'll have a fever over 101 degrees Fahrenheit, much more abdominal pain and cramping, and, often, blood in your stools, says David A. Sack, M.D., associate professor in the School of Public Health and director of the International Travel Clinic at Johns Hopkins University in Baltimore.

The following are prevention and treatment options that can help save your vacation or business trip.

PREVENTION STRATEGIES

Here's what you can do to try to prevent a case of traveler's diarrhea from spoiling your trip. "A lot of it involves using your head about your eating or drinking," says Sack.

GIVE UP ICE CUBES FOR THE DURATION.

They're made with tap water, and despite some people's beliefs, freezing will not kill the bacteria. Neither will floating those cubes in an alcoholic drink; the alcohol isn't strong enough to kill the bugs.

DRINK BOTTLED WATER.

Don't drink water delivered to your table in a glass and don't drink water straight from a tap. And if you don't like the looks of the water in the bottle, "if it looks scummy," don't drink it, advises Peter A. Banks, M.D., director of the Clinical Gastroenterology Service at Brigham and Women's Hospital in Boston.

OPEN YOUR OWN BOTTLES.

Whether it's water, a soft drink, or beer, open the bottle yourself. Otherwise, says Banks, "you don't know whether someone took an empty bottle and filled it up at the back sink." What's more, Banks adds, "Some people are not terribly clean and may rub their grimy hand or a dishtowel over the top of a bottle that's been opened to theoretically clean it."

USE CAUTION WITH OTHER BEVERAGES.

Fresh lemonade may sound appealing, but you don't know the source of the water. Boiled beverages are OK—that means tea and coffee can be safe.

WHAT IF THERE IS NO BOTTLED WATER?

If you're roughing it in the wilds of some under-developed nation, bottled or even boiled water may not be a practical option. You've got two alternatives, says David A. Sack, M.D.:

• **Purify the water.** Add iodine drops or chlorine tablets, which can be purchased at a camping-supply store in the United States before your departure.

• **Pack a water purifier.** The type with both a filter and iodine resin has been tested and shown to remove bacteria, viruses, and parasites.

KNOW YOUR DAIRY PRODUCTS.
Don't drink unpasteurized milk and dairy products.

STICK TO COOKED FOODS.
This is not the time to indulge in raw oysters. You'll have to pass on that green salad, too. Avoiding raw vegetables is one of the most important things you can do, stresses Sack.

EAT YOUR COOKED FOODS WHILE THEY'RE HOT.
If they have time to sit around and cool off, bacteria-carrying flies have time to visit your food before you even touch it.

EAT ONLY FRUITS YOU PEEL YOURSELF.

"Pass up that pretty grapefruit salad and get a grapefruit you can peel yourself," says Banks. The same advice goes for hard-boiled eggs. Sack points out that the bacteria isn't *in* the food, it's *on* the food.

TAKE YOUR OWN CARE PACKAGE.

"Bring along some granola bars, tea bags, packets of instant cocoa," says Banks. You can make your own tea, for example, if you boil the water *thoroughly*.

"You can ruin a vacation with one bad meal," Banks says. "You're entitled to be careful."

COPING TIPS

If, despite your precautions, you still get sick, take steps for diarrhea that you would at home:

BEWARE OF BECOMING DEHYDRATED.

The danger in diarrhea is in losing both fluids and electrolytes, minerals like sodium and potassium that regulate many different functions in the body.

TRY ORAL REHYDRATION THERAPY (ORT).

"You can usually buy a packet of oral rehydration solution to mix with water in a drugstore in any country except the United States," says Sack. "Mix it with the best water available, but don't worry if you have to mix it with tap water. It's important to get fluids, and besides, the horse is already out of the barn at this stage."

MAKE YOUR OWN ORT.

If you can't get to a drugstore, you can use common kitchen ingredients to make your own oral rehydration

TAKE A SUITCASE OF PEPTO-BISMOL

Researchers have found that taking Pepto-Bismol can prevent traveler's diarrhea. In fact, they managed to reduce the frequency anywhere from 23 to 61 percent.

The only problem: You've got to take a bottle of the stuff a day (that's two ounces, four times daily). And there's no guarantee you still won't be in the percentage that gets sick, points out David A. Sack, M.D.

therapy solution. Mix four tablespoons of sugar, one-half teaspoon of salt, and one-half teaspoon of baking soda in one liter of water. "Be sure to eat lots of oranges and bananas for potassium with this," points out Sack. "There's no common kitchen ingredient with potassium to include."

DRINK A COMBINATION OF FLUIDS.

Remember, the biggest danger in diarrhea is becoming dehydrated. You're also losing electrolytes, so drink a combination of liquids besides water, such as weak tea with sugar, broth, moderate amounts of fruit juices (be careful—some have a laxative effect), defizzed nondiet and noncaffeinated soda pop, or Gatorade.

SIP, DON'T GUZZLE.

Frequent small drinks are less irritating to your gut.

EAT A BLAND DIET.

Forget the enchiladas and salsa. This is the time for toast, rice, noodles, bananas, gelatin, soups, boiled potatoes, cooked carrots, and soda crackers.

PACK THE PINK STUFF.

Pepto-Bismol is definitely the first choice when it comes to treating traveler's diarrhea. "It actually has a mild antibacterial effect, so it's especially useful in traveler's diarrhea," says Rosemarie L. Fisher, M.D., professor of medicine in the Division of Digestive Diseases at Yale University School of Medicine in New Haven, Connecticut.

DON'T RELY ON OVER-THE-COUNTER MEDICINES THAT DECREASE MOTILITY.

In plain English, avoid Imodium and Kaopectate; they slow down the movement of the bowel. "That can have serious consequences, especially if you've got dysentery [signified by bloody diarrhea]," says Fisher.

BRING ALONG AN ANTIBIOTIC—JUST IN CASE.

Visit your doctor *before* you leave on vacation and get a prescription antibiotic such as doxycycline, sulfamethoxazole, or quinolones (Sack's first choice). "If you start taking it early in the disease, you'll shorten the duration [the average duration is four to five days] to one to two days," says Sack. He stresses the need to visit your doctor or a travel clinic before leaving. "I've heard too many horror stories about tourists calling the hotel doctor and what kind of remedies he's given them. It's worth the expense to see a doctor ahead of time when you've invested so much in a trip."

PREVENTIVE ANTIBIOTICS

One possibility: Take antibiotics along to take every day as a preventive measure. That's usually not recommended for most people, although there are exceptions:
• If you're over 65 or have a history of heart disease or stroke so that diarrhea could compromise your health.
• If you're a businessman on a tight schedule.
• If you're on your honeymoon. "It's just not nice to have diarrhea on your honeymoon," says David A. Sack, M.D.

Don't be alarmed if your diarrhea waits until you get home to show up. If you've picked up a parasite like giardia, its appearance may be delayed. And some travelers relax their restrictions on the plane home—forgetting the food was prepared in the country they just left.

Varicose veins

16 Coping Techniques

The circulatory system could be compared to a big city's freeways, where the bumper-to-bumper cars, in this case the frenetic blood cells, are delivering oxygen and nutrients to every part of the body. The pumping heart maintains the pulse of the "traffic" by pushing the blood cells on their way through the arteries.

On the cells' return trip to the heart and lungs, the veins have a harder time of it. For one thing, the pressure caused by the pumping heart is decreased. For another, the veins below the heart, in the legs and torso, must work against gravity, as the blood makes its way up from the feet. So these vessels depend more on the leg muscles to help pump the blood back to the heart. The veins also contain valves to help keep the blood moving along. The valves work like locks in a canal. As blood flows through a valve, its "doors" slam shut so the blood can't go backward.

When any one of these valves fails, blood can seep back and begin to pool, often in the lower legs. The extra pressure of the increased volume of pooling blood can, over time, cause subsequent valves to fail. Then the vein's walls begin to bulge and become misshapen. At this point, the vein may show through the skin surface, looking knotty and gnarled, blue and bumpy.

It's estimated that 25 percent of all women and 10 percent of all men are affected by varicose veins. Fortunately, there are ways to prevent or, at the very least, postpone, their development and decrease their severity. Here's how:

CHECK YOUR FAMILY TREE.

"The tendency to develop varicose veins can run in families," says Hugh Gelabert, M.D., assistant professor of surgery in the Section of Vascular Surgery at the University of California at Los Angeles School of

Medicine. The reason for this is unknown. Some experts believe there is a weakness in the gene that governs the development of the veins. This may lead to defects in the structure of valves and veins or, in some people, a decrease in the number of valves in the veins, causing the few that are there to get overloaded in their duties. If you do find a history of varicose veins in your family, the sooner you follow preventative measures the better.

GET MOVING.

"Exercise works by keeping the veins empty of pooling blood," says Gelabert. "Every time a muscle contracts in the buttocks, thighs, or lower legs, blood is helped on its way back to the heart." However, it's hard to say if exercise will only postpone, or if it can prevent, varicose veins. "If there's a strong family history of the condition present, then exercise will probably only postpone the condition," says Gelabert. To get your legs moving, almost any exercise that involves the legs will do, from aerobics to strengthening to spot-toning activities, say the experts. Ride a bike, take an aerobics class, go for a walk or a run, use the stair machine in the gym—these are all good exercises for the legs. Spot-toning exercises, such as leg raises, that specifically build up the muscles in the buttocks, thighs, and lower legs are also recommended.

LOSE WEIGHT.

Obesity "puts a strain on every part of the body," explains Luis Navarro, M.D., founder and director of the Vein Treatment Center in New York and author of *No More Varicose Veins*. "Furthermore, people who are overweight tend to be more immobile and get less exercise." As a result, overweight people usually have muscles that can't as efficiently help the veins pump their blood back to the heart. In addition, an overweight person's blood vessels carry more blood than a thinner person's, so the strain is greater on the vessels themselves.

EAT A BALANCED DIET.

Besides helping you to maintain proper weight, a balanced diet can give you nutrients that may actually help prevent varicose veins. Protein and vitamin C are both components of collagen, part of the tissue in the veins and valves. If the collagen is in good shape, the tissues may not fall apart as readily. However, "diet will not reverse a case of varicose veins," says Frank J. Veith, M.D., professor of surgery and chief of Vascular Surgical Services at Montefiore Medical Center–Albert Einstein College of Medicine in New York.

TAKE A BREAK FROM STANDING.

"When you're upright, the feet are the furthest possible distance away from the heart, so the blood has far to go, against gravity no less, to get back to the heart," says Gelabert. As a result, the blood can have a tendency to pool in the lower legs, leading to the development of varicose veins.

BUT DON'T SIT TOO LONG, EITHER.

Some experts theorize that even sitting can contribute to varicose veins. "They believe since the knees and groin are bent while sitting, the blood flow has a difficult course back to the heart," says Navarro. So it's very important on a long car or plane ride or during a day of sitting at the office that you get up and stretch your legs once in a while. Navarro suggests this rejuvenator: Stand on your toes and flex the heel up and down ten times.

GET SUPPORT FROM YOUR STOCKINGS.

Support panty hose is better than regular hosiery for helping to control the development of varicose veins. Better yet are the support stockings available by prescription. These stockings help by keeping the veins in the legs from bulging, and as a result, keeping fluids from collecting in the legs. How do they work? They apply more pressure to the lower legs than to the thigh area. Since more pressure is exerted on the lower legs, blood is more readily pushed up toward the heart. The stockings' compression on the legs is measured in millimeters of mercury, called mm Hg, and ranges from 20 mm Hg for milder cases to 60 mm Hg for severe varicosity. (In comparison, support panty hose from a department store has a strength of 14 mm Hg to 17 mm Hg.) The prescription stockings also come in a variety of lengths: below the knee, midthigh, full thigh, and waist high. The lower-strength stockings are sometimes recommended for pregnant women (see "Advice for Moms-to-Be"). Since the stockings are only available in a few colors, some women prefer to wear them under pants. The downside: The stockings have a tendency to feel hot.

SLIP INTO SPANDEX PANTS.

Like store-bought support panty hose, this type of stretch pant applies pressure to the legs, says Gelabert.

COVER UP THE BLUES.

If you've stopped wearing shorts or going to the beach because you're embarrassed about your varicose veins,

ADVICE FOR MOMS-TO-BE

Pregnancy can also lead to the development of varicose veins and spider veins. Surging hormones weaken collagen and connective tissues in the pelvis in preparation for giving birth. Unfortunately, as a side effect, the hormones may also weaken the collagen found in the veins and valves of the body. These weakened tissues have a more difficult time standing up to the increased blood volume that comes with carrying a baby. In addition, the weight of the fetus itself may play a role in the development of varicose veins and spider veins in the legs, says Hugh Gelabert, M.D. Elevating the legs whenever possible can be helpful, and compression stockings in the 20 mm Hg to 30 mm Hg range may be prescribed. The good news is that for many women, the swollen veins subside after the baby is born.

make them "disappear." There are products specially made to cover the blue vein lines that are causing you to take cover. Available in a variety of shades to match your skin, the cream is applied by hand and blended. Leg Magic by Covermark Cosmetics is waterproof and even has a sun protection factor (SPF) of 16 to protect your legs from the sun's harmful rays. Wearing stockings over the cover-up won't make it fade or rub off, and you can even go for a swim, says Richard Ottaviano, president of Covermark Cosmetics in Moonachie, New Jersey.

SPIDER VEINS: "COUSIN" TO VARICOSE VEINS

Eighty percent of varicose-vein sufferers will also develop spider veins, says Luis Navarro, M.D. And half of all spider-vein sufferers also have varicose veins. But unlike knotty varicose veins, spider veins are thin and weblike in appearance (thus the name) and most often show up on the legs, neck, and face. These veins are actually dilated blood vessels that appear no thicker than a thread or hair. Except for their link to pregnancy and hormones (see "Advice for Moms-to-Be"), no one knows for sure why they crop up. Because the cause hasn't been pinpointed, the veins can't be prevented. But on the plus side, they rarely cause problems—perhaps only a little itching now and again.

While these types of products obviously won't fix the veins, they may make you feel better about yourself.

CONSIDER THE EFFECTS OF ESTROGEN.
Estrogen is believed to have a detrimental effect on the collagen and connective tissue of the veins. It may also have an indirect effect on varicose veins, says Gelabert. "The Pill may lead to the development of embolisms, or clots in the blood, which can interfere with blood flow" (see "Clots: Be Careful!").

CLOTS: BE CAREFUL!

Though thankfully rare, clots can form in varicose veins. Thrombophlebitis, the inflammation of a vein caused by a clot, can be potentially dangerous if the clot begins to travel through the veins. The traveling clot, then called an embolism, can end up blocking part of the blood flow in the heart or lungs, possibly resulting in a pulmonary (lung) embolism or heart failure.

If the clot forms in what's called the superficial venous system, "you may see localized redness at the site, as well as tenderness and pain," says Alan M. Dietzek, M.D. If the clot forms in what's known as the deep venous system, you won't be able to see the clot, but you may have swelling and tenderness in all or part of either leg, he says. If you experience any of these symptoms, see your doctor.

Some of the best measures to help prevent clotting: Keep active; maintain a desirable weight; and take breaks from sitting, especially on long car and plane rides and during long hours of sitting at work.

PROP UP YOUR LEGS.

Elevating the legs is good, but raising them above your heart is even better. By doing this, you're working with gravity to help get the blood out of the ankles and back to the heart. "This is the oldest and most successful way to alleviate discomfort and facilitate drainage and reduce swelling," says Gelabert. As a matter of fact, Hippocrates in ancient Greece wrote of its benefits, he notes. Lie down on a couch and put your feet on the back of it. "If you can, elevate the legs for ten minutes every hour," recommends Alan M. Dietzek, M.D., vascular surgeon at North Shore University Hospital in Manhasset, New York, and assistant professor of surgery at Cornell Medical College in New York.

FLEX YOUR FEET.

"Flexing might help by making the muscles contract, which in turn helps squeeze the blood out of the veins," explains Gelabert. While your legs are elevated, try these three exercises to keep the blood pumping out of your feet and back to your heart:

- **The Ankle Pump:** Flex your foot up and down as you would when you pump a piano pedal or gas pedal.
- **Ankle Circles:** Rotate your feet clockwise and counterclockwise.
- **Heel Slips:** With your knees bent, slide your heels back and forth.

SLEEP WITH ELEVATED FEET.

For those with chronic swelling in the lower legs, it may help to put a few pillows under your feet while sleeping, says Gelabert.

WEAR TENNIS SHOES.

If your feet habitually swell, it may be worthwhile to wear tennis shoes or other lace-up shoes that can be opened up or loosened in order to alleviate some of the pressure.

Warts

11 Ways to Wipe Them Out

Most of us have had one of these ghastly bumps at one point or another. Warts are caused by the human papilloma virus (HPV). Because they're brought on by a virus, they are contagious. That's why an initial wart can create a host of other ones. Common warts are the rough-looking lesions most often found on the hands and fingers. The much smaller, smoother flat wart can also be found on the hand but may show up on the face, too. Warts that occur on the soles of the feet are called plantar warts and can sometimes be as large as a quarter. Genital warts, which have become a growing problem, develop in the genital and anal areas (see "Caution: Genital Warts"). If you suspect that you have a genital wart, see your doctor; do not try the remedies suggested here.

No one knows why warts occur and disappear and later recur in what appears to be a spontaneous fashion. Andrew Lazar, M.D., assistant professor of clinical dermatology at Northwestern University School of Medicine in Chicago, tells a story to typify how warts remain a medical mystery. A woman came to him about the warts on her feet. As common practice, he asked her if she was on any medications or pregnant. She said she and her husband were trying to have a baby. Soon after, the woman found out she was pregnant. After she had the baby, the warts disappeared. About two years later, the

CAUTION: GENITAL WARTS

The number of cases of genital warts is growing at a phenomenal rate, says the American Academy of Dermatology. The reason: Genital warts are extremely contagious. The usual mode of transmission is through sexual contact. It's also possible for an infected woman to pass on the virus to her fetus during pregnancy or birth.

The use of condoms can help protect against sexually transmitted diseases, including genital warts, says Joseph P. Bark, M.D. Yet, he says, many people still choose not to protect themselves. He points to "the immediacy-of-death rule" as the reason. "For instance, if someone was told that the next time they go out in the sun they would get skin cancer, they would be very careful about their exposure. The same goes for sexually transmitted diseases. Many people still believe it can't happen to them." One incentive for using protection may lie in the fact that certain strains of HPV have now been linked to cancer.

woman came back to Lazar again with warts on her feet. Later she got the news she was pregnant for the second time. A few years after that, the woman called one day and told the doctor she had warts on her feet for the third time. "Doctor," she asked, "do you think I'm pregnant?" Sure enough, she was. (Of course, not all pregnant women get warts, nor are pregnant women the only people plagued by warts.)

A medical mystery also surrounds the fact that researchers have yet to find a way to get rid of warts for good. The solution may lie in developing a wart vaccine, but an approved, safe vaccine has yet to be developed. That leaves the wart sufferer with two options: Having a dermatologist or podiatrist treat the warts or trying a few methods on their own. As for home remedies, some people swear by certain tactics, while others will never have any success with them. This has led Jerome Z. Litt, M.D., a dermatologist in private practice in Beachwood, Ohio, and an assistant clinical professor of dermatology at Case Western Reserve University School of Medicine in Cleveland, to observe: "Everything works and nothing works." And it seems that in some cases, prevention may be the best medicine. Here are some tips to help you be wart free.

MAKE SURE IT'S A WART.

First and foremost, before you try any type of treatment, know whether your skin eruption is a wart or another condition. Warts (except the small, smooth flat wart) commonly have a broken surface filled with tiny red dots. (Some people mistakenly call these dots seeds, when in reality they are the blood vessels that are supplying the wart.) Moles, on the other hand, are usually smooth, regularly shaped bumps that are not flesh-colored (as flat warts can be). Rough and tough patches with the lines of the skin running through them may be a corn or a callus. There is also a chance that the lesion could be skin cancer. You may be able to recognize skin cancer by its irregular borders and colors. When in doubt, see your doctor. In addition, if you are diabetic, do not try any home therapy for wart removal; see your doctor.

DON'T TOUCH.

The wart virus can spread from you to others, and you can also keep reinfecting yourself. The virus develops into a wart by first finding its way into a scratch in the skin's surface—a cut or a hangnail or a wound, for instance. Even the everyday task of shaving can spread the flat warts on a man's face. Inadvertently cutting a wart as you trim your cuticles can cause an infection. So keep the virus's travels to a minimum by not touching your warts at all, if possible. If you do come in contact with the lesions, wash your hands thoroughly in hot water. Children should also be told that picking or chewing their warts can cause them to spread.

STICK TO IT.

Adhesive tape has shown to be especially successful on finger warts. Litt has been using this method with success since the 1950s. Here's how he does it: Wrap the wart completely with four layers of adhesive tape. The first piece goes over the top of the finger; the second around the finger. Repeat these two steps with two more pieces of tape. Wrap the wart snugly but never too tightly. Leave the tape on for six and a half days. Then remove the tape for half a day. You may need to repeat the procedure for about three to four weeks before the wart disappears. You can try the procedure on a plantar wart, notes Litt, but use strips of tape that are long enough to properly secure the adhesive. "What's so good about this approach is that it's inexpensive and leaves no scar," says Litt.

TRY CASTOR OIL.

The acid in castor oil probably does the trick by irritating the wart. The oil treatment works best on small, flat warts on the face and on the back of the hands, says Litt. He recommends applying the castor oil to the wart with a cotton swab twice a day.

"C" WHAT YOU CAN DO.

Vitamin C is mildly acidic, so it may irritate the wart enough to make it go away, says Litt. Apply a paste made of crushed vitamin C tablets and water. Apply the paste only to the wart, not to the surrounding skin. Then cover the paste with gauze and tape.

HEAT IT UP.

One study found that having patients soak their plantar warts in very hot water was helpful because it softens the wart and may kill the virus. Make sure the water is not too hot, cautions Litt, or you may burn yourself.

TAKE PRECAUTIONS WITH OVER-THE-COUNTER PREPARATIONS.

The Food and Drug Administration (FDA) recently approved wart-removal medications made with 26 percent salicylic acid, reports Litt. Typically, remedies have contained about 16 percent. While the stronger formulas may work well for adults (except for those who have sensitive skin), Litt does not suggest using them on children. Salicylic acid works because it's an irritant, so no matter which strength of solution you use, try to keep it from irritating the surrounding skin. If you're using a liquid medication, do this by smearing a ring of petroleum jelly around the wart before using the medication.

If you're applying a medicated wart pad or patch, cut it to only the size of the wart. Litt suggests applying over-the-counter medications at night and then leaving the area uncovered.

CHALK IT UP TO THE POWER OF SUGGESTION.

Some physicians use this technique on children, who are still impressionable. The doctor tells the child that if the doctor rubs chalk on the child's warts, they will disap-

CAN YOU WISH YOUR WARTS AWAY?

Some dermatologists agree that the power of suggestion, especially when used on children, can be very effective in making warts disappear. It may be that the warts were about to vanish anyway (children's warts usually disappear more quickly than warts in adults), or perhaps positive thoughts boost the immune system. No one knows for sure.

Taking the power of suggestion one step further, there have been studies of the use of hypnosis in the treatment of warts. At the mention of the word hypnosis, many people conjure up images of a magician gently swaying a crystal bauble in the face of an unwilling suspect who, unbeknownst to him, is about to cluck like a chicken. Unlike popular myth, hypnosis can't make you do something you don't want to do. Today, it's an acceptable way to quit smoking and can be used as an adjunct to losing weight.

pear. There are variations on this, including: Coloring the warts with crayon or drawing a picture of a child's hand with the warts crossed out and throwing the picture in the garbage (see "Can You Wish Your Warts Away?").

DON'T GO BAREFOOT.

"Millions of virus particles leak out of a wart," says Joseph P. Bark, M.D., chairman of dermatology at St.

Owen S. Surman, M.D., C.M., F.A.P.A., associate professor of psychiatry at Massachusetts General Hospital in Boston, used hypnosis to see if it would make warts go away. His study was done on 17 people who were treated with hypnosis once a week for five weeks. Seven other patients were not treated with hypnosis. Both groups were asked to abstain from any wart treatment, including home remedies. The patients who underwent hypnosis were told that they would experience a tingling sensation in the warts on one side of their body and only those warts would disappear. Nine patients lost more than three-quarters of all their warts, and four of them lost all the warts on both sides of their body. Meanwhile, the untreated group showed no improvement. Surman can only speculate on why the hypnosis may have worked. "Perhaps, a belief in the power of suggestion enhanced the activity of the body's T-cells, which combat viruses."

Joseph Hospital in Lexington, Kentucky. That fact puts people in public places at high risk for plantar, or foot, warts. The best protection: footwear. Locker rooms, pools, showers in fitness centers, even the carpets in hotel rooms harbor a host of viruses—not just wart viruses. You can catch any of a number of infections, from scabies to herpes simplex, says Bark. Never go barefoot, and at least, wear a pair of flip-flops, or thongs.

KEEP DRY.
Warts, especially plantar warts, tend to flourish in an environment that's damp. That's why people who walk or exercise extensively may be more prone to foot warts, says the American Academy of Dermatology in Schaumburg, Illinois. So change your socks any time your feet get sweaty, and use a medicated foot powder.

COVER YOUR CUTS AND SCRAPES.
The wart virus loves finding a good scratch so it can make its way under your skin. By keeping your cuts and scrapes covered, you'll be helping to keep out the wart virus.

Yeast infections
12 Strategies to Beat Them

M ost women are bothered at one time or another by the itching, burning, pain, and discharge that comes with a vaginal infection. Yeast infections can be caused by a number of organisms, many of which inhabit the healthy vagina. One of the most common causes of vaginitis is the fungus *Candida albicans*.

"Yeast infections are characterized by itching, caked discharge that smells like baking bread, and reddening of the labia and sometimes upper thighs," says Felicia Stewart, M.D., a gynecologist in Sacramento, California.

Yeast infections, especially recurrent ones, are a signal that your body is out of balance. *Candida* normally grows in a healthy vagina, but the slightly acid pH environment keeps *Candida* and other microorganisms from multiplying rapidly enough to cause infection. However, a variety of factors can make the body go "tilt" and alter the vaginal pH enough to allow one or more microorganisms to grow unchecked. The itching, burning, pain, and discharge are caused by the waste products of rapidly multiplying *Candida* (or other) organisms.

There are plenty of things that can throw your body out of balance. Many women find they are more vulnerable to yeast infection under these conditions:

• **Pregnancy.** The hormonal changes associated with pregnancy alter the vaginal pH and increase carbohydrate (glycogen) production, which provides food for infectious organisms.

• **Menstruation.** Some women report more yeast flareups just before or just after their menstrual period.

• **Antibiotics.** *Candida* live in the healthy vagina in balance with other microorganisms, especially lactobacilli. Tetracycline, ampicillin, and other antibiotics kill the vagina's lactobacilli and allow *Candida* to multiply, says Sadja Greenwood, M.D., assistant clinical professor in the Department of Obstetrics, Gynecology, and Reproductive Sciences at the University of California at San

Francisco. Some antibiotics, especially tetracycline, also appear to stimulate the growth of yeast organisms.

• **Diabetes or a high-sugar diet.** High blood sugar caused by diabetes or by a high-sugar diet can change vaginal pH and contribute to yeast infections. "Some women," says Stewart, "drink lots of fruit juice to prevent bladder infections. But fruit juice contains so much sugar, it may promote yeast infections."

• **Stressful times.** Doctors don't fully understand the stress/yeast connection, but many women report an increase in yeast infections during times of high stress.

While yeast infections can often be treated successfully at home, be sure yeast is the culprit. Other organisms, which require medical treatment, may be causing your symptoms. If the discharge is foul-smelling, yellowish, and frothy, you may be infected by one-celled protozoans called *trichomonas* or "trick." If you have a heavy discharge without much irritation and notice a fishy odor, particularly after intercourse, your symptoms may be caused by a bacterial infection doctors call "bacterial vaginosis." Bacterial infections are the most common cause of vaginitis. Both of these infections require treatment with prescription medication. In addition, symptoms similar to those of vaginitis may be caused by sexually transmitted diseases such as gonorrhea or chlamydia. *It's important to have your vaginal symptoms evaluated by a physician to ensure proper treatment.*

Many women who suffer from recurrent yeast infections have had their symptoms diagnosed by a doctor and know all too well the signs and symptoms of a yeast flare-up. If you're sure your vaginitis is caused by a yeast infection, try these home remedies:

HELLO, DOCTOR?

While mild cases of yeast infection can be effectively treated at home, Sadja Greenwood, M.D., says it's important to see a physician if:

• You have abdominal pain.

• You have recurrent or significant amounts of bloody discharge between periods.

• The discharge gets worse or persists for two weeks or more despite treatment.

• You may have been exposed to a sexually transmitted disease.

• You have recurrent yeast infections. You may have diabetes or a prediabetic condition that is contributing to your yeast infections.

• Your discharge is thin, foamy, and grey or yellowish green in color.

USE A VINEGAR DOUCHE.

At the first sign of infection, try douching with a mild vinegar douche, suggests Stewart. Use one to three tablespoons of white vinegar to one quart of warm water (see "Self-Care Douche").

BRING ON THE BORIC.

Several studies have shown boric acid to be a safe, inexpensive, and effective yeast remedy. Amanda Clark,

M.D., assistant professor of obstetrics and gynecology at Oregon Health Sciences University in Portland, suggests using boric-acid capsules as a suppository. "You can't buy the capsules already made up," she says. "Buy size 'O' gelatin capsules and fill them with boric acid. Then insert one per day vaginally for seven days." (Check with your pharmacist for the gelatin capsules and boric acid.)

Boric acid hasn't been studied among pregnant women. If you're pregnant, Clark says to skip the boric acid. Instead, talk with your physician about other treatment options.

USE AN OVER-THE-COUNTER ANTIFUNGAL.

Stewart says both miconazole (Monistat) and clotrimazole (Gyne-Lotrimin) are effective in treating yeast infections. They've recently become available in pharmacies without prescription. Use the suppositories nightly for three days or the cream once daily for one week. Don't stop using the medication when your symptoms subside. Use it for the full course. If recurrent yeast infections are a problem, try using one of these antifungal creams a few days before and/or after your menstrual period.

TRY YOGURT TABS.

"Some women find relief using Lactinex (lactobacillus) tablets vaginally once or twice a day and douching with vinegar twice a day for two days," says Greenwood.

WASH OUT THE SECRETIONS.

The organisms that cause yeast infection produce secretions that are irritating to the genital tissues, says

SELF-CARE DOUCHE

Routine douching isn't a good idea if you don't have vaginal symptoms. However, for women who are experiencing yeast-infection symptoms, a mild vinegar douche can help restore the vagina's normal pH (which is about 4.5). Douching with yogurt that contains live lactobacillus or acidophilus bacteria may help restore the friendly microorganisms lost during infection or because of the use of an antibiotic medication. For the best douche results, follow these easy steps:

1. Prepare the douche solution as outlined in the first remedy.

2. Make sure the container, tube, and irrigation nozzle are very clean. If not, clean them with a good antiseptic solution.

3. Lie in the tub with a folded towel under your buttocks and with your legs parted.

4. Suspend the container 12 to 18 inches above the hips.

5. Insert the nozzle into the vagina with a gentle rotating motion until it encounters resistance (approximately two to four inches).

6. Allow the douching solution to flow in slowly. Use your fingers to close the vaginal lips until a little pressure builds up inside. This allows the solution to reach the entire internal surface. An effective douche should take about ten minutes or so.

Clark. The nerve endings that sense the presence of the yeast are located at the vaginal opening. Although you may have an infection inside the vagina, you can often get symptomatic relief, she says, by simply washing away the secretions with water or with a douche.

STAY DRY AND LOOSE.

Yeast organisms like warm, moist conditions, where there is little or no oxygen. In order to deny them the perfect growing medium, be careful to dry your vaginal area thoroughly after bathing or showering. Avoid wearing tight, restrictive clothing that can hold in heat and moisture, and avoid lounging around in a wet bathing suit for long periods of time. Opt for loose clothing and "breathable" cotton underwear and, if you must wear nylons, wear the type that has a cotton-lined panty or cotton-lined crotch.

AVOID HARSH SOAPS, "FEMININE HYGIENE" SPRAYS, AND PERFUMED PRODUCTS.

"Harsh soaps and hygiene sprays irritate the vagina and throw off its natural balance," says Susan Woodruff, B.S.N., childbirth and parenting education coordinator for Tuality Community Hospital in Hillsboro, Oregon. "Perfumed products contain alcohol that is drying to the tissues and hundreds of other chemicals that can cause irritation."

RETHINK YOUR CONTRACEPTION.

Women who take birth control pills or use contraceptive sponges appear to be at greater risk for developing yeast infections. While researchers haven't established a cause-and-effect relationship between the Pill and yeast, some studies have shown that oral contraceptives increase the glycogen in the vagina (which provides more food for yeast reproduction).

Contraceptive sponges seem to be a yeast culprit, too. "We don't know exactly why contraceptive sponges increase yeast infections," says Stewart, "but we know they alter the vagina's normal ecology." If recurrent yeast infections are a problem for you, Stewart suggests considering an alternative birth control method like condoms, a diaphragm, a cervical cap, or an intrauterine device (IUD).

HAVE BOTH PARTNERS TREATED.

Sexual partners can play "Ping-Pong" with yeast infections by passing the infection back and forth unless both partners are treated. Often, men harbor yeast organisms, especially in the foreskin of an uncircumcised penis, but show no symptoms. When one partner is treated, the other should be treated to avoid reinfection, advises Woodruff.

WASH UP AND USE CONDOMS.

Women with yeast infections should ask their lovers to wash up extra carefully before lovemaking. Couples who make love before the infection is completely cured should use condoms during intercourse.

AVOID ROUTINE DOUCHING.

"The American culture is into cleansing," says Woodruff. "But the vagina doesn't need to be cleaned. It does that naturally. Routine douching upsets the vaginal pH and can actually cause yeast infections" (see "Douche Danger").

DOUCHE DANGER

The ads for douches admonish women to "feel fresh." And some women erroneously believe that douching after intercourse will prevent pregnancy (it doesn't). But new evidence shows that routine douching may be too much of a good thing and may actually do more harm than good.

Routine douching has been associated with an increased risk of pelvic inflammatory disease," says Felicia Stewart, M.D. "I don't recommend it."

Pelvic inflammatory disease, or PID, is an infection of the uterus, fallopian tubes, or ovaries. It can cause scarring of the fallopian tubes and result in infertility. If the infection spreads to the circulatory system, it can cause death.

According to a 1990 study in **The Journal of the American Medical Association**, women who douched three or more times per month were three-and-a-half times more likely to have PID than women who douched less than once a month.

PRACTICE GOOD HYGIENE.

While yeast is usually passed between sexual partners, Woodruff says it can also be passed to others like children through activities such as shared baths. To ensure you're not passing yeast, she recommends not bathing or sharing towels with your children, washing your hands frequently with soap and water, and washing your clothing in hot water. "The hot water in your washing ma-

The symptoms of PID include fever, chills, lower abdominal pain or tenderness, back pain, spotting, pain during or after intercourse, and puslike vaginal discharge. In most cases, a woman does not show all of the symptoms listed. If you have any PID symptoms, consult a physician immediately.

Not only has routine douching been associated with an increased risk of PID, some researchers believe it may increase a woman's risk of developing cervical cancer. A study that appeared in **The American Journal of Epidemiology** showed that women who douched more than once a week were nearly five times as likely to develop cervical cancer as women who douched less often. The researchers suspect that vaginal secretions and normal vaginal bacteria may somehow protect the pelvic area and that routine douching may invite microbes that trigger cancer.

The message is clear: While an occasional douche during an infection might be a good idea, don't make a habit of douching.

chine should kill the yeast organisms present in your clothes," says Woodruff. "But if you're really worried about it, toss a cup of white vinegar into your rinse water."

MEDICAL AND TECHNICAL ADVISORS

Sabiha Ali, M.D. Neurologist, Houston Headache Clinic, Houston, Texas **David Alpers, M.D.** Professor of Medicine and Chief of the Gastroenterology Division, Washington University School of Medicine, St. Louis, Missouri **Philip C. Anderson, M.D.** Chairman of Dermatology, University of Missouri–Columbia School of Medicine, Columbia, Missouri **Covert Bailey** Fitness/Weight Expert; Author, *Fit or Fat* and *The New Fit or Fat* **Diane Baker, M.D.** Clinical Professor of Dermatology, Oregon Health Sciences University, Portland, Oregon; Advisor, National Psoriasis Foundation **Peter A. Banks, M.D.** Director, Clinical Gastroenterology Service, Brigham and Women's Hospital; Lecturer on Medicine, Harvard Medical School, Boston, Massachusetts **Joseph P. Bark, M.D.** Chairman of Dermatology, St. Joseph Hospital, Lexington, Kentucky; Author, *Retin-A and Other Youth Miracles* and *Skin Secrets* **Andrew Baron, D.D.S.** Clinical Associate Professor, Lenox Hill Hospital, New York, New York **Ronald G. Barr, M.D.C.M.** Associate Professor of Pediatrics and Psychiatry, McGill University; Director of the Child Development Program, Montreal Children's Hospital, Montreal, Quebec, Canada **Erwin Barrington, D.D.S.** Professor of Periodontics, University of Illinois in Chicago, Chicago, Illinois **Rodney Basler, M.D.** Chairman, Task Force on Sports Medicine, American Academy of Dermatology; Assistant Professor of Internal Medicine, University of Nebraska Medical Center, Omaha, Nebraska **Evan T. Bell, M.D.** Specialist in Infectious Diseases, Lenox Hill Hospital, New York, New York **Loomis Bell, M.D.** Chief, Pulmonary–Critical Care Medicine, St. Luke's–Roosevelt Hospital Center; Clinical

Professor of Medicine, Columbia University College of Physicians and Surgeons, New York, New York **Richard Bennett, M.D.** Assistant Professor of Medicine, Johns Hopkins School of Medicine, Baltimore, Maryland **Michael S. Benninger, M.D.** Chairman, Speech, Voice, and Swallowing Disorders Committee, American Academy of Otolaryngology–Head and Neck Surgery; Vice-Chairperson, Department of Otolaryngology, Henry Ford Hospital, Detroit, Michigan **Wilma Bergfeld, M.D., F.A.C.P.** Head, Clinical Research, Department of Dermatology, Cleveland Clinic Foundation, Cleveland, Ohio **Cheston M. Berlin, Jr., M.D.** Professor of Pediatrics and Professor of Pharmacology, Pennsylvania State University College of Medicine, Milton S. Hershey Medical Center, Hershey, Pennsylvania **Lawrence H. Bernstein, M.D.** Family Physician, Storrs, Connecticut **Henry J. Bienert, Jr., M.D.** Orthopedic Surgeon, Tulane University School of Medicine, New Orleans, Louisiana **Henry Blackburn, M.D.** Mayo Professor of Public Health and Professor of Medicine, University of Minnesota, Minneapolis, Minnesota **Zachary T. Bloomgarden, M.D.** Assistant Clinical Professor of Medicine, Mount Sinai School of Medicine, New York, New York **Larry Borish, M.D.** Staff Physician, National Jewish Center for Immunology and Respiratory Medicine, Denver, Colorado **Jon H. Bosland, M.D.** General Ophthalmologist, Bellevue, Washington **Charles Boylan, M.D.** Specialist in Pediatric Ophthalmology, A Children's Eye Clinic, Seattle, Washington **Richard C. Bozian, M.D.** Director of Research, Monarch Foundation, Cincinnati, Ohio; Professor of Medicine, Assistant Professor of Biochemistry, Director, Division of Nutrition, University of Cincinnati, Cincinnati, Ohio **Earl J. Brewer, Jr., M.D.** Former Head, Rheumatology Division, Texas Children's Hospital, Houston, Texas; Former Clinical Professor, Former Head, Rheumatology Division, Department of Pediatrics, Baylor College of Medicine; Author, *Parenting a Child with Arthritis* **James E. Bridges, M.D.** Family Physician, Fremont, Nebraska **Vera Brown** Skin-Care Expert; Author, *Vera*

Clark, M.D. Assistant Professor of Obstetrics and Gynecology, Oregon Health Sciences University, Portland, Oregon **Jack W. Clinton, D.M.D.** Associate Dean of Patient Services, Oregon Health Sciences University School of Dentistry, Portland, Oregon **Peter F. Cohn, M.D.** Chief of Cardiology, State University of New York at Stony Brook Health Sciences Center, Stony Brook, New York **Cheryl Coleman, R.N., B.S.N., I.C.C.E.** Director, Public Relations, International Childbirth Education Association; Childbirth Educator, Hillcrest Medical Center, Tulsa, Oklahoma **Sonja Connor, M.S., R.D.** Coauthor, *The New American Diet*; Research Associate Professor, School of Medicine, Oregon Health Sciences University, Portland, Oregon **Paul Contorer, M.D.** Chief of Dermatology, Kaiser Permanente; Clinical Professor of Dermatology, Oregon Health Sciences University, Portland, Oregon **James R. Couch, Jr., M.D., Ph.D.** Professor and Chairman, Department of Neurology, University of Oklahoma Health Sciences Center, Oklahoma City, Oklahoma **Donald R. Coustan, M.D.** Professor and Chair, Obstetrics and Gynecology, Brown University School of Medicine; Chief, Obstetrics and Gynecology, Women and Infants Hospital of Rhode Island, Providence, Rhode Island **Mick Crowley, R.N., B.S.N.** Department Manager, Burn Care Center/Neurosurgical Unit, University of Missouri Hospital and Clinics, Columbia, Missouri **Jeffrey A. Cutler, M.D.** Hypertension Specialist and Chief, Prevention and Demonstration Research Branch, National Heart, Lung, and Blood Institute, National Institutes of Health, Bethesda, Maryland **Joseph C. D'Amico, D.P.M.** Podiatrist, New York, New York **C. Ralph Daniel III, M.D.** Clinical Professor of Medicine (Dermatology), University of Mississippi Medical Center, Jackson, Mississippi **John Staige Davis IV, M.D.** Margaret Trolinger Professor of Medicine, University of Virginia School of Medicine, Charlottesville, Virginia **Vincent A. DeLeo, M.D.** Assistant Professor of Dermatology, Columbia–Presbyterian Medical Center, New York, New York **William C. Dement, M.D., Ph.D.**

Medical Center, New York, New York **Rosemarie L. Fisher, M.D.** Professor of Medicine, Division of Digestive Diseases, Yale University School of Medicine, New Haven, Connecticut **Michael O. Fleming, M.D., F.A.A.F.P.** Family Physician, Shreveport, Louisiana **Sharon Fleming, Ph.D.** Associate Professor of Food Science, Department of Nutritional Sciences, University of California at Berkeley, Berkeley, California **Patricia Fosarelli, M.D.** Assistant Professor of Pediatrics, Johns Hopkins School of Medicine, Baltimore, Maryland **Raven Fox, R.N., I.B.C.L.C.** Registered Nurse and Lactation Consultant, Evergreen Hospital Medical Center, Kirkland, Washington **Phyllis Frey, A.R.N.P.** Nurse Practitioner, Bellevue, Washington **Lawrence S. Friedman, M.D.** Associate Professor of Medicine, Jefferson Medical College, Thomas Jefferson University, Philadelphia, Pennsylvania **Clifton T. Furukawa, M.D.** Past Chairman, Professional Education Council, American Academy of Allergy and Immunology; Clinical Professor of Pediatrics, University of Washington School of Medicine, Seattle, Washington **Kathleen Galligan, D.C.** Chiropractor, Lake Oswego, Oregon **Glenn B. Gastwirth, D.P.M.** Deputy Executive Director, American Podiatric Medical Association, Bethesda, Maryland **Hugh Gelabert, M.D.** Assistant Professor of Surgery, Section of Vascular Surgery, University of California at Los Angeles School of Medicine, Los Angeles, California **Ruby Ghadially, M.D.** Assistant Clinical Professor, Department of Dermatology, University of California at San Francisco, San Francisco, California **David N. Gilbert, M.D.** Director, Chiles Research Institute; Director, Department of Medical Education, Providence Medical Center, Portland, Oregon **J. Christian Gillin, M.D.** Professor of Psychiatry, Director, Mental Health Clinical Research Center, University of California at San Diego; Staff Psychiatrist, Veterans Administration Medical Center; Adjunct Professor in the Department of Psychology, San Diego State University, San Diego, California **Donald Girard, M.D.** Head, Division of General Internal Medicine,

Oregon Health Sciences University, Portland, Oregon **W. Paul Glezen, M.D.** Pediatrician, Influenza Research Center, Professor of Microbiology and Immunology, Professor of Pediatrics, Chief Epidemiologist, Baylor College of Medicine, Houston, Texas **Billy Glisan, M.S.** Director, Injury Prevention Program, Texas Back Institute, Dallas, Texas **Alan H. Gluskin, D.D.S.** Associate Professor and Chairperson, Department of Endodontics, University of the Pacific School of Dentistry, San Francisco, California **David Golden, M.D.** Chair, Insect Committee, American Academy of Allergy and Immunology; Assistant Professor of Medicine, Johns Hopkins University, Baltimore, Maryland **Howard Goldin, M.D.** Clinical Professor of Medicine, The New York Hospital–Cornell Medical Center, New York, New York **Arthur I. Grayzel, M.D.** Senior Vice-President for Medical Affairs, Arthritis Foundation, Atlanta, Georgia **Sadja Greenwood, M.D.** Assistant Clinical Professor, Department of Obstetrics, Gynecology, and Reproductive Sciences, University of California at San Francisco, San Francisco, California **Fredric Haberman, M.D.** Author, *The Doctor's Beauty Hotline* and *Your Skin: A Dermatologist's Guide to a Lifetime of Beauty and Health*; Teaching Faculty, Montefiore Medical Center–Albert Einstein School of Medicine, New York, New York **Jon M. Hanifin, M.D.** Professor of Dermatology, Oregon Health Sciences University; Board Member, Eczema Association for Science and Education, Portland, Oregon **Terry L. Hankey, M.D.** Clinical Associate Professor of Family Practice, University of Wisconsin School of Medicine, Madison, Wisconsin **Richard E. Hannigan, M.D.** Specialist in Internal Medicine, Helotes, Texas **Peter Hauri, Ph.D.** Author, *No More Sleepless Nights*; Professor of Psychology, Director, Mayo Clinic Insomnia Program, Rochester, Minnesota **Gregory F. Hayden, M.D.** Professor of Pediatrics, Attending Pediatrician, University of Virginia Health Sciences Center, Charlottesville, Virginia **Sandra Hazard, D.M.D.** Managing Dentist, Willamette Dental Group, Inc., Oregon **Robert P. Heaney, M.D.** John A.

Creighton University Professor, Creighton University, Omaha, Nebraska **James A. Hearn, M.D.** Assistant Professor of Medicine, University of Alabama at Birmingham, Birmingham, Alabama **Michael J. Henehan, D.O.** Director of the Sports Medicine Department, Stanford/San Jose Family Practice Residency Program, San Jose, California **Mindy Hermann, R.D.** Spokesperson for the American Dietetic Association **Sherman Hess, B.S., R.Ph.** Registered Pharmacist and Manager, Hillsdale Pharmacy, Portland, Oregon **John W. House, M.D.** Associate Clinical Professor, Department of Otolaryngology, Head and Neck Surgery, University of Southern California at Los Angeles; President, House Ear Institute; Otologist–Neurotologist, House Ear Clinic, Los Angeles, California **Ellen Nona Hoyven, P.T.** Owner and Director, Ortho Sport Physical Therapy P.C., Clackamas, Oregon **Rose Hust** Osteoporosis Coordinator, Knoxville Orthopedic Clinic, Knoxville, Tennessee **Pascal James Imperato, M.D.** Professor and Chairman, Department of Preventive Medicine and Community Health, State University of New York Health Science Center, Brooklyn, New York **Janna Jacobs, P.T., C.H.T.** President, Section on Hand Rehabilitation, American Physical Therapy Association (APTA) **Katherine Jeter, Ed.D., E.T.** Executive Director, Help for Incontinent People (HIP), Union, South Carolina **John C. Johnson, M.D.** Past President, American College of Emergency Physicians; Director, Emergency Department, Porter Memorial Hospital, Valparaiso, Indiana **Lanny L. Johnson, M.D.** Clinical Professor of Surgery, Michigan State University, East Lansing, Michigan **Conrad Johnston, M.D.** Chief, Division of Endocrinology and Metabolism, Indiana University School of Medicine, Indianapolis, Indiana **James F. Jones, M.D.** Professor of Pediatric Medicine, University of Colorado School of Medicine; Staff Member, National Jewish Center for Immunology and Respiratory Medicine, Denver, Colorado **Stephen R. Jones, M.D.** Chief of Medicine, Good Samaritan Hospital and Medical Center; Associate Professor of Medicine, Oregon Health

Sciences University, Portland, Oregon **Judy Jordan, M.D.** Spokesperson, American Academy of Dermatology; Dermatologist, San Antonio, Texas **Donald B. Kamerer, M.D., F.A.C.S.** Professor, Department of Otolaryngology, University of Pittsburgh School of Medicine; Staff Physician, Pittsburgh Eye and Ear Hospital, Pittsburgh, Pennsylvania **Chrissy Kane, L.P.T.** Physical Therapist, Outpatient Physical Therapy Department, Providence Medical Center, Portland, Oregon **Marcia Kielhofner, M.D.** Clinical Assistant Professor of Medicine, Baylor College of Medicine, Houston **Alan D. Klein, M.D.** Spokesperson, American Academy of Dermatology; Teaching Staff, Ventura County Medical Center, Ventura, California **Albert M. Kligman, M.D., Ph.D.** Emeritus Professor of Dermatology, University of Pennsylvania School of Medicine, Philadelphia, Pennsylvania **Matthew J. Kluger, Ph.D.** Professor of Physiology, University of Michigan Medical School, Ann Arbor, Michigan **Albert B. Knapp, M.D., F.A.C.P.** Adjunct Assistant Attending Physician, Lenox Hill Hospital, New York, New York; Instructor in Medicine, New York Medical College, Valhalla, New York **Zeb Koran, R.N., C.E.N., C.C.R.N.** Director, Educational Services, Emergency Nurses Association, Chicago, Illinois **Kermit E. Krantz, M.D.** University Distinguished Professor, Professor of Gynecology and Obstetrics, Professor of Anatomy, University of Kansas Medical Center, Kansas City, Kansas **Stephen Kriebel, M.D.** Family Physician, Forks, Washington **Daniel Kuriloff, M.D.** Associate Director, Department of Otolaryngology–Head and Neck Surgery, St. Luke's–Roosevelt Hospital Center; Associate Professor, Columbia University College of Physicians and Surgeons, New York, New York **Jerold Lancourt, M.D.** Orthopedic Surgeon, North Dallas Orthopedics & Rehabilitation, P.A., Dallas, Texas **Robert P. Langlais, D.D.S., M.S.** Spokesperson for the American Academy of Oral Medicine; Professor, Department of Dental Diagnostic Science, University of Texas Health Science Center at San Antonio School of Dentistry, San Antonio,

Texas **Daniel M. Laskin, D.D.S., M.S.** Professor and Chairman, Department of Oral and Maxillofacial Surgery, Director, TMJ and Facial Pain Research Center, Medical College of Virginia, Richmond, Virginia **Ira J. Laufer, M.D.** Clinical Associate Professor of Medicine, New York University School of Medicine; Medical Director, The New York Eye and Ear Infirmary Diabetes Treatment Center, New York, New York **Andrew Lazar, M.D.** Assistant Professor of Clinical Dermatology, Northwestern University School of Medicine, Chicago, Illinois **Paul Lazar, M.D.** Professor of Clinical Dermatology, Northwestern University School of Medicine, Chicago, Illinois **Harold E. Lebovitz, M.D.** Professor of Medicine, Chief of Endocrinology and Diabetes, Director, Clinical Research Center, State University of New York Health Science Center, Brooklyn, New York **Mark Lebwohl, M.D.** Medical Advisor, National Psoriasis Foundation; Director of Clinical Dermatology, Mount Sinai School of Medicine, New York, New York **Theodore Lehman, M.D.** Associate Clinical Professor of Surgery (Urology), Oregon Health Sciences University; Director, The Oregon Impotence Center, Portland, Oregon **Suzanne M. Levine, D.P.M.** Podiatrist, New York, New York **Alan S. Levy, D.D.S.** Clinical Instructor, University of Southern California School of Dentistry, Los Angeles, California **Jerome Z. Litt, M.D.** Author, *Your Skin: From Acne to Zits*; Assistant Clinical Professor of Dermatology, Case Western Reserve University School of Medicine, Cleveland, Ohio **Allan L. Lorincz, M.D.** Professor of Dermatology, University of Chicago Medical Center, Chicago, Illinois **Irwin D. Mandel, D.D.S.** Professor Emeritus of Dentistry, Columbia University School of Dental and Oral Surgery, New York, New York **Michael Martindale, L.P.T.** Physical Therapist, Sports Medicine Center, Portland Adventist Medical Center, Portland, Oregon **Robert Matheson, M.D.** Dermatologist, Portland, Oregon **Raymond Merkin, D.P.M.** Podiatrist, Rockville, Maryland **V.E. Mikkelson, M.D.** Retired General Practitioner, Hayward, California **Marilyn C.**

Miller, D.D.S., F.A.G.D. Codirector, Princeton Dental Resource Center, Princeton, New Jersey **Anthony Montanaro, M.D.** Associate Professor of Medicine, Division of Allergy and Immunology, Oregon Health Sciences University, Portland, Oregon **H. Christopher Moore III, M.D.** Assistant Professor, Department of Otolaryngology/Head and Neck Surgery, University of California at Irvine, Irvine, California **Gregg R. Morris, D.C.** Chiropractor, Beaverton, Oregon **Michael S. Morris, M.D.** Otolaryngologist and Assistant Professor, Georgetown University School of Medicine, Washington, D.C. **Alan N. Moshell, M.D.** Director, Skin Disease Program, National Institute of Arthritis and Musculoskeletal and Skin Diseases, National Institutes of Health, Bethesda, Maryland **Willibald Nagler, M.D.** Anne and Jerome Fisher Physiatrist-in-Chief, Chairman of the Department of Rehabilitation Medicine, The New York Hospital–Cornell Medical Center, New York, New York **Charlie Nardozzi** Horticulturist, National Gardening Association, Burlington, Vermont **Luis Navarro, M.D.** Author, *No More Varicose Veins*; Founder and Director, Vein Treatment Center, New York, New York **Harold Neu, M.D.** Professor of Medicine and Pharmacology, Columbia University College of Physicians and Surgeons, New York, New York **Michael G. Newman, D.D.S.** President of the American Academy of Periodontology; Adjunct Professor of Periodontology, University of California at Los Angeles School of Dentistry, Los Angeles, California **Noreen Heer Nicol, M.S., R.N., F.N.C.** Senior Clinical Instructor, University of Colorado Health Sciences Center School of Nursing; Dermatology Clinical Specialist/Nurse Practitioner, National Jewish Center for Immunology and Respiratory Medicine, Denver, Colorado **Linda Niessen, D.M.D., M.P.H.** Associate Professor and Chair, Geriatric Oral Medicine, Department of Community Health and Preventive Dentistry, Baylor College of Dentistry, Dallas, Texas **German Nino-Murcia, M.D.** Founder and Medical Director, Sleep Medicine and Neuroscience Institute, Palo Alto, California **Lawrence A. Norton,**

M.D. Clinical Professor of Dermatology, Boston
University School of Medicine, Boston, Massachusetts
Nelson Lee Novick, M.D. Author, *Super Skin: A
Leading Dermatologist's Guide to the Latest
Breakthroughs in Skin Care*; Associate Clinical
Professor of Dermatology, Mount Sinai School of
Medicine, New York, New York **Edward J. O'Connell,
M.D.** Past President, American College of Allergy and
Immunology; Professor of Pediatrics,
Allergy/Immunology, Mayo Clinic, Rochester, Minnesota
Carole Palmer, Ed.D., R.D. Associate Professor and
Cochair, Division of Nutrition and Preventive Dentistry,
Tufts University School of Dental Medicine, Boston,
Massachusetts **Mary Papadopoulos, D.P.M.** Podiatrist,
Alexandria, Virginia **Frank Parker, M.D.** Professor and
Chairman, Department of Dermatology, Oregon Health
Sciences University, Portland, Oregon **Nalin M. Patel,
M.D.** Author of *The Doctor's Guide to Your Digestive
System*; Clinical Instructor, University of Illinois at
Urbana–Champaign, Champaign, Illinois **Hillard H.
Pearlstein, M.D.** Assistant Clinical Professor of
Dermatology, Mount Sinai School of Medicine, New York,
New York **Jeannette M. Pergam, M.D.** Assistant
Professor of Pediatrics, University of Nebraska Medical
Center, Omaha, Nebraska **Henry D. Perry, M.D.** Clinical
Associate Professor of Ophthalmology, Cornell Medical
College, New York, New York **Robert A. Phillips, M.D.,
Ph.D.** Director, Hypertension Section, Associate
Director, Cardiovascular Training Program, Division of
Cardiology, Mount Sinai Medical Center, New York, New
York **Neville R. Pimstone, M.D.** Chief of Hepatology,
Division of Gastroenterology, University of California
Davis, Davis, California **Rock G. Positano, D.P.M.,
M.Sc., N.P.H., F.A.C.P.R.** Codirector, Foot and Ankle
Orthopedic Institute, Hospital for Special Surgery, New
York, New York **David Posner, M.D.** Assistant Professor
of Medicine, University of Maryland School of Medicine,
Baltimore, Maryland **Arnold Prywes, M.D.** Head,
Glaucoma Clinic, Long Island Jewish Medical Center,
New Hyde Park, New York; Assistant Clinical Professor

of Ophthalmology, Albert Einstein Medical College, New York, New York; Chief of Ophthalmology, Mid-Island Hospital, Bethpage, New York **Deborah Purcell, M.D.** Past Chair, Department of Pediatrics, St. Vincent Hospital and Medical Center, Portland, Oregon **Gayle Randall, M.D.** Assistant Professor of Medicine, Department of Medicine, University of California, Los Angeles, School of Medicine, Los Angeles, California **David Rempel, M.D.** Assistant Professor of Medicine, Director, Ergonomics Laboratory, University of California at San Francisco, San Francisco, California **Basil M. Rifkind, M.D., F.C.R.P.** Chief, Lipid Metabolism and Atherogenesis Branch, National Heart, Lung and Blood Institute, National Institutes of Health, Bethesda, Maryland **Margaret Robertson, M.D.** Staff Physician, St. Vincent Hospital and Medical Center, Portland, Oregon **Robert S. Robinson, M.D.** General Practitioner, Metter, Georgia **Norton Rosensweig, M.D.** Associate Clinical Professor of Medicine, Columbia University College of Physicians and Surgeons, New York, New York **Donald Rudikoff, M.D.** Assistant Clinical Professor of Dermatology, Mount Sinai School of Medicine, New York, New York **John D. Rugh, Ph.D.** Professor, Department of Orthodontics, Director of Research for the Dental School, University of Texas Health Science Center at San Antonio, San Antonio, Texas **Paul S. Russell, M.D.** Past Officer, American Academy of Dermatology; Clinical Professor of Dermatology, Oregon Health Sciences University, Portland, Oregon **David A. Sack, M.D.** Associate Professor, School of Public Health, Director, International Travel Clinic, Johns Hopkins University, Baltimore, Maryland **Peter K. Sand, M.D.** Associate Professor of Obstetrics and Gynecology, Northwestern University School of Medicine; Director, Evanston Continence Center, Evanston Hospital, Evanston, Illinois **Gordon Scarbrough** Owner and Instructor, Moler Barber College, Portland, Oregon **Richard K. Scher, M.D.** Professor of Clinical Dermatology, Columbia University School of Medicine, New York, New York **Andrew Schink, D.P.M.** Past President, Oregon

Podiatric Medical Association **Alexander Schleuning, M.D.** Professor and Chairman, Department of Otolaryngology/Head and Neck Surgery, Oregon Health Sciences University, Portland, Oregon **Marvin Schuster, M.D.** Professor of Medicine with Joint Appointment in Psychiatry, Johns Hopkins University School of Medicine; Chief, Division of Digestive Diseases, Francis Scott Key Medical Center, Baltimore, Maryland **Alan R. Shalita, M.D.** Chairman, Department of Dermatology, State University of New York Health Science Center at Brooklyn, Brooklyn, New York **Gary Y. Shaw, M.D.** Associate Professor of Otolaryngology, Head and Neck Surgery, University of Kansas Medical Center, Kansas City, Kansas **James Shaw, M.D.** Chief, Division of Dermatology, Good Samaritan Hospital and Medical Center; Associate Clinical Professor of Medicine, Oregon Health Sciences University, Portland, Oregon **James E. Sheedy, O.D., Ph.D.** Associate Clinical Professor, School of Optometry, University of California at Berkeley, Berkeley, California **Fred D. Sheftell, M.D.** Director and Founder, The New England Center for Headache, Stamford, Connecticut **Martyn Shorten, Ph.D.** Former Director, NIKE's Sports Research Laboratory **Louisa Silva, M.D.** General Practitioner, Osteopath, Acupuncturist, Salem, Oregon **Herbert Silverstein, M.D.** President, Ear Research Foundation and Florida Otologic Center, Sarasota, Florida **Karl Singer, M.D., F.P., I.M.** Family Practitioner and Internist, Exeter, New Hampshire **Donald Skwor, D.P.M.** Past President, American Podiatric Medical Association; Podiatrist, Memphis, Tennessee **Elyse Sosin, R.D.** Supervisor of Clinical Nutrition, Mount Sinai Medical Center, New York, New York **Frank Spano, M.D.** Internist, Bridgeport, Connecticut **Thomas J. Stahl, M.D.** Assistant Professor of General Surgery, Georgetown University Medical Center, Washington, D.C. **James Stankiewicz, M.D.** Professor and Vice-Chairman, Department of Otolaryngology–Head and Neck Surgery, Loyola University Medical School, Maywood, Illinois **Michael R. Stefan, M.D.** Internist, Los Angeles,

California **Felicia Stewart, M.D.** Coauthor, *My Body, My Health* and *Understanding Your Body*; Gynecologist, Sacramento, California **William E. Straw, M.D.** Team Physician, San Francisco Giants; Clinical Associate Professor of Medicine, Stanford University School of Medicine, Stanford, California **Owen Surman, M.D., C.M., F.A.P.A.** Associate Professor of Psychiatry, Massachusetts General Hospital, Boston, Massachusetts **Mark Tager, M.D.** Coauthor, *Working Well*; President, Great Performance, Inc., Beaverton, Oregon **Jeffrey L. Tanji, M.D.** Associate Professor of Family Practice, Director, Sports Medicine Program, University of California Davis Medical Center, Davis, California **David M. Taylor, M.D** Author, *Gut Reactions: How to Handle Stress and Your Stomach*; Assistant Professor of Medicine, Emory University, Atlanta, Georgia; Assistant Professor of Medicine, Medical College of Georgia, Augusta, Georgia **Joseph Tenca, D.D.S., M.A.** Past President, American Association of Endodontists; Professor and Chairman, Department of Endodontics, Tufts University School of Dental Medicine, Boston, Massachusetts **Abba I. Terr, M.D.** Clinical Professor of Medicine, Director, Allergy Clinic, Stanford University Medical Center, Stanford, California **William R. Treem, M.D.** Associate Professor of Pediatrics, University of Connecticut School of Medicine; Pediatric Gastroenterologist, Division of Pediatric Gastroenterology and Nutrition, Hartford Hospital, Hartford, Connecticut **George Triadafilopoulos, M.D.** Associate Professor of Medicine, University of California Davis; Staff Physician, VA Northern California Systems of Clinics, Venicia, California **Thomas F. Truhe, D.D.S.** Codirector, Princeton Dental Resource Center, Princeton, New Jersey **Joan Ullyot, M.D.** Author, *Running Free* and *Women's Running*; Sports Medicine Physician, World-Class Runner, San Francisco, California **Frank J. Veith, M.D.** Professor of Surgery, Chief, Vascular Surgical Services, Montefiore Medical Center–Albert Einstein College of Medicine, New York, New York **Ken Waddell, D.M.D.** Dentist, Tigard, Oregon **Douglas C.**

Walta, M.D. Gastroenterologist, Portland, Oregon **John R. Ward, M.D.** Professor of Medicine, University of Utah School of Medicine, Salt Lake City, Utah **Kimra Warren, R.D.** Outpatient Dietitian, St. Vincent Hospital and Medical Center, Portland, Oregon **Jack J. Wazen, M.D.** Associate Professor of Otolaryngology, Director, Department of Otology and Neurotology, Columbia University College of Physicians and Surgeons, New York, New York **Miles M. Weinberger, M.D.** Director, Pediatric Allergy and Pulmonary Division, University of Iowa Hospitals and Clinics, Iowa City, Iowa **Allan M. Weinstein, M.D.** Asthma and Allergy Specialist, Washington, D.C. **Thelma Wells, Ph.D., R.N., F.A.A.N., F.R.C.N.** Professor of Nursing, University of Rochester School of Nursing, Rochester, New York **Sally Wenzel, M.D.** Assistant Professor of Medicine, National Jewish Center for Immunology and Respiratory Medicine, Denver, Colorado **Ronald Wismer, D.M.D.** Past President, Washington County Dental Society; Dentist, Beaverton, Oregon **Susan Woodruff, B.S.N.** Childbirth and Parenting Education Coordinator, Tuality Community Hospital, Hillsboro, Oregon **Virginia L. Woodward, R.D.H.** Past President, American Dental Hygienists' Association; Private Practice Clinician, Louisville, Kentucky **Stuart Young, M.D.** Director of Allergy Fellows, Clinical Education, Mount Sinai Medical Center, New York, New York **John Youngblood, M.D.** Associate Professor, University of Texas Health Science Center, San Antonio, Texas; President, Austin Ear Clinic, Austin, Texas **Carol Ziel, M.D.** Ophthalmologist, Wausau, Wisconsin **Harold Zimmer, M.D.** Obstetrician and Gynecologist, Bellevue, Washington **Jane Zukin** Author, *The Dairy-Free Cookbook* and *The Newsletter for People with Lactose Intolerance and Milk Allergies*

INDEX